Intensive Care Management of
Post-Transplant Patients
A Guide for Critical Care Specialists

VOLUME 3

Liver, Kidney, Pancreas and Small Bowel Transplant

Intensive Care Management of
Post-Transplant Patients
A Guide for Critical Care Specialists

VOLUME 3

Liver, Kidney, Pancreas and Small Bowel Transplant

Editors

Aklesh Tandekar
MD EDIC IDCCM FIMSA
Head and Consultant
Department of Critical Care
Wockhardt Hospitals
Mumbai, Maharashtra, India

Suvadeep Sen
MD FNB EDIC
Consultant
Critical Care Unit
Apollo Hospital
Navi Mumbai, Maharashtra, India

Mentors

Lakshmi Kumar
MD FCCM
Professor and Head
Department of Anesthesiology and Critical Care
Amrita Institute of Medical Sciences and Research Centre
Kochi, Kerala, India

Ravi Mohanka
MBBS MS DNB MSc MBA FASTS FACS
Director
Department of Liver Transplant and Hepato-Biliary Surgery
Sir HN Reliance Foundation Hospital
Mumbai, Maharashtra, India

Ravindra V Nikalji
DM (Nephrology) MD (Internal Medicine)
Consultant Nephrologist (Kidney Specialist)
and Kidney Transplant Physician
Apollo Hospital
Navi Mumbai, Maharashtra, India

Forewords
Ravi Mohanka
Lakshmi Kumar

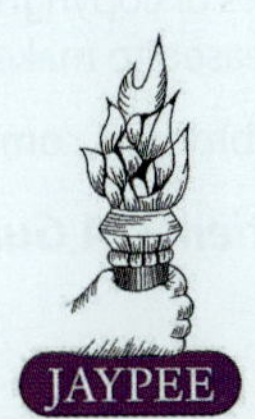

JAYPEE BROTHERS MEDICAL PUBLISHERS
The Health Sciences Publisher
New Delhi | London

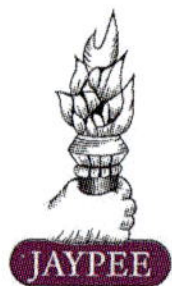

Jaypee Brothers Medical Publishers (P) Ltd

Headquarters
EMCA House, 23/23-B
Ansari Road, Daryaganj
New Delhi 110 002, India
Landline: +91-11-23272143, +91-11-23272703
+91-11-23282021, +91-11-23245672
e-mail: jaypee@jaypeebrothers.com

Corporate Office
4838/24, Ansari Road, Daryaganj
New Delhi 110 002, India
Phone: +91-11-43574357
Fax: +91-11-43574314
e-mail: jaypee@jaypeebrothers.com

Overseas Office
JP Medical Ltd.
83, Victoria Street, London
SW1H 0HW (UK)
Phone: +44-20 3170 8910
e-mail: info@jpmedpub.com

EU GPSR Authorised Representative
Logos Europe, 9 rue Nicolas Poussin
17000, La Rochelle, France
Phone: +33 (0) 6 67 93 73 78
e-mail: contact@logoseurope.eu

Website: www.jaypeebrothers.com
Website: www.jaypeedigital.com

Inquiries for bulk sales may be solicited at: jaypee@jaypeebrothers.com

Intensive Care Management of Post-Transplant Patients: A Guide for Critical Care Specialists (Volume 3)

First Edition: **2026**

ISBN: 978-93-6616-094-8

Printed at: Samrat Offset Pvt. Ltd.

Contributors

Aaditya A Prabhudesai DNB DESAIC (Brussels, EU) Fellow Liver Transplantation Anesthesiology and Critical Care (CLBS, New Delhi)
Consultant Anesthesiologist
Gleneagles Hospital
Mumbai, Maharashtra, India

Abdul S Ansari MD FNB IDCCM
Director
Department of Critical Care Services
Nanavati Max Super Speciality Hospital
Mumbai, Maharashtra, India

Aditya Kunte
MBBS MS Mch (Surgical oncology)
Department of Liver Transplant and HPB Surgery
Sir HN Reliance Foundation Hospital and Research Centre
Mumbai, Maharashtra, India

Akash Shukla MBBS MD (Medicine) DM
Consultant
Department of Hepatology
Sir HN Reliance Foundation Hospital and Research Centre
Mumbai, Maharashtra, India

Akila Rajakumar MD FRCA
Clinical Lead
Department of Liver Intensive Care and Anesthesia
Rela Institute and Medical Centre
Chennai, Tamil Nadu, India

Aklesh Tandekar MD EDIC IDCCM FIMSA
Head and Consultant
Department of Critical Care
Wockhardt Hospitals
Mumbai, Maharashtra, India

Amal Francis Sam MD DM
Consultant
Department of Liver Intensive Care and Anesthesia
Rela Institute and Medical Centre
Chennai, Tamil Nadu, India

Ambreen Sawant
MD Fellow Solid Organ Transplant Anesthesia (AIMS, Kochi)
Consultant Transplant Anesthesiologist
Clinical Lead
Department of Pediatric Transplant and Perioperative Care
Ruby Hall Clinic
Pune, Maharashtra, India

Amey Sonavane
DNB (Med) DNB (Gastro) MRCP (SCE-Gastro)
Fellowship in Clinical and Transplant Hepatology
Medanta—The Medicity
Consultant
Department of Gastroenterology, Hepatology and Liver Transplantation
Apollo Hospital
Navi Mumbai, Maharashtra, India

Amit C Langote
MD (Int Med) DNB (Nephrology)
Hypertension Specialist (ASH)
Kidney Transplant Physician (AST)
Home Dialysis Physician (Canada)
Consultant
Nephrologist and Kidney Transplant Physician
Apollo Hospital
Navi Mumbai, Maharashtra, India

Amruthraj C
MBBS MS MCh (GI Surgery AIIMS) Fellowship in Robotic Surgery (FARIS)
Consultant HPB and Liver Transplant Surgeon
Apollo Hospital
Navi Mumbai, Maharashtra, India

Anant Vikram Pachisia MBBS MD FNB
Consultant
Department of Critical Care Medicine
Medanta Institute of Critical Care and Anaesthesiology
Medanta—The Medicity
Gurugram, Haryana, India

Bharat V Shah MD DrNB (Nephrology)
Consultant Nephrologist
Institute of Renal Sciences
Gleneagles Hospital
Mumbai, Maharashtra, India

Bhushan Shah MD DNB (Cardiology) FESC
Assistant Professor
Department of Cardiology
All India Institute of Medical Sciences
Bhopal, Madhya Pradesh, India

Binoj ST
MS (General Surgery) DNB (Surgical Gastroenterology) Fellowship in Minimal Access Surgery
Clinical Professor
Amrita Hospital
Kochi, Kerala, India

Deepak Govil MD EDIC FCCM
Vice Chairman
Department of Critical Care Medicine
Medanta Institute of Critical Care and Anaesthesiology
Medanta—The Medicity
Gurugram, Haryana, India

Gaurav Gupta MBBS MS ASTS
Co-Director
Department of HPB and Liver Transplant Surgery
Sir HN Reliance Foundation Hospital and Research Centre
Mumbai, Maharashtra, India

Guhan Venkatakrishnan
MS Mch (Gastrosurgery) FRCS
Assistant Professor
Department of GI Surgery and Solid Organ Transplantation
Amrita Institute of Medical Sciences and Research
Kochi, Kerala, India

Guruprasad Shetty
MBBS MS (General Surgery) DNB (Surgical Gastroenterology) Fellowship in HPB
Surgery Fellowship in HPB and Liver Transplantation
Lead
Department of HPB and Liver Transplantation Surgery
Apollo Hospitals
Mumbai, Maharashtra, India

Hirak Pahari MBBS DNB FLT
Consultant
Institute of Surgical Gastroenterology
Department of GI and HPB Oncosurgery and Liver Transplantation
Sir Ganga Ram Hospital
New Delhi, India

Johann Paulo Guzman
Division of Transplantation
University of Tennessee Health Science Center
University of Tennessee
Memphis, Tennessee

Kalpana Tathe
MBBS MD PDCC Organ Transplant Anesthesia
Consultant
Apollo Hospital
Navi Mumbai, Maharashtra, India

Kelika Prakash
MD (Anesthesiology) DM (Organ Transplant Anesthesia and Critical Care)
Associate Professor
Department of Anesthesiology, Pain Medicine and Critical Care
All India Institute of Medical Sciences
New Delhi, India

Ketul Shah MBBS MS Mch GI Surgery
Consultant
Department of GI and Transplant Surgery
Apollo Hospital
Navi Mumbai, Maharashtra, India

Krishnanunni Nair
Associate Professor
Department of GI and Solid Organ Transplant
Amrita Institute of Medical Sciences and Research Centre
Amrita Vishwa Vidyapeetham
Kochi, Kerala, India

Lakshmi Kumar MD FCCM
Professor and Head
Department of Anesthesiology and Critical Care
Amrita Institute of Medical Sciences and Research Centre
Kochi, Kerala, India

Madhavi A Dadwe
MD DrNB (Nephrology)
Department of Nephrology
Ruby Hall Clinic
Pune, Maharashtra, India

Makrand Karpe
MBBS FCPS (SURG) Fellow Surgical Oncology
Consultant Liver Transplant
Apollo Hospital
Navi Mumbai, Maharashtra, India

Neha Bhatt
MBBS MS (Gen Surg) MCh (Surg Gastroenterology)
Associate Consultant
Department of HPB Surgery and Liver Transplantation
Hepato-Pancreato-Biliary Surgery and Liver Transplantation
Kokilaben Dhirubhai Ambani Hospital
Mumbai, Maharashtra, India

Pooja Lakhani
MSc RD CNSC-ASPEN PhD Scholar
Founder and Consultant Dietitian—Poshan Mantra, Dubai, UAE

Prabha Ranjana MBBS DNB (Radiology)
Consultant
Department of Fetal Medicine
DNB consultant Radiologist
Apollo Hospital
Navi Mumbai, Maharashtra, India

Pramod Kumar Guru
MBBS DM (Neph) MD
Professor of Medicine
Nephrology and Critical Care Medicine
Professor of Medicine
Mayo Clinic Florida
Jacksonville, Florida, USA

Prashant Kadam
MBBS MS MCh MRCSEd FRCSEd FEBS (Transplant Surgery)
Senior Consultant
Department of HPB and Liver Transplant Surgery
Sir HN Reliance Foundation Hospital and Research Centre
Mumbai, Maharashtra, India

Puneet Bhuwania
MD DNB (Med) DrNB (Nephrology) MNANS FASN
Consultant
Nephrologist and Transplant Physician
Department of Nephrology
Wockhardt Hospitals
Mumbai, Maharashtra, India

Ravi Mohanka
MBBS MS DNB MSc MBA FASTS FACS
Director
Department of Liver Transplant and Hepato-Biliary Surgery
Sir HN Reliance Foundation Hospital
Mumbai, Maharashtra, India

Rohan J Chaudhary
MBBS MS FACS Fellowship Liver Transplant Surgery
Associate Director
Department of HPB and Liver Transplant Surgery, Gleneagles (Global) Hospital
Mumbai, Maharashtra, India

S Sudhindran
MS (General Surgery) FRCS (Glasgow) FRCS (Eng) FRCS (General Surgery)
Head
Department of Digestive Diseases, Surgical Oncology, Solid Organ Transplantation and HPB Surgery
Gastrointestinal Surgery
Amrita Institute of Medical Sciences and Research Centre
Kochi, Kerala, India

Samiran Nundy
MA Mchir FRCS FRCP DSc (Hon)
Emeritus Consultant
Institute of Surgical Gastroenterology, GI and HPB Oncosurgery and Liver Transplantation
Sir Ganga Ram Hospital
New Delhi, India

Sanjay Chaudhary MD
Assistant Professor of Medicine
Critical Care Medicine, Nephrology
Assistant Professor of Medicine
Mayo Clinic Florida
Jacksonville, Florida, USA

Shabala Paul
MBBS MD (Anesthesiology) Fellowship in Solid Organ Transplant Anesthesia
Consultant
Department of Transplant Anesthesia
SPARSH Hospitals
Bengaluru, Karnataka, India

Shikhar Tripathi MBBS
Fellow
Institute of Surgical Gastroenterology, GI and HPB Oncosurgery and Liver Transplantation
Sir Ganga Ram Hospital
New Delhi, India

Shweta Mallick
Associate Professor
Department of GI Surgery and Solid Organ Transplantation
Amrita Hospital
Kochi, Kerala, India

Somnath Chattopadhyay
MBBS MS (Gen Surg) MCh (Surg Gastroenterology)
Consultant and Head
Department of HPB Surgery and Liver Transplantation
Hepato-Pancreato- Biliary Surgery and Liver Transplantation
Kokilaben Dhirubhai Ambani Hospital
Mumbai, Maharashtra, India

Sunaina Tejpal Karna
MD (Anesthesiology) PDCC (Liver Transplant Anesthesia)
Additional Professor
Department of Anesthesiology
All India Institute of Medical Sciences
Bhopal, Madhya Pradesh, India

Suvadeep Sen MD FNB EDIC
Consultant
Critical Care Unit
Apollo Hospital
Navi Mumbai, Maharashtra, India

Sweta J Patel MBBS DA IDCCM
Associate Director
Department of Critical Care Medicine
Medanta Institute of Critical Care and Anaesthesiology
Medanta—The Medicity
Gurugram, Haryana, India

Tushar Parmar DM
Chief Intensivist
Head
Department of Emergency
Sir HN Reliance Foundation Hospital
Mumbai, Maharashtra, India

Vaishali Solao
MD (Medicine) FNB (Critical Care)
Director
Department of Critical Care
Fortis Hospital
Mumbai, Maharashtra, India

Zubair Umer Mohamed
BA MD FRCA FCARSCI EDIC FFICM Pg. Dip
Associate Professor
Department of Anesthesia and Critical Care
Amrita Institute of Medical Sciences and Research Centre
Kochi, Kerala, India

Editorial

Organ transplantation stands as one of modern medicine's most profound achievements, offering a second chance at life to those who once faced insurmountable odds. The journey from diagnosis to transplantation—and beyond—is not merely a clinical process but an emotional, ethical, and deeply personal odyssey. This book seeks to illuminate that journey, shedding light on the advancements, challenges, and human stories that define transplantation today.

The progress in transplant medicine has been nothing short of extraordinary. From pioneering surgical techniques to groundbreaking immunosuppressive therapies and advances in intensive care, we have witnessed a revolution that has increased survival rates and enhanced quality of life for countless individuals. Yet, for all its triumphs, the field continues to grapple with significant hurdles: Organ shortages, ethical dilemmas, and the lifelong complexities of post-transplant care.

At the heart of every transplant is a narrative of hope—patients who persevere against the odds, families who make profound decisions in the face of grief, and healthcare professionals who dedicate their lives to saving others. These stories remind us that transplantation is more than science; it is a testament to human resilience, generosity, and innovation.

For intensive care physicians, the role in transplantation is pivotal. As frontline providers, they manage critically ill patients awaiting transplants, optimize donor organ function, and navigate the intricate postoperative care that determines long-term success. Their expertise in hemodynamic management, infection control, and immunosuppression protocols are crucial in ensuring favorable outcomes. Moreover, intensivists serve as advocates, guiding families through difficult decisions and supporting patients through the complexities of recovery.

This book brings together experts, patients, and advocates to explore the ever-evolving landscape of transplantation. It delves into the latest research, examines the ethical considerations that shape policy, and celebrates the individuals who make transplantation possible—donors, recipients, and medical professionals alike.

As we turn the pages, we are reminded that transplantation is not simply about replacing organs—it is about restoring lives, rekindling hope, and redefining what is possible in transplant medicine. May this book serve as a source of knowledge, inspiration, and a call to action for continued progress in the field of transplantation, particularly for intensive care physicians whose dedication is integral to every stage of the transplant journey.

Aklesh Tandekar
Suvadeep Sen

Foreword

I am happy to write a foreword for this book on *Intensive Care Management of Post-Transplant Patients: A Guide for Critical Care Specialists* edited by Dr Aklesh Tandekar and Dr Suvadeep Sen. While they are both very accomplished critical care experts specializing in the care of transplant patients, they are also close friends and professional colleagues. We have discussed several complex clinical situations among us and with several authors of this book over years and in international and national meetings, especially during my tenure as the President of the Liver Transplant Society of India (LTSI) and the Vice President of the Indian Society of Organ Transplantation (ISOT).

This book consists of three volumes. The first volume, covering aspects common for all types of transplants, includes topics such as setting up a unit, history, brain death, immunology and immunotherapy, pretransplant evaluation, and future of transplantation. The second volume covering thoracic organ transplants includes indications and selection, pretransplant evaluation and care, organ preservation, surgical techniques, postoperative care, the role of extracorporeal membrane oxygenation (ECMO) as a bridge, postoperative complications and their management, and future directions for both heart and lung transplants. The third volume covers abdominal organ transplantation, which includes all pre- and postoperative aspects of both living donor and deceased donor liver and kidney, pancreas, and intestinal transplants. A detailed account of postoperative ICU care, complications and their management, and complex situations such as ABO incompatible transplants, makes it a compelling read.

Having contributed two chapters myself, I attest that both editors have contributed a lot of dedicated time and effort to have it published in a very short time. Perspectives relevant to the Indian context in individual chapters make this book a very strong read. This book is a first of its kind in India and will serve as a comprehensive guide and reference for critical care physicians taking care of transplant patients and other transplant professionals.

Ravi Mohanka
MBBS MS DNB MSc MBA FASTS FACS
Director
Department of Liver Transplant and Hepato-Biliary Surgery
Sir HN Reliance Foundation Hospital
Mumbai, Maharashtra, India

Foreword

There has been an exponential growth in transplants in India with a large number of centers developing transplant units in the last two decades. Training programs are few and are limited to large-volume centers that perform transplants. Most of the training centers focus largely on preoperative evaluation and anesthesia management, and few have dedicated training in postoperative critical care management.

It is well recognized that intraoperative management is challenging and crucial in determining outcomes after transplantation. However, the role of the intensivist in postoperative management of patients, to oversee the subtle perturbations during recovery while managing immunosuppression, is equally challenging and also contributes substantially to the outcomes after surgery.

A dedicated book that provides a comprehensive overview of preparation of patients for surgery, relevant anesthetic management, and surgical steps as well as postoperative care is the need of the hour for intensivists in India.

This book has been the brainchild of Dr Suvadeep Sen, an intensivist who works at the Apollo Group of Hospitals at Navi Mumbai, and the content has largely been supported by authors in India who have described the management of these patients as per the conditions that exist in our country today for the care of such patients.

The first volume dwells briefly on guidelines to start an ICU that can assist new centers which are likely to find this information useful. Declaration of brain death, support of the organ system to ensure an optimal management of the organ donor, and immunosuppressive protocols are described here. Prehabilitation and rehabilitation of the potential solid organ transplant recipient as well as psychological aspects in transplantation that are pertinent in selection and outcomes have been addressed. The authors have also brought out the role of ECMO in the setting of solid organ transplants as well as ex-vivo organ preservation techniques.

The second volume is dedicated to the performance of lung and heart transplants. The first section on lung transplants describes donor procurement and surgical techniques in lung transplants. It describes ventilatory strategies, organ procurement, hemodynamic management, and post-transplant management. The role of ECMO as a bridge to heart and lung transplants, management of lung graft dysfunction, and rehabilitation to normal recovery following lung transplant have been addressed while the authors have drawn attention to the scope and future in lung transplants.

The section on heart transplant also provides insights into recipient evaluation and organ procurement as well as surgical techniques. The authors have described hemodynamic and ventilatory strategies, mechanical circulatory assist devices, and ECMO in heart transplant recipients. I believe that this volume may be a primer for intensivists who deal with heart and lung transplants in the future.

The third volume focuses on liver transplants and describes donor selection and cardiac evaluation of liver recipients. This volume has described the management of patients with acute liver failure and acute on chronic liver failure. The authors of this section, while highlighting indications for transplant, have described situations that may not be suitable for transplant. The surgical steps in liver transplant and hemodynamic management and pertinent anesthetic issues have been highlighted. Post-transplant surgical complications, rejection, and infectious and noninfectious complications have been addressed by authors. Management of hypoxemia following transplant for hepatopulmonary syndrome has also been described and the role of extracorporeal machine perfusion has been addressed. The impact of frailty on surgical outcomes following transplant has been described. This volume also briefly describes the management of pancreatic, intestinal, and renal transplants today.

The comprehensive and structured coverage of various facets of transplant intensive care is a commendable effort and I would whole-heartedly recommend this book as a guide for intensivists and teams working in the care of transplant patients.

Lakshmi Kumar
MD FCCM
Professor and Head
Department of Anesthesiology and Critical Care
Amrita Institute of Medical Sciences and Research Centre
Kochi, Kerala, India

Preface

The field of transplantation medicine stands as one of the most remarkable achievements in modern health care, offering patients with end-stage organ failure a new lease on life. However, the journey for post-transplant patients does not end with surgery; it extends into a complex and often precarious phase of care that demands meticulous management in the intensive care setting. This book, *Intensive Care Management of Post-Transplant Patients: A Guide for Critical Care Specialists,* is crafted as a trusted resource for critical care students, residents, and physicians who are navigating the challenges of managing these vulnerable patients.

As critical care physicians, we stand on the frontlines of a delicate balance—responsible for recognizing early signs of complications, preventing organ dysfunction, and optimizing patient outcomes. Our conviction in creating this book stemmed from the desire to remove the fear and uncertainty that often surrounds post-transplant care while guiding physicians through the intricate principles, protocols, and nuances involved in caring for transplant patients in the intensive care unit (ICU).

Whether you are assessing a newly transplanted patient or managing long-term complications, this book offers a robust framework to guide your decision-making process. We have structured the book to begin with the preoperative identification of patients with end-stage organ failure who will require transplants, emphasizing the optimization of patients in their acute stages. Understanding their overall medical, physical, and functional status is a fundamental aspect of managing them in the postoperative period. The intraoperative aspect is addressed in a dedicated chapter. The focus of the book remains on the intensive care unit (ICU) management of post-transplant patients. The book provides a detailed and practical discussion on the immunosuppression strategies, infectious complications, and organ-specific challenges that follow liver, kidney, small bowel, and pancreas transplants. Special emphasis has been placed on prehabilitation, immunology, extracorporeal support, and other critical aspects essential for optimal care. Additionally, we have covered simultaneous liver–kidney transplantation, offering insights into multivisceral organ transplants.

This three-volume work is the first of its kind to comprehensively cover the full spectrum of post-transplant management. Each chapter has been meticulously written by distinguished transplantation specialists, ensuring that the content is evidence-based and to the point. We have worked to seamlessly integrate the perspectives of transplant surgeons, anesthesiologists, hepatologists, nephrologists, and other specialists involved in the care of these patients. As perioperative care providers and critical care specialists, it is crucial to understand the perspectives of various medical fields. This integrated approach is key to delivering comprehensive care to post-transplant patients.

As guardians of these patients' new beginnings, our expertise and vigilance play a pivotal role in ensuring the long-term success of transplantation, particularly in India. With this book, we aim to equip our readers with the knowledge, tools, and confidence necessary to provide the highest standard of care, making every transplant a lasting triumph.

Aklesh Tandekar
Suvadeep Sen

Acknowledgments

The completion of *Intensive Care Management of Post-Transplant Patients: A Guide for Critical Care Specialists* has been an immensely rewarding journey, made possible through the collective contributions and unwavering support of many individuals and institutions. We are deeply grateful for their involvement and would like to take this opportunity to acknowledge their invaluable contributions.

First and foremost, our heartfelt gratitude goes to the patients facing end-stage organ failure and undergoing transplant surgery during one of the most critical stages of their lives. Their resilience, strength, and unwavering resolve in the face of adversity have been a constant source of inspiration and learning. This book is dedicated to them, as their experiences are central to its creation.

We are especially indebted to Lakshmi Kumar, Professor and Head of the Department of Anesthesiology and Critical Care at the Amrita Institute of Medical Sciences and Research Centre; Dr Ravi Mohanka, a distinguished liver transplant surgeon; and Dr Ravindra V Nikalji, a renowned nephrologist and kidney transplant physician. Their mentorship, guidance, and unwavering support have been instrumental in shaping the content and direction of this book.

Our sincere thanks also go to Dr Prakash Jiandani, an esteemed critical care physician and educator, whose exceptional knowledge and dedication to teaching have profoundly impacted on our professional journey. His mentorship has significantly enhanced our understanding of critical care and transplant medicine, and we are deeply appreciative of his influence.

We would like to extend our sincere thanks to our respective institutions for providing us with the opportunity to contribute meaningfully to patient care. The hospital's commitment to excellence has fostered an environment conducive to continuous learning and improvement, empowering us to deliver the highest standard of care.

We must also acknowledge the tireless dedication of the nurses, sisters, and fellow physicians who work tirelessly to provide compassionate care to our patients. Their teamwork and commitment form the foundation of quality care, and this book would not have been possible without their unwavering support.

We are deeply thankful to the esteemed authors who contributed to the preparation of this manuscript, despite their busy schedules. Their expertise, insights, and thoughtful contributions have greatly enriched the content of this work, and we are sincerely grateful for their collaboration.

Our heartfelt thanks go to M/s Jaypee Brothers Medical Publishers (P) Ltd, New Delhi, India, for their consistent professionalism and support throughout the publication process. We would like to extend special appreciation to Mr Akhilesh Saxena and Ms Kritika Dua for their meticulous attention to detail, guidance, and invaluable support during the manuscript preparation and editing phases. Their efforts have been crucial in bringing this project to fruition.

Finally, we are deeply grateful to our families for their unwavering love, understanding, and support. Their constant encouragement has been a pillar of strength, enabling us to navigate the challenges of balancing professional and personal responsibilities with dedication and purpose.

This book is the result of a collective effort, and we are profoundly grateful to everyone who has contributed to its creation. Their expertise, encouragement, and support have been essential to this project, and we are honored to share it with the medical community.

Aklesh Tandekar
Suvadeep Sen

Contents

VOLUME 3: LIVER, KIDNEY, PANCREAS AND SMALL BOWEL TRANSPLANT

SECTION 1: Liver Transplant

SECTION 1

Liver Transplant

CHAPTER

Indications of Liver Transplantation in the Setting of Acute Liver Failure, Acute-on-Chronic Liver Failure, and Chronic Liver Disease

Aditya Kunte, Johann Paulo Guzman, Akash Shukla, Ravi Mohanka

INTRODUCTION

Liver disease is a significant global health challenge, accounting for nearly 2 million (4% of all) deaths, two third of them occurring in men.[1] It also contributes to high disability-adjusted life years (DALYs), especially in the young population, and poses an economic burden of more than 30 billion USD in the US alone. There has been a consistent increase in the incidence of liver disease and liver-related deaths over the past decade, thus necessitating a coordinated response to improve prevention, early detection, and treatment strategies.[1,2]

Dr Thomas Starzl performed the first successful liver transplantation (LT) from a deceased (cadaveric) donor liver transplantation (DDLT) in 1968.[3] Initial challenges with high rates of surgical complications, rejection, and graft loss have improved with advances in surgical techniques, safety of anesthesia, specialty critical care, diagnostic and immunological tests, organ allocation systems, better organ preservation methods, immuno-suppressive, antimicrobial and other medicines, leading to excellent short- and long-term outcomes. Currently, LT is the standard of care for end-stage liver disease (ESLD) treatment, with 34,694 liver transplants performed globally in 2023, an increase of 6.5% from 2020 and 20% from 2015.[4] Although there is high variability between countries, LT continues to increase globally **(Figs. 1 and 2)**.

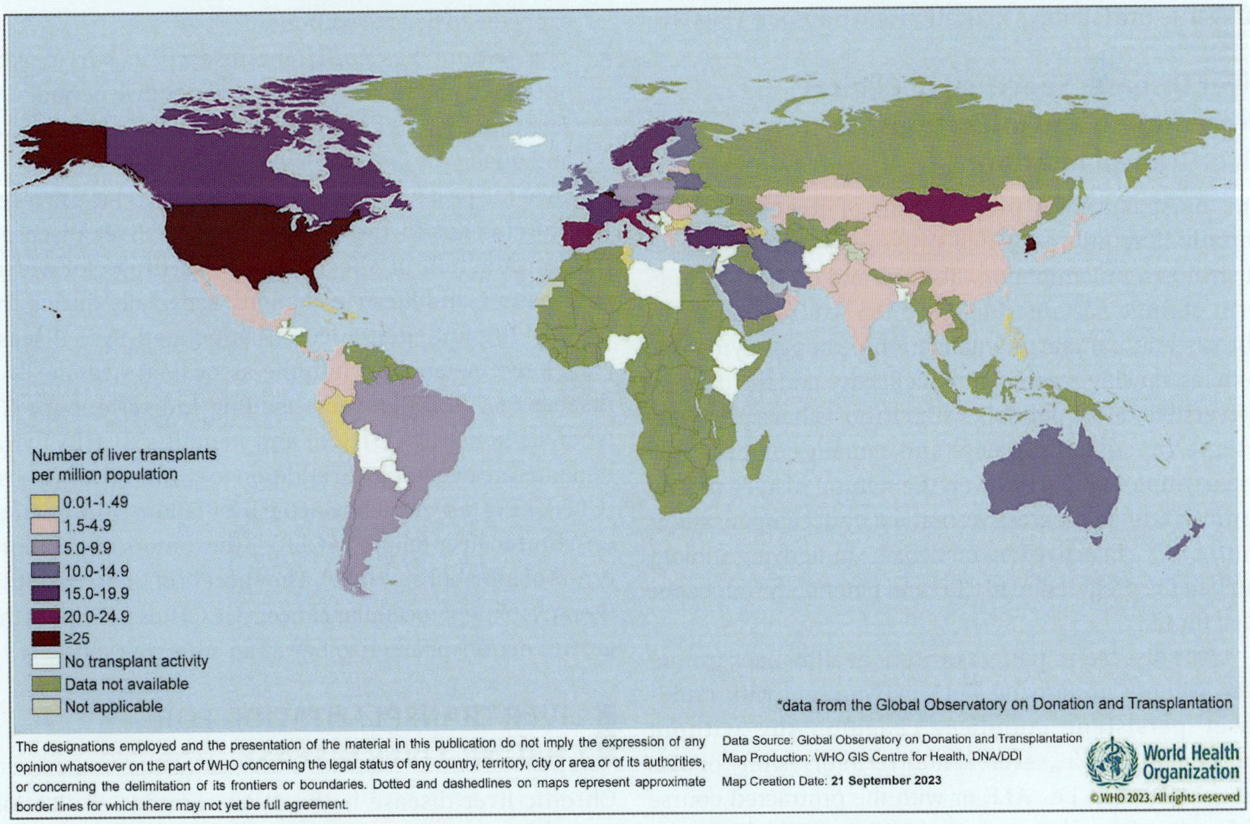

Number of liver transplants per million population
- 0.01-1.49
- 1.5-4.9
- 5.0-9.9
- 10.0-14.9
- 15.0-19.9
- 20.0-24.9
- ≥25
- No transplant activity
- Data not available
- Not applicable

*data from the Global Observatory on Donation and Transplantation

The designations employed and the presentation of the material in this publication do not imply the expression of any opinion whatsoever on the part of WHO concerning the legal status of any country, territory, city or area or of its authorities, or concerning the delimitation of its frontiers or boundaries. Dotted and dashedlines on maps represent approximate border lines for which there may not yet be full agreement.

Data Source: Global Observatory on Donation and Transplantation
Map Production: WHO GIS Centre for Health, DNA/DDI
Map Creation Date: **21 September 2023**

World Health Organization

Fig. 1: Global liver transplant activity in 2022 per million population.[4]

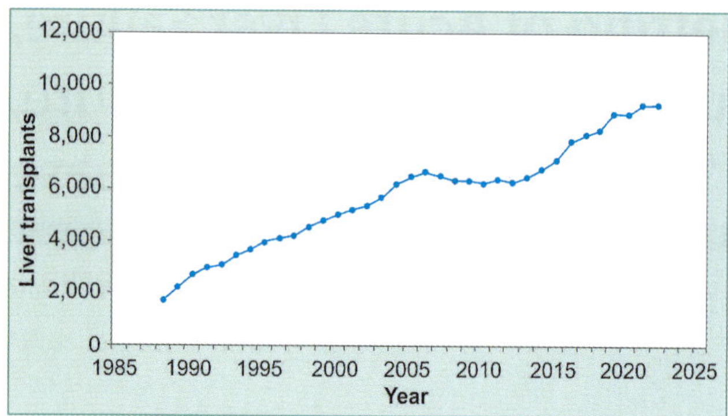

Fig. 2: Globally increasing number of transplants.
Source: OPTN/SRTR Annual Data Reports: Liver. Scientific Registry of Transplant Recipients. U.S. Department of Health and Human Resources (Kwong).[5]

The demand for LT far exceeds available organs, leading to a huge and widening gap. This has been partially addressed by expanding the donor pool using livers from extended criteria donors (ECD), donation after circulatory death (DCD), and living donor liver transplant (LDLT). Almost 90% of LTs in Western countries are DDLT, whereas the majority in Asian countries are LDLT,[4] which may be because of deceased donor organ availability, cultural and religious beliefs, and availability of surgical expertise and infrastructure for organ allocation and transport **(Fig. 3)**.

Liver Disease: Spectrum of Clinical Presentation and Indications for Liver Transplantation

The most common presentation of liver disease is chronic liver failure, which progresses through stages of steatosis, inflammation, fibrosis, and cirrhosis. Long-term chronic sustained injury often leads to repair by fibrosis and compartmentalization of hepatocytes into nodules, making regeneration ineffective and the damage irreversible. Most patients with cirrhosis have adequate reserve/functional capacity and remain compensated and asymptomatic. However, the natural history of liver cirrhosis is often progressive, marked by decompensations and/or HCC. Effective treatment of the underlying etiology can halt the progression of CLD and potentially reduce the need for LT.

Liver disease in patients with a healthy background liver, without underlying CLD, may present with rapid-onset persistent jaundice, coagulopathy without encephalopathy, i.e., severe acute liver injury (sALI), or with encephalopathy, i.e., ALF, or with the protracted course and ascites, i.e., subacute hepatic failure (SHF) **(Table 1)**. Even if the injury/damage/inflammation/necrosis is widespread/extensive, spontaneous recovery with regeneration is common if there is adequate hepatocyte mass. If the magnitude of injury is overwhelming and hepatocyte mass is inadequate for regeneration, and/or there is failure of regeneration, it may lead to rapid deterioration, severe systemic inflammatory response syndrome (SIRS), multiorgan dysfunction syndrome (MODS), or cerebral edema, which could be fatal within days to weeks. Historically, ALF patients had >80% risk of mortality, whereas an emergency LT is often life-saving. When a stable CLD patient deteriorates rapidly due to acute events such as infection, variceal bleeding, acute HBV flare, or others, it is called ACLF **(Table 1 and Fig. 4)**.[6]

Liver transplantation should be offered to patients at an optimum time in the course of their liver disease and performed at the most appropriate time when the expected risk of mortality due to the natural progression of liver disease is higher than the risk of LT. If done too early, the patient may be deprived of a chance at spontaneous recovery, and if delayed beyond a point, they may be too sick and have lower chances of success of LT.[7] LT should be done when:

- The recipient has irreversible acute or CLD that is expected to be fatal without LT.
- The patient has sufficient reserve to survive the operation and recover in the perioperative period.
- The candidate is expected to have significant survival and quality-of-life (QoL) benefits from LT.

Over the past few decades, LT indications have evolved due to changes in the epidemiology of liver diseases, the introduction of effective antiviral drugs, universal vaccination, and lifestyle changes, especially during the COVID-19 pandemic. Alcohol-associated liver disease (ALD) and metabolic syndrome-associated steatotic liver disease (MASLD) are now leading indications for LT, whereas hepatitis C (HCV) and hepatitis B (HBV) viral hepatitis are declining.[2] In addition to chronic liver disease (CLD), LT is performed for acute liver failure (ALF), acute-on-chronic liver failure (ACLF), liver tumors, and inborn errors of metabolism (IEM). The success of LT as a curative therapy for hepatocellular cancer (HCC) has prompted the growth of transplant oncology as an emerging specialty.

LIVER TRANSPLANTATION FOR CHRONIC LIVER DISEASE

Chronic liver disease is the most common indication for LT. Cirrhosis has increased by 74.5% from 1990 to

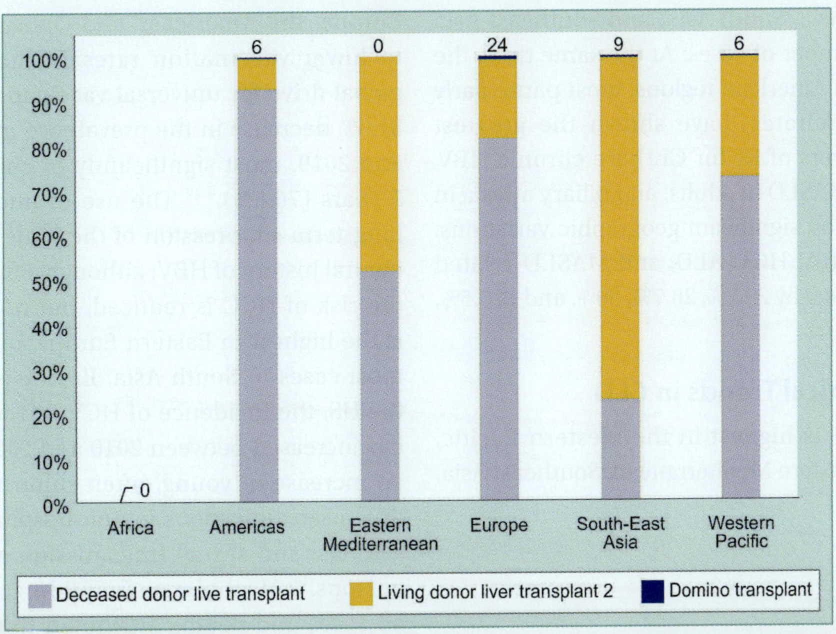

	African region	Region of the Americas	Eastern Mediterranean region	European region	South-East Asian region	Western Pacific region
Number of liver transplants: Absolute per million population (PMP)	0 (0.0)	13,387 (13.6)	1,817 (3.9)	9,840 (14.3)	4,067 (2.5)	8,325 (4.7)
% DDLT	0	88	59	82	19	71
Countries with liver TX activity/ (total countries in the region)	0 (46)	15 (35)	7 (22)	36 (53)	2 (11)	8 (27)
Liver TX centers (millions of inhabitants/center)	0	404 (2.4)	35 (13.2)	229 (3.0)	247 (6.7)	231 (7.7)

Fig. 3: Variations in liver transplant practices in different WHO regions globally.[4] (PMP: per million population; WHO: World Health Organization)

TABLE 1: Phenotypic spectrum of liver failure.

Liver failure syndrome	*Definition/description*	*Outcome*
Severe acute liver injury (sALI)	Jaundice and prolonged PT/INR >1.5 over days/weeks	Usually recovers spontaneously, some may progress to ALF
Acute liver failure (ALF)	• Encephalopathy associated with jaundice and PT/INR >1.5 occurring over hours/days (up to 26 weeks) • In children, sALI with PT-INR >2 is classified as ALF, even without encephalopathy	Associated with a high 15-day mortality
Subacute hepatic/liver failure (SHF)	*A variant of ALF:* Persistent jaundice and progressive followed by ascites beyond 4 and within 24 weeks	High mortality over 6 months
Chronic liver disease (decompensated cirrhosis)	Cirrhosis and portal hypertension, characterized by progressive ascites, jaundice, encephalopathy, and coagulopathy	Mortality is often proportional to disease severity
Acute-on-chronic liver failure (ACLF)	Acute deterioration of chronic liver disease leading to multiorgan failure	High mortality in 4 and 12 weeks

(INR: international normalized ratio; PT: prothrombin time)

2017 **(Fig. 4)**. East Asia, South Asia, and Southeast Asia have the highest number of cases. At the same time, the Caribbean and Latin American regions, most particularly the United Arab Emirates, have shown the greatest increase. Major drivers of LT for CLD are chronic HBV, chronic HCV, ALD, MASLD in adults, and biliary atresia in children. These exhibit significant geographic variations. The prevalence of HBV, HCV, ALD, and MASLD-related liver cirrhosis increased by 29.2%, 28.7%, 80%, and 125.6%, respectively **(Fig. 5)**.

Global Geographical Trends in CLD

The burden of HBV is highest in the Western Pacific, followed by Africa, Eastern Mediterranean, Southeast Asia, Europe, the Americas,[3] and Qatar, which corresponds to lower vaccination rates in these regions. With a global drive for universal vaccination, there has been a 31.3% decrease in the prevalence of HBV between 1990 and 2019, most significantly in children younger than 5 years (76.8%).[8-10] The use of nucleoside analogs for long-term suppression of the virus has also altered the natural history of HBV; although a functional cure is rare, the risk of HCC is reduced, but not eliminated.[11] HCV is the highest in Eastern Europe and Central Asia, with most cases in South Asia, East Asia, and the UAE.[12] In the US, the incidence of HCV infections among donors has increased between 2010 and 2021,[13] probably due to an increase in young, often suburban heroin injection drug users; infections in non-hospital healthcare (clinic) settings; and sexual transmission among HIV-infected persons.[14] Alcohol consumption caused almost half of all cases and deaths attributed to CLD in 2016. While the burden of ALD impacts most regions of the world, in 2019, Mongolia, Kazakhstan, El Salvador, Guatemala, Greenland, Kyrgyzstan, Poland, Rwanda, Ireland, and Brazil were most affected by ALD.[8,9] MASLD is the most common cause of CLD in many regions of the world,[2] with a 15.78% prevalence in North America, an estimated 42.4%, and a projected prevalence of >55% by 2040.[15] There is a shift in the disease burden to Middle Eastern and North African, Asian, and Latin American countries, with 26.5% prevalence in the Middle East. In Asia, the increase in MASLD is driven by China, India, and Indonesia.[16]

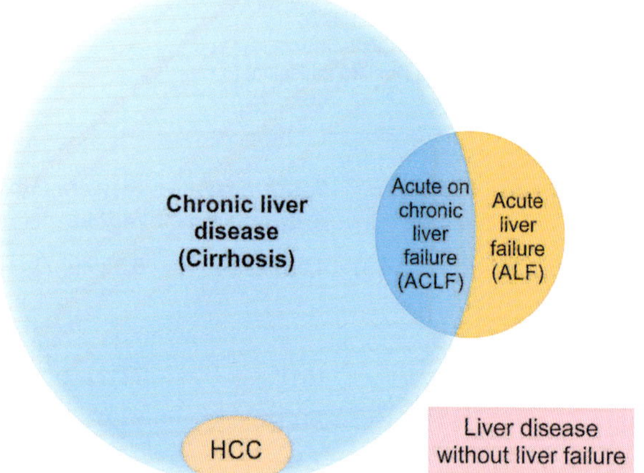

Fig. 4: Clinical presentations of liver diseases requiring a liver transplant.

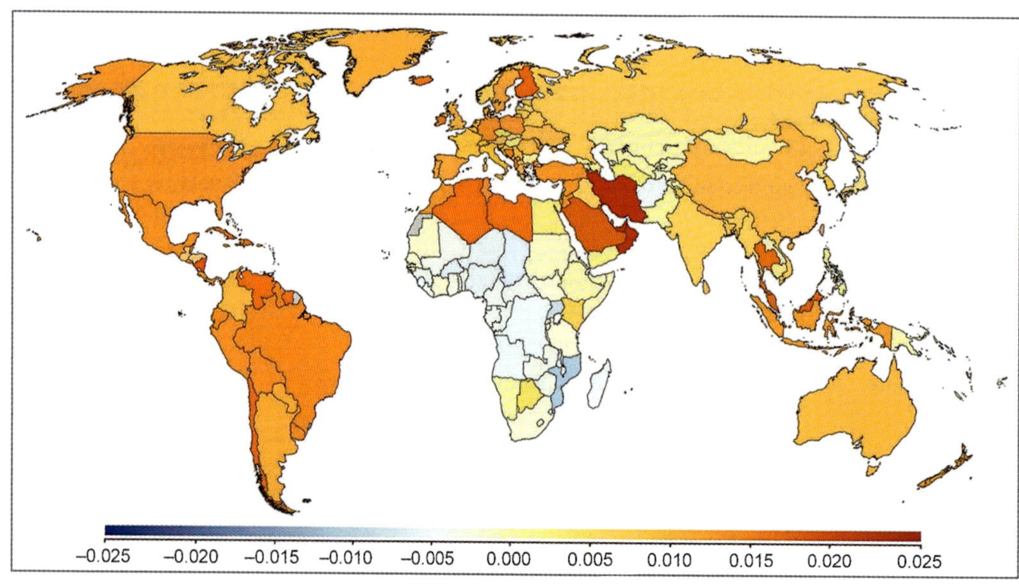

Fig. 5: Annual percentage change of cirrhosis from 1990 to 2017.[7]

Globally, nonalcoholic fatty liver disease (NAFLD) has increased at an annual rate of 1.47%/year from 10.5% in 1990 to 16.0% in 2019[17] **(Figs. 6 to 8)**.

With the increasing burden of cirrhosis worldwide, the need for LT and its activity has increased and its etiologies have changed **(Fig. 9)**.

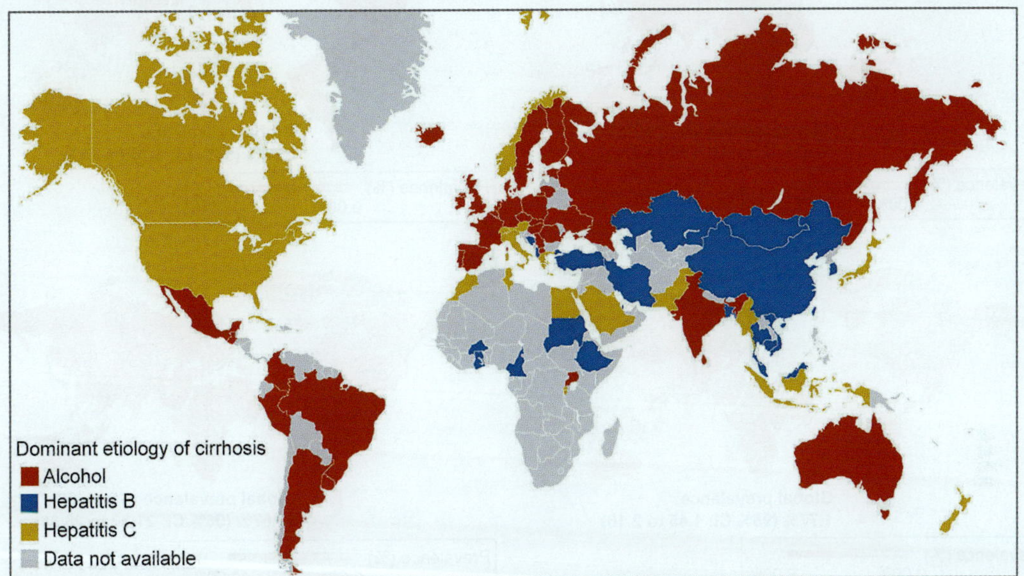

Fig. 6: Geographic variations in the dominant etiology of cirrhosis.[18]

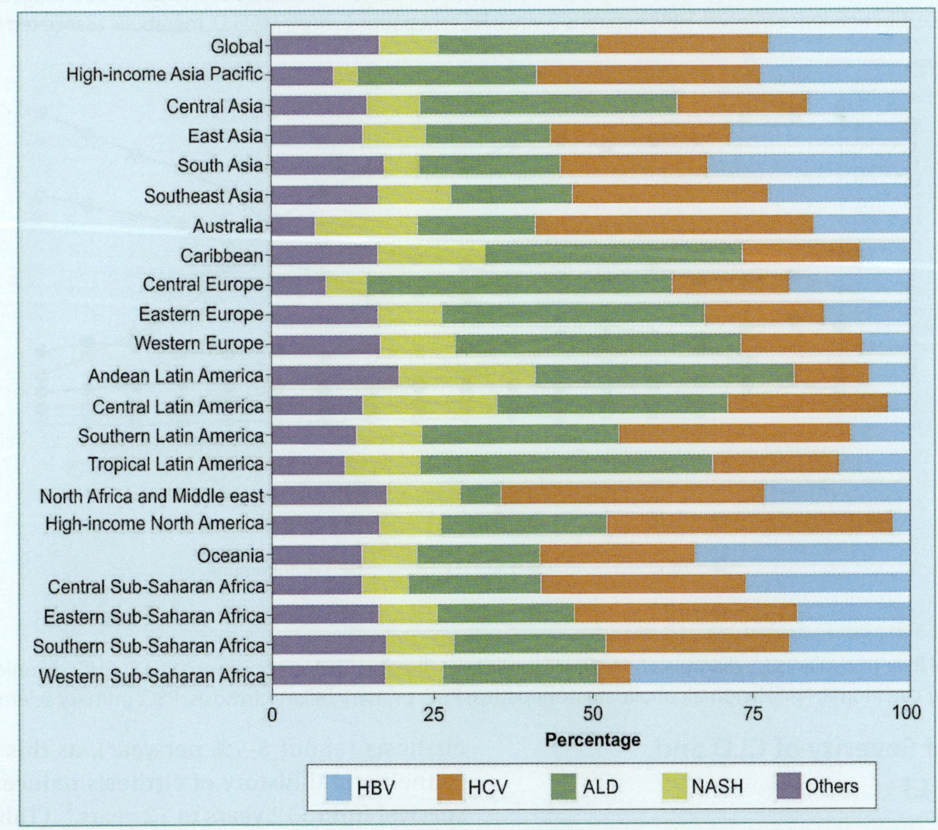

Fig. 7: Variations in dominant etiology of cirrhosis in various WHO regions.[19] (ALD: alcoholic liver disease; HBV: hepatitis B virus; HCV: hepatitis C virus; NASH: non-alcoholic steatohepatitis; WHO: World Health Organization)

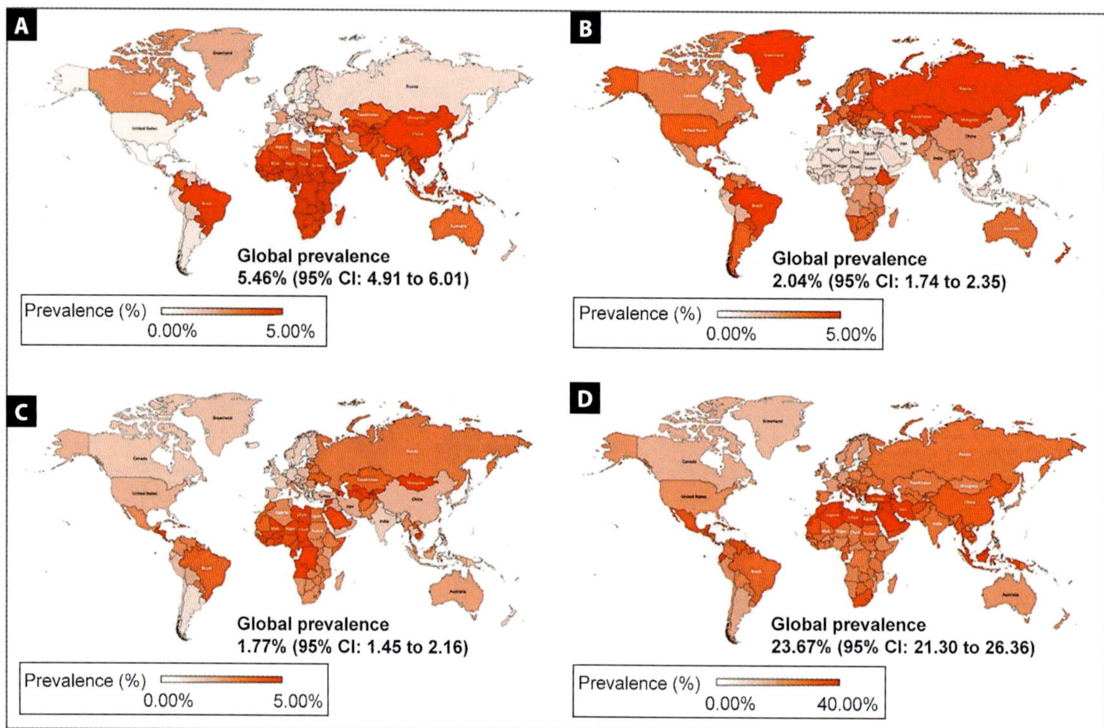

Figs. 8A to D: (A) Prevalence of HBV; (B) Prevalence of HCV; (C) Prevalence of ALD; (D) Prevalence of MAFLD (in adults aged ≥20 years).[4] (ALD: alcoholic liver disease; CI: confidence interval; HBV: hepatitis B virus; HCV: hepatitis C virus; MAFLD: metabolic associated fatty liver disease)

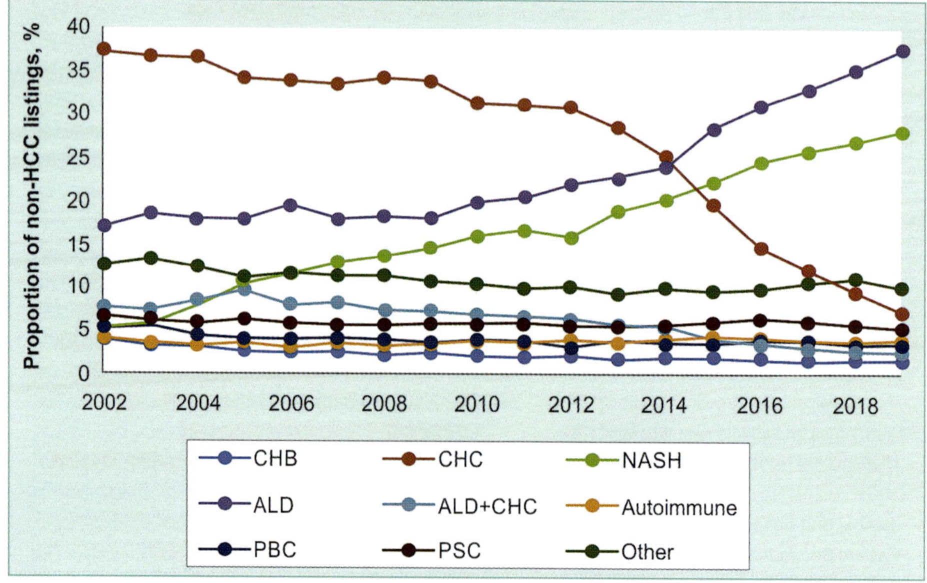

Fig. 9: US total liver transplants by diagnosis.[20] (ALD: alcoholic liver disease; CHB: chronic hepatitis B; CHC: chronic hepatitis C; HCC: hepatocellular carcinoma; NASH: non-alcoholic steatohepatitis; PBC: primary biliary cirrhosis; PSC: primary sclerosing cholangitis)

Assessment of Severity of CLD and Indication for LT

Liver transplantation in CLD is generally considered when patients transition from compensated to decompensated cirrhosis (about 5–7% per year), as this seminal event in the natural history of cirrhosis reduces their median survival from >12 years to ~2 years.[21] **(Table 2)**. Children with liver disease may also experience growth failure and benefit from LT before puberty to enable catch-up growth.

TABLE 2: Complications/decompensations of CLD and their prognosis.

Complications/Decompensation	*Incidence*	*Expected median survival*	*Mortality risk*
Hepatic encephalopathy		6–9 months	
Variceal bleed		• CTP-A: 5 years • CTP-B: 3 years • CTP-C: 3 months	
Ascites	5–10%/year	20 months	
Refractory ascites	10–15% from ascites	6 months	50% at 6–12 months
Spontaneous bacterial peritonitis (SBP)	• Outpatient: 1.5–3.5% • In-patient: 10%	9 months	In each episode 20%
HRS-1 (HRS-AKI)		2 weeks	
HRS-2 (HRS-CKD)		6 months	
Hepatic hydrothorax			
Hepatopulmonary syndrome	10–17%	Severe: 10.5 months	
Portopulmonary hypertension		2.8 years	
Malnutrition, sarcopenia, and frailty		8.5 months	

(CLD: chronic liver disease; CTP: Child-Turcotte-Pugh; HRS-AKI: hepatorenal syndrome–acute kidney injury; HRS-CKD: hepatorenal syndrome–chronic kidney disease)

Decompensation is more commonly, objectively, and comprehensively classified using the Child-Turcotte-Pugh (CTP) and Model for End-Stage Liver Disease (MELD) scores for comparison between patients **(Tables 3 and 4)**.[22]

The CTP score is subjective and has limited discriminatory power; therefore, it was replaced by the MELD score for organ allocation in 2002 in the USA, which is more objective and reliable for predicting mortality. Subsequent modifications of the MELD score have addressed some of its deficiencies; the MELD-Na incorporates hyponatremia as a surrogate marker for the degree of ascites, and the more recent MELD 3.0 accounts for interactions between bilirubin, sodium, and albumin and has a better predictive value.[23] Several countries have adopted the MELD score or its modifications for organ allocation in their systems.

Liver transplantation improves survival and quality of life for CTP >7.[21] DDLT confers a survival advantage compared to continuing medical management at a MELD cutoff of >14, and with an LDLT, the benefit may accrue at a score >10.[24] LT candidates with stage 3 acute kidney injury (AKI), needing dialysis, with estimated glomerular filtration rate (eGFR) <35 by MDRD-6 (modification of diet in renal disease-6) for >4 weeks or with evidence of structural renal disease should be considered for simultaneous liver-kidney transplant (SLKT).[25]

TABLE 3: Child-Turcotte-Pugh (CTP) score.

	Points		
Parameters	*1*	*2*	*3*
Encephalopathy	None	Grade 1–2	Grade 3–4
Ascites	None	Mild to moderate (diuretic responsive)	Severe (diuretic refractory)
Serum albumin (g/dL)	>3.5	2.8–3.5	<2.8
Total bilirubin (mg/dL)	<2	2–3	>3
PT (sec prolonged) or INR	<4	4–6	>6
	<1.7	1.7–2.3	>2.3

CTP classification is based on the sum of all the above components
Class A = 5–6 points, *Class B* = 7–9 points, *Class C* = 10–15 points

CTP classification and prognosis

Class	***Score***	***Expected 1-year survival***	***Expected 5-year survival***
A	5–6	90%	90%
B	7–9	80%	70%
C	10–15	45%	38%

(INR: international normalized ratio; PT: prothrombin time)

TABLE 4: Model for End-Stage Liver Disease (MELD) score, its variations, and prognosis.

MELD	*MELD Na*	*UK MELD*	*MELD 3.0*
9.57 × Log_e (creatinine) + 3.78 × Log_e (bilirubin) + 11.20 × Log_e (INR) + 6.43	MELD + 1.32 × (137 – Na) – 0.033 × MELD × (137 – Na)	1.485 × Log_e (creatinine) + 3.13 × Log_e (bilirubin) + 5.395 × Log_e (INR) + 81.565 × Log_e (Sodium) + 435	1.33 (if female) + 4.56 × Log_e (bilirubin) + 0.82 × (137 – Na) – 0.24 × (137 – Na) × Log_e (bilirubin) + 9.09 × Log_e (INR) + 11.14 × Log_e (creatinine) + 1.85 × (3.5 – albumin) – 1.83 × (3.5 – albumin) × Log_e (creatinine) + 6
125 < Na <137 mmol/L, and MELD Na is applied when MELD >11. A value of 4.0 is assigned if serum creatinine ≥4.0 or if the patient received ≥2 dialysis sessions within the prior week. The maximum serum creatinine has been lowered from 4.0 to 3.0 in the MELD 3.0			

Survival MELD score	*3 months*	*1 year*
0–9	98%	90%
10–19	94%	80%
20–29	81%	66%
30–39	48%	33%
>40	29%	<5%

(INR: international normalized ratio)

In addition to these common etiologies, CLD maybe caused by autoimmune, cholestatic, metabolic, vascular, and other etiologies. In about 20% of cases, the etiology may not be identified, i.e., cryptogenic. In some diseases, these scores do not accurately reflect the severity of their liver disease, and alternative scoring systems are used and indications for LT may be different **(Table 5)**.

LIVER TRANSPLANTATION FOR ACUTE LIVER FAILURE

Common Etiologies of ALF

- *Hepatitis A:* <1% of acute hepatitis A virus (HAV) infections result in ALF. HAV generally causes subclinical hepatitis in children and more severe infection in adults.
- *Hepatitis B:* This is an uncommon cause of ALF, caused by acute infection or reactivation in chronic HBV, both of which can be differentiated by IgM anti-HBc titers and HBV viral load and have markedly different prognoses.
- *Hepatitis E:* This is the most common cause of acute sporadic and epidemic hepatitis and accounts for 10–40% of acute hepatitis and 15–45% of ALF in India, with high mortality.
- *Toxins/drug-induced liver injury (DILI):* Paracetamol toxicity constitutes nearly half of all ALF in the West, others being antibacterials, anti-tuberculosis (TB) drugs, herbal and dietary supplements, antiepileptics, nonsteroidal anti-inflammatory drugs (NSAIDs), mushrooms (Amanita), and others. In India, paracetamol only constitutes ~1% of all drug-induced ALF, the more common ones being anti-TB drugs, complementary and alternative medicines (CAM), antiepileptic drugs (first generation), sulfonamides, antiretroviral drugs, yellow phosphorus (rat poison), and others **(Box 1)**.
- *Pregnancy:* Pregnant women are more likely to have ALF than other women and men. It is more common in the third trimester and is most commonly caused by viral hepatitis, hepatitis E virus (HEV) (60%), HBV, HAV, and rarely herpes simplex virus (HSV) and varicella-zoster virus (VZV). Acute fatty liver of pregnancy (AFLP) and hemolysis, elevated liver enzymes, and low platelets (HELLP) syndromes are specific for pregnancy and may improve with termination.
- *Vascular causes:* ALF may be seen in shock liver after cardiac arrest, significant hypovolemia/hypotension, or severe congestive heart failure. About 1% of cases of Budd–Chiari syndrome present with ALF.

TABLE 5: Scoring systems and indications for liver transplantation in selected chronic liver diseases.[25-29]

Disease	*Scoring system*	*Indication for LT*
Primary sclerosing cholangitis (PSC)	*Mayo PSC risk score:* 0.03 × (*age* in years) + 0.54 × log (*bilirubin* in mg/dL) + 0.54 × log (*AST* in IU/L) + 1.24 × (history of *variceal bleeding*) – 0.84 × (*albumin* in g/dL)	• Decompensated CLD • Recurrent cholangitis (≥2 episodes in 1 year requiring hospitalization) • Intractable pruritus with an unacceptable quality of life
Primary biliary cirrhosis (PBC)	*Mayo PBC risk score:* 0.871 × $\log_e$ (*bilirubin* in mg/dL) – 2.53 × $\log_e$ (*albumin* in g/dL) + 0.039 × (*age* in years) + $\log_e$ × (*prothrombin time* in seconds) + 0:859 (if *edema* is present)	• MRS ≥7.8 • Decompensated cirrhosis • Intractable pruritus • Profound disabling fatigue • Severe osteoporosis
	• UK-PBC score • *Baseline values:* Albumin, platelet count • *Values after 12 months of UDCA therapy:* Bilirubin, transaminases, alkaline phosphatase	Continuous score estimating 5-, 10-, and 15-year risk of death or liver transplant
	GLOBE score: Bilirubin, alkaline phosphatase, albumin, platelet count at 12 months, age at baseline	A score >0.3 is associated with significantly lower transplant-free survival
Alcoholic hepatitis	*Maddrey discriminant function (DF):* 4.6 × (prolongation of *prothrombin time* in seconds) + serum *bilirubin* (mg/dL)	DF >32 with hepatic encephalopathy >50% mortality within 28 days
	Glasgow Alcoholic Hepatitis Score (GAHS): Based on age, serum bilirubin, blood urea nitrogen, prothrombin time, and the peripheral leukocyte count	GAHS ≥9 predicts 28- and 84-day mortality
	Lille model: Age, renal insufficiency, albumin, prothrombin time, bilirubin, and the evolution of bilirubin on day 7 in response to steroids	Predicts 6-month mortality

(AST: aspartate aminotransferase; CLD: chronic liver disease; LT: liver transplantation; MRS: Mayo risk score; UDCA: ursodeoxycholic acid)

BOX 1: Drugs causing idiosyncratic reactions leading to acute liver failure.

Single agents causing heapatotoxicity		
Isoniazid: • Valproic acid • Carbamazepine • Efavirenz • Methyldopa • Dapsone • Labetalol • Disulfiram • Gemtuzumab • Propylthiouracil • Phenytoin	*Pyrazinamide:* • Diclofenac • Abacavir • Ketoconazole • Etodolac • Tolcapone • MDMA (Ecstasy) • Terbinafine • Ciprofloxacin • Nicotinic acid • Sulfasalazine	*Isoflurane:* • Itraconazole • Doxycycline • Didanosine • Allopurinol • Amiodarone • Cocaine • Nitrofurantoin • Imipramine • Statins
Combination agents with enhanced toxicity		
• Trimethoprim-sulfamethoxazole	• Rifampin–Isoniazid	• Amoxicillin–clavulanate
Herbal products/dietary supplements associated with hepatotoxicity		
• Kava • Herbalife • Comfrey	• Greater celandine • LipoKinetix • Senecio	• He Shon Wu • Hydroxycut • Ma Huang

(MDMA: 3,4-methylenedioxymethamphetamine)

- *Autoimmune hepatitis* (AIH) may account for 8–30% of all ALFs. It should be suspected in patients with autoantibodies, high globulins, and other autoimmune diseases. A liver biopsy is required for diagnosis. Patients with high-grade hepatic encephalopathy, high MELD scores, and/or lack of improvement within 7 days of steroids should be considered for LT.
- *Rare diseases* such as Reye's syndrome, hemophagocytic lymphohistiocytosis (HLH), and extensive malignant infiltration of the liver may also present with ALF.
- *Indeterminate/seronegative (non-A-E) hepatitis*: All etiological workup may be negative in about 15–47% of adult and 13–20% of children with ALF. They are generally tested for hepatitis A–E, although rare viruses [dengue, HSV, Epstein–Barr virus (EBV), VZV, and others] may be responsible.

Prognostication and Classification in Acute Liver Failure

Several factors, such as age, severity of insult, organ failure, and comorbidities, have been identified to predict spontaneous recovery in ALF, although etiology and rapidity of progression [measured by jaundice-encephalopathy interval (JEI)] are most significant. JEI is most often used for the subclassification of ALF **(Table 6)**. Counterintuitively, the highest rate of spontaneous recovery is seen in patients with rapidly progressive (shorter JEI) ALF, whereas a slower clinical course (longer JEI), with modest coagulopathy and lower incidence of cerebral edema, exhibits much lower rates of spontaneous recovery and is most likely to require LT **(Fig. 10)**.

Several scores have been described to prognosticate disease progression in ALF; King's College criteria is the most widely used tool, although several etiology-specific and dynamic scoring systems have also been described **(Table 7)**. They are aimed at differentiating patients into one of the following categories:

TABLE 6: Subclassifications of ALF based on jaundice–encephalopathy interval (JEI).

Classification system	*Jaundice–encephalopathy interval*
Trey and Davidson[25]	≤8 weeks
Fulminant hepatitis[26]	≤8 weeks
• Acute	≤10 days
• Subacute	11–56 days
• Fulminant hepatic failure[27]	≤2 weeks
• Subfulminant hepatic failure	2 weeks–to 3 months
British classification[28]	
• Hyperacute liver failure	≤7 days
• Acute liver failure	8–28 days
• Subacute liver failure	29–72 days
• Late-onset	56–182 days
International Association for Study of the Liver (IASL)[29]	
• Hyperacute	≤10 days
• Fulminant	10–30 days
• Subacute	5–24 weeks (with ascites and/or HE)
AASLD[30]	≤26 weeks
Intractable Hepato-Biliary Diseases Study Group of Japan[31]	
• ALF without hepatic coma	≤8 weeks
• ALF with hepatic coma	
– Acute	≤10 days
– Subacute	11–56 days

(AASLD: American Association for the Study of Liver Diseases; ALF: acute liver failure; HE: hepatic encephalopathy)

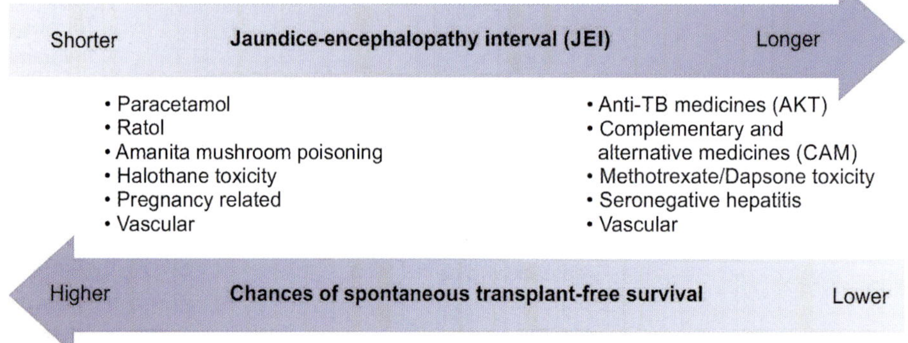

Fig. 10: Inverse relationship of spontaneous recovery to encephalopathy interval.

TABLE 7: Prognostic scores in acute liver failure.

Criteria, year, etiologies	*Prognostic parameters*	*Criteria performance*
King's College Criteria for paracetamol toxicity[31]	Arterial pH <7.3 (independent of HE grades) OR Grade 3 or 4 encephalopathy and PT >100 seconds and Serum creatinine >3.4 mg/dL	Sensitivity 69%, specificity 92%
King's College Criteria for nonparacetamol etiologies[31]	PT >100 seconds (independent of HE grades) OR Any three of the following variables (independent of HE grades): 1. *Age:* <10 or >40 years 2. *Etiology:* Non-A, non-B, halothane hepatitis, idiopathic drug reactions 3. Duration of jaundice before onset of encephalopathy >7 days 4. PT >50 seconds 5. Serum bilirubin >18 mg/dL	
Bernuau et al.[32] HBV	Age, factor V levels	
Bismuth et al.[33] Mixed etiologies	Age, factor V levels, HE grades 3–4	
Hadem et al.[34] BiLE score Mixed etiologies	Etiology, bilirubin, lactate	
Dhiman et al.[35] Mixed etiologies	Any three of the six parameters: 1. Age >50 years 2. Prothrombin time >35 seconds 3. Creatinine >1.5 mg/dL 4. Jaundice to encephalopathy >7 days 5. HE grades 3–4 6. Cerebral edema	Superior to KCH and MELD
Kumar et al.[36] ALFED dynamic criteria Indian, HAV, HEV	• Age >50 years, time from JEI > 7 days • PT >35 seconds, serum creatinine >1.5 mg/dL	Late clinical complications associated with poor outcomes
Bechmann et al.[37] Mixed etiologies	Creatinine, INR, cytokeratin 18	Superior to KCH and MELD
Bernal et al.[38] Paracetamol	Serum lactate (early 3.5 mmol/L, postresuscitation 3.0 mmol/L)	
Schmidt and Dalhoff[39] Paracetamol	Serum phosphate (1.2 mmol/L, 48–96 hours after overdose)	Not superior to KCH
Schmidt and Larsen[40] Paracetamol	MELD score	• Sensitivity 60% • Not superior to KCH
Rutherford et al.[41] ALFSG index Mixed etiologies	INR, serum bilirubin, phosphate, M30, encephalopathy grade	• Sensitivity 86% • Superior to KCH and MELD
Taylor et al.[42] HAV	ALT <2,600 IU/L, creatinine >2.0 mg/dL Mechanical ventilation, inotropes	Superior to KCC and MELD
Ganzert et al.[43] Amanita phyllodes	Prothrombin index <25%, creatinine >106 µmol/L Applicable from day 3	Sensitivity 100%, specificity 98%

Contd...

Contd…

Criteria, year, etiologies	***Prognostic parameters***	***Criteria performance***
Westbrook et al.[44] Pregnancy-related	Lactate >2.8 mg/dL, HE	*Lactate*: Sensitivity 73%, specificity 75% *Lactate + HE:* Sensitivity 90%, specificity 86% Predicting death and LT
Nonparacetamol	MELD >32	Sensitivity 76%, specificity 67% Not superior to KCC
Clichy criteria[45] (Paracetamol/HBV)	Factor VIII/V ratio >30, factor V <10%	Sensitivity 91%, specificity 91% Superior to KCC
Paracetamol	Arterial lactate 3.5 mmol/L on admission, 3 mmol/L postresuscitation	Sensitivity 81%, specificity 95% Superior to KCC
Paracetamol	Serum phosphate 1.2 mmol/L, 48–96 hours after overdose	Sensitivity 89%, specificity 100% Superior to KCC
Paracetamol	MELD >33 at onset of HE	Sensitivity 60%, specificity 69% Not superior to KCC
NHS criteria for paracetamol toxicity	• pH <7.25 >24 hours after overdose and after fluid resuscitation • Significant liver injury and coagulopathy following exclusion of other causes of hyperlactatemia (e.g., pancreatitis, intestinal ischemia) after adequate fluid resuscitation – Arterial lactate >5 mmol/L on admission – Arterial lactate >4 mmol/L after 24 hours of fluid resuscitation – Clinical hepatic encephalopathy • *All three criteria fulfilled:* – Prothrombin time >100 seconds or INR >6.5 – Serum creatinine >300 μmol/L (3.39 mg/dL) or anuria – Grade 3–4 encephalopathy • Two of the above three criteria from the category with clinical evidence of deterioration (e.g., increased ICP, FiO_2 >50%, increasing inotrope requirements) in the absence of clinical sepsis	
NHS criteria for favorable etiologies (HAV, HEV, Ecstasy, Cocaine toxicity, etc.)	• Clinical hepatic encephalopathy is mandatory • Prothrombin time >100 seconds or INR >6.5 or • Any three of the following: – Age >40 or <10 years – Prothrombin time >50 seconds or INR > 3.5 – Any grade of hepatic encephalopathy with jaundice to encephalopathy time >7 days – Serum bilirubin >300 mol/L (17.54 mg/dL)	
NHS criteria for unfavorable etiologies [seronegative hepatitis, idiosyncratic drug reactions, drug-induced liver injury (DILI), others]	• Prothrombin time >100 seconds or INR >6.5 or • In the absence of clinical hepatic encephalopathy – INR >2 after vitamin K repletion is mandatory and – Any two of the following - Age >40 years - Age <10 years - Prothrombin time >50 seconds or INR >3.5 • If hepatic encephalopathy is present – Jaundice to encephalopathy time >7 days – Serum bilirubin >17.54 mg/dL (>300 mmol/L)	

Contd…

Contd...

Criteria, year, etiologies	*Prognostic parameters*	*Criteria performance*
Yellow phosphorus (rodenticide)	*Three of the following four criteria:* 1. Prothrombin time >100 seconds or INR >6.5 after vitamin K repletion. In patients undergoing plasmapheresis, 12 hours after the second set of plasmapheresis, if INR >2.5 2. MELD > 37 3. HE ≥ grade II 4. Arterial lactate (24 hours after admission) ≥6 mmol/L after fluid resuscitation No active cardiac dysfunction (EF <50%)	
AIH	Histology showing: • Confluent or massive hepatic necrosis (AIH/DILI) • Marked microvesicular steatosis (DILI) • Cholestatic hepatitis with ductopenia (DILI) MELD >28 No improvement in bilirubin/INR with steroids for 5 days	
Pediatric	Any one of the below: • INR >4 or • Grade 3–4 encephalopathy Multisystem disorders such as leukemia, lymphoma, hemophagocytosis, and disseminated intravascular coagulopathy are excluded	

(ALFSG: acute liver failure study group; ALFED: acute liver failure early dynamic; AIH: autoimmune hepatitis; BILE: Bilirubin Lactate and Etiology; DILI: drug-induced liver injury; EF: ejection fraction; HAV: hepatitis A virus; HBV: hepatitis B virus; HE: hepatic encephalopathy; HEV: hepatitis E virus; ICP: intracranial pressure; JEI: jaundice-encephalopathy interval; KCC: King's College Criteria; KCH: King's College Hospital; LT: liver transplantation; MELD: model for end-stage liver disease; NHS: National Health Service; INR: international normalized ratio; PT: prothrombin time)

- *Patients unlikely to survive without transplant:* Need urgent LT (prognostic models should have high sensitivity and specificity to predict death).
- *Patients with a high likelihood of spontaneous recovery and functionality with medical management*: Do not need LT.
- *Patients too sick to transplant*: LT is likely to be futile.

The decision for LT is often a dynamic one based on:

- Persistence of accepted ALF criteria is associated with a poor prognosis.
- Patients with sustained improvement in prognostic criteria and an absence of clinical deterioration should wait
- Patients with favorable etiologies such as paracetamol, HAV, HEV, and others have a good chance of spontaneous recovery
- Comorbidities and conditions independent of ALF that would impact survival, such as active infection, sepsis, invasive fungal infection, rapidly escalating inotropes, severe pancreatitis (usually in paracetamol-related ALF)
- Complications of ALF associated with reduced survival, especially compromised brainstem function, especially fixed and dilated pupils
- Psychosocial profile suggestive of poor adaptation of rigor of post-transplant survival
- Availability of a suitable donor for LT. Marginal livers from the elderly, steatotic, ABO incompatible, and others should preferably be avoided.

Most organ allocation systems prioritize ALF over CLD due to higher short-term mortality risk. Patients with Wilson's disease, AIH, or Budd–Chiari syndrome with ALF phenotype are also prioritized for LT despite having underlying CLD.

LIVER TRANSPLANTATION FOR ACUTE-ON-CHRONIC LIVER FAILURE

Acute-on-chronic liver failure is the syndrome of acute decompensation in a patient with CLD or cirrhosis characterized by rapidly progressive deterioration and high short-term mortality **(Table 8)**.

Acute-on-Chronic Liver Failure: Definitions

A global consensus on the definition of acute-on-chronic liver failure has not yet been reached. Three definitions are most widely used; the APASL/AARC (Asian Pacific Association for the Study of the Liver/APASL ACLF Research Consortium) definition, which is followed in the regions of South East Asia and South Asia, the EASL-CLIF (European Association for the Study of the Liver—Chronic Liver Failure) definition, which is followed in Europe, and the North American Consortia for the Study of End-Stage Liver disease (NASCLED) definition, which is followed in North America. The key differences between the definitions are summarized in **Table 8**.

TABLE 8: Acute triggers for acute-on-chronic liver failure.

	APASL (Asian Pacific Association for the Study of the Liver)/AARC (APASL ACLF Research Consortium)	***EASL-CLIF (European Association for the Study of the Liver-Chronic Liver Failure)***	***NACSELD (North American Consortia for the Study of End-Stage Liver Disease)***
Definition	Acute hepatic insult manifesting as jaundice (total bilirubin ≥5 mg/dL) and coagulopathy (INR of ≥1.5, or prothrombin activity <40%) complicated by ascites and/or encephalopathy in a patient with previously diagnosed or undiagnosed CLD associated with high mortality	Acute deterioration of pre-existing CLD is usually related to a precipitating event and associated with increased mortality at 3 months due to multisystem organ failure	A syndrome characterized by acute deterioration in a patient with cirrhosis due to infection, presenting with two or more extrahepatic organ failures
Inclusion	• Compensated cirrhosis (diagnosed or undiagnosed) • CLD but not cirrhosis • Acute insult directed at the liver • Presentation with liver failure • Index presentation	• Cirrhosis (compensated or decompensated) • Renal failure is mandatory • Presentation is not necessarily associated with liver failure • Can be repeated episodes of ACLF	• Cirrhosis (compensated or decompensated) • Two extrahepatic organ failures • Presentation is not necessarily associated with liver failure • Can be repeated episodes of ACLF
Time frame	4 weeks	4–12 weeks (variable)	Not defined
Precipitating factors	Intrahepatic	Intrahepatic (alcoholic hepatitis), extrahepatic (infection, gastrointestinal bleed), or both	Extrahepatic (infection)
Major organ systems considered for definition	Liver	One of the six major organ systems (liver, kidney, brain, coagulation, circulation, and respiration)	Two to four organ systems (kidney, brain, circulation, and respiration)
Exclusion criteria for the absence of ACLF	• Acute decompensation of cirrhosis • Prior decompensation HCC	• HCC • No organ system failure • Single organ failure (liver, coagulation, circulation, respiration) without kidney or brain dysfunction • Cerebral failure without kidney dysfunction	• Infections not requiring hospitalization • Cirrhosis without infection • *Immune-compromised patients:* HIV, prior organ transplant, disseminated malignancies • None of the four organ failures used to define ACLF • Single organ system failure
Homogeneity	More homogeneous patients	Heterogeneous patients (40% have unknown acute insult), extrahepatic organ failure, and systemic inflammation may confound comparative studies	Heterogeneous patients, extrahepatic organ failure, and systemic inflammation may confound comparative studies

(ACLF: acute-on-chronic liver failure; CLD: chronic liver disease; HCC: hepatocellular carcinoma; HIV: human immunodeficiency virus; INR: international normalized ratio)

Acute-on-Chronic Liver Failure Precipitants/Triggers

Acute-on-chronic liver failure is often triggered by identifiable acute events, with bacterial infections such as spontaneous bacterial peritonitis (SBP), secondary peritonitis, and pneumonia being the most common, in addition to alcohol and HBV exacerbation (few eastern countries) **(Table 9)**.

Prognostication and Indication for LT

Acute-on-chronic liver failure offers a very narrow therapeutic window for LT. The prognosis depends on the number of hepatic and extrahepatic organ failures. However, if infection is the trigger for ACLF, it may preclude an LT. Different scoring systems for the prognostication of ACLF are outlined in **Table 10**.

For patients not meeting the ACLF definition, the CLIF-C AD (acute decompensation) score is used for prognostication. The CLIF-C ACLF score of >65 is associated with 100% mortality in 3–7 days, and LT may be futile.

LIVER TRANSPLANTATION FOR LIVER TUMORS

Hepatocellular Carcinoma

Liver transplantation may be curative for liver cirrhosis with HCC since it removes the tumor with the widest possible margin and reduces the risk of new tumors. Most HCC patients have compensated cirrhosis or early decompensation and, therefore, have CTP/MELD scores. Since their mortality risk is dominantly determined by the progression of HCC rather than cirrhosis, criteria based on tumor characteristics are used for organ allocation. Milan and University of California San Francisco (USCF) criteria are most commonly used, although several other/expanded criteria have been described **(Table 11)**. Patients may require locoregional or systemic therapy to prevent tumor progression while waiting for a transplant (bridging) or to downstage them to within the criteria.

Cholangiocarcinoma

Cholangiocarcinoma (CCA) is an aggressive tumor with a poor prognosis. Radical surgical resection with clear

TABLE 9: Acute triggers for acute-on-chronic liver failure.

Triggers	*Common*	*Uncommon*
Infections	• Bacterial infections – Spontaneous bacterial peritonitis – Spontaneous bacterial empyema – Spontaneous/secondary bacteremia – Urinary tract infection – Pneumonia – Bronchitis – Skin and soft-tissue infection – Cholangitis – Secondary peritonitis – *Clostridium difficile* infection • Fungal infections – Invasive candidiasis – Invasive aspergillosis • Hepatotropic viral infections – Hepatitis B virus (HBV) infection or reactivation – Superimposed hepatitis A – Superimposed hepatitis E	• Hepatotropic viral infections – Superimposed hepatitis D in patients with chronic HBV – Superimposed hepatitis C • Systemic viral infections – Epstein–Barr virus (EBV) – Cytomegalovirus (CMV) – Herpes simplex virus (HSV 1, 2, 6) – Varicella zoster virus (VZV) – Human immunodeficiency virus (HIV) – Parvovirus B19 – Severe acute respiratory syndrome coronavirus 2 (SARS-CoV-2) – Influenza A, influenza B, and syncytial respiratory virus • *Parasitic infection:* Visceral Leishmaniasis
Toxin/drugs	• Alcoholic hepatitis • Drug-induced acute kidney injury • Drug-induced encephalopathy	Drug-induced liver injury (DILI)
Others	Gastrointestinal hemorrhage ± shock	• Wilson's disease • Flare of autoimmune hepatitis (AIH) • Ischemic hepatitis • Surgical or radiological intervention

Note: 20–40% of cases have no identifiable trigger, possibly linked to bacterial translocation or hepatocyte damage.[46]

TABLE 10: Scoring systems for acute-on-chronic liver failure and mortality risk.

CLIF-C OF score				
		Scale		
System	***Variable***	***1 point***	***2 points***	***3 points***
Liver	Bilirubin (mg/dL)	<6.0	6.0–12	≥12
Kidney	Creatinine (mg/dL)	<1.5 ≥1.5 to <2.0	≥2.0–<3.5	≥3.5 or use of RRT
Cerebral	HE grade (West Haven)	0	I–II	III–IV or endotracheal intubation for HE
Coagulation	INR	<2.0	≥2.0–<2.5	≥2.5
Circulation	MAP (mm Hg)	≥70	<70	Use of vasopressors
Respiration	PaO_2/FiO_2	>300	>200 to ≤300	≤200
	SpO_2/FiO_2	>357	>214 to ≤357	≤214 or use of mechanical ventilation
Grade	***Definition***			***28-day mortality risk***
ACLF-1	Single organ failure (coagulation, liver, circulation, respiration) in patients with creatinine 1.5–1.9 and/or HE grade 1–2			20%
ACLF-2	2 organ failures			30%
ACLF-3	≥3 organ failures			80%
NASCELD definitions of organ failure				
System	***Definition of organ failure***			
Kidney	Need for dialysis or other forms of renal replacement therapy			
Brain	HE grade III or IV			
Circulation	Shock: MAP <60 mm Hg or a reduction of 40 mm Hg in systolic blood pressure from baseline, despite adequate fluid resuscitation and cardiac output			
Respiration	Need for mechanical ventilation			
	Mortality risk in 30 days	***30-day mortality risk***		
	2 organ failures	49%		
	3 organ failures	64%		
	4 organ failures	77%		
APASL definition				
AARC score	AARC score comprises bilirubin, grade of hepatic encephalopathy, PT-INR, lactate, and creatinine. This liver failure grading system classifies patients into one of three categories[47]			
AARC Grade	***Score***	***28-day mortality***	***Expected action/outcome***	
Grade 1	5–7	13%	Potentially recoverable group	
Grade 2	8–10	45%	Requires critical monitoring	
Grade 3	11–15	86%	Requires immediate intervention for improved outcomes	

(ACLF-1: acute-on-chronic liver failure grade 1; CLIF-C OF: Chronic Liver Failure Consortium Organ Failure; HE: hepatic encephalopathy; INR: international normalized ratio; MAP: mean arterial pressure; NASCELD: North American Consortium for the Study of End-Stage Liver Disease; PT–INR: prothrombin time–international normalized ratio; RRT: renal replacement therapy)

margins offers the best chance of cure, but is frequently not possible due to locally advanced disease or underlying cirrhosis. LT has good outcomes in early intrahepatic CCA (<2 cm). Unresectable perihilar CCA responding to neoadjuvant chemoradiation has satisfactory outcomes, the largest experience with the Mayo protocol **(Table 12)**.

Colorectal Liver Metastases

Radical liver resection offers the best chance for long-term survival for patients with colorectal liver metastases (CRLM). Unfortunately, up to 50% of patients have unresectable disease, and 5-year survival is <20% with systemic therapies. Many studies over the last 20 years

TABLE 11: Commonly used selection criteria for liver transplantation in hepatocellular carcinoma.

Standard criteria		
Criteria	***Milan criteria***[48]	***UCSF criteria***[49]
	• Solitary lesion >2 and ≤5 cm • ≤3 lesions with size • Largest ≤3 cm • No gross portal vein invasion • No extrahepatic metastases	• Solitary lesion ≤6.5 cm • <3 lesions with size • Largest ≤4.5 cm • Total ≤8 cm • No gross portal vein invasion • No extrahepatic metastases
Post-LT survival (patients within criteria)	• 4-year survival: Overall survival 85% • Recurrence-free survival: 92%	• 90% at 1 year • 75.2% at 5 years
Post-LT survival (patients beyond criteria)	4-year survival: Overall 50% Recurrence-free survival: 59%	50% at 1 year

Expanded criteria					
		Multiple lesions			
Criteria	***Single lesion (cm)***	***No.***	***Size (cm)***	***Nonsize criteria***	***Survival***
Pittsburgh[50]	Modified TNM staging				
Barcelona[51]	<7	3	<5		
		5	<3		
Kyoto[52]		≤10	≤5	PIVKA II ≤400 mAU/mL	Beyond Milan 5-year survival rate: 65%
Hong Kong	≤6.5	3	≤4.5		
Shanghai criteria[53]	≤9 cm	≤3	≤5	No macrovascular or lymph node invasion or extrahepatic metastasis	• 5-year OS: 78.1% • 5-year RFS: 52.6%
Tokyo (5-5 rule)[54]		5	≤5		5-year: 75%
Kneteman, Canada[55]	<7.5	Any	<5		
Fukuoka, Japan[56]		Any	Any	No gross vascular invasion or extrahepatic spread	
Hangzhou criteria[57]	≤8 cm				
	>8 cm			Grade I or II and AFP ≤400	
New Milan (up to 7)[58]	The sum of the number of tumors + the diameter of the largest tumor ≤7				• 5-year • Within Milan: 73.3% • Beyond Milan: 71.2%
Edmonton criteria[59]	Total tumor volume ≤115 mL, AFP ≤400 ng/mL				5-year: 80%
Asan criteria (LDLT)[60]		≤6	≤5	No gross vascular invasion	
Extended Toronto Criteria (ETC)[61]	• No limit in size and number • No vascular invasion or extrahepatic disease • No cancer-related symptoms • Biopsy of the largest tumor, not poorly differentiated				Beyond Milan 5-year survival rate: 68%

(AFP: alpha-fetoprotein; LT: liver transplantation; LDLT: living donor liver transplant; OS: overall survival; PIVKA II: protein induced by vitamin K absence or antagonism II; RFS: recurrence-free survival; UCSF: University of California, San Francisco) have observed a 5-year survival of 50–60% with LT for CRLM, leading to scores to select patients for LT **(Table 13)**.

The International Hepato-Pancreato-Biliary Association (IHPBA) consensus guidelines require the removal of primary tumors, no extrahepatic disease, fulfillment of molecular criteria (tumors should have microsatellite stability, mismatch repair proficiency, and no *BRAFV600E* mutation), and appropriate response to at least 6 months of bridging therapy before consideration for LT.[67] Patient selection is guided by both tumor biology and resectability **(Table 14)**.

Metastatic Neuroendocrine Tumors

Selected neuroendocrine tumor (NET) cases after removal/treatment of the primary tumor with regional lymph nodes (LNs) and extrahepatic disease, with favorable pathological grade and stable post-treatment course, have excellent outcomes with LT **(Table 15)**. Metastatic NETs

TABLE 12: Mayo protocol for liver transplantation in perihilar cholangiocarcinoma.

Inclusion criteria	*Exclusion criteria*	*Neoadjuvant protocol*
• Pathologic diagnosis of cholangiocarcinoma • Transcatheter biopsy or brush cytology OR • Malignant-appearing biliary stricture with CA 19-9 >100 ng/mL OR positive FISH OR • Mass at the stricture site • Lesion size <3 cm • Tumor unresectable by conventional liver resection	• Metastatic disease • Intrahepatic or extrahepatic metastases • Lymph node metastases • Prior chemoradiotherapy or attempted resection • Uncontrolled sepsis • Intrahepatic cholangiocarcinoma • Previous malignancy in the last 5 years	• EUS and FNA of regional periportal nodes • EBRT for 3 weeks to a target dose of 45 Gy with continuous infusion of 5-Fluorouracil • Brachytherapy for 2 weeks after EBRT • Administered by transcatheter irradiation (20–30 Gy) with iridium Ir 192 wires • These wires are placed by ERCP or PTC • Oral capecitabine continued until the transplant • Elective staging laparotomy before transplant, including biopsy of at least one lymph node along the proper hepatic artery and another along the common bile duct, as well as any lymph nodes or nodules suspicious of the tumor

(EBRT: external beam radiotherapy; ERCP: endoscopic retrograde cholangiopancreatography; EUS: endoscopic ultrasound; FNA: fine needle aspiration; FISH: fluorescent in situ hybridization; PTC: percutaneous transhepatic cholangiography)

TABLE 13: Risk stratification for liver transplantation for colorectal liver metastasis

Score	*Criteria*	*Risk stratification*
Nordlinger et al.[62]	• Age >60 years • Serosal invasion of primary (pT3) • DFI <24 months • Liver lesions> 3 • Largest liver lesion >5 cm	• Low: 0–2 • Intermediate: 3–4 • High: 5–6
Fong Clinical Risk Score[63]	• Synchronous disease (DFI <12 months) • Number of lesions >1 • Preoperative CEA >200 ng/mL • Largest liver lesion >5 cm • Lymph node-positive primary tumor	• Low: 0–2 • High: 3–5
Nagashima et al.[64]	• Serosal invasion of primary tumor (pT3) • Lymph node positive primary tumor • Number of liver metastases ≥2 • Largest liver lesion <5 cm • Resectable extrahepatic metastases	• Low: 0–1 • Intermediate: 2–3 • High: 4–5
Konopke et al.[65]	• Number of liver metastases ≥4 • CEA ≥200 ng/mL • Synchronous liver metastases	• Low: 0 • Intermediate: 1 • High: 2–3
GAME score[66]	• *KRAS* mutation • CEA ≥20 ng/mL • Tumor burden score 3–8 (1 point) or ≥9 (2 points) • Extrahepatic disease (2 points)	

Contd...

Contd...

Score	Criteria	Risk stratification
Modified FCRS, 2019	• Largest liver lesion > 5cm • Lymph node positive tumor • *RAS* mutation	
Oslo score, 2020	• Tumor diameter >5.5 cm • CEA >80 ng/mL • <2-year interval between primary resection and LT • Progressive disease at the time of LT	• Low: 0–2 • High: 3–4

(CEA: carcinoembryonic antigen; DFI: disease-free interval; LT: liver transplantation)

TABLE 14: Factors associated with biological unresectability.

Factor	Evidence	Rational for transplantation
Potential transplant benefit		
• Tumor burden score (TBS) >9[68] • Increasing number and size of metastases[69]	• A TBS > 9 has been associated with reduced OS • An increasing number (HR 1.3, 1.1–1.6) and diameter (HR 1.1, 1–1.2) are associated with reduced OS	Recurrence in the presence of these factors is likely to be due to microscopic, undetectable diseases left behind during resection. The complete hepatectomy performed during LT may reduce this recurrence risk by eliminating all intrahepatic disease
Need for intraoperative ablation[70]	Associated with early recurrence (OR 1.6, 1.1–2.5)	
Surgical margin 0 mm[70]	Associated with early recurrence (OR 1.5, 1–2.2)	
R1 resection[71]	Associated with early recurrence (HR 2.2, 1.2–4.2)	
Need for PVE[72,73]	Associated with reduced OS (HR 1.48, 1.09–1.98) In patients with high tumor load, median OS 19.2 months (95% CI 0.0–39.5 months) after PVE vs. 40.5 months (95% CI 26.3–54.7 months) after LT ($p = 0.007$)	
Initially unresectable disease[71]	Associated with early recurrence (HR 1.9, 1.02–3.7)	
More metastases were detected intraoperatively[74]	Associated with reduced OS (HR 3.19, 1.28–7.97)	
Need for preoperative chemotherapy[69]	Associated with reduced OS (HR 1.7, 1.2–2.5)	
Transplant benefit unlikely		
More than 1 preoperative chemotherapy line[73]	Associated with early recurrence (RR 1.6, 1.1–2.4)	Recurrence in the presence of these factors is likely to be due to aggressive biological characteristics; thus, a liver transplant is unlikely to change the prognosis
Progression during last-line chemotherapy[73]	Associated with early recurrence (RR 2.18, 1.11–4.47)	
Higher CEA levels[71]	CEA > 30 ng/mL associated with early recurrence (HR 2.3, 1.2–4.7)	
Higher CA 19-9 levels[73]	CA 19-9 levels >60 U/mL associated with early recurrence (RR 2.21, 1.44–3.43). CA 19-9 levels >100 U/mL associated with reduced OS (HR 1.86, 1.37–2.48)	
Primary tumor T stage >2[69,70]	• Associated with reduced OS (HR 1.4, 1.1–2) Associated with early recurrence (OR 2.6, 1.4–4.8)	
Right-sided primary tumor[69]	Associated with reduced OS (HR 1.5, 1–2.1)	
Primary tumor lymphovascular invasion[71]	Associated with early recurrence (HR 2.5, 1.3–4.8)	
Nodal positive primary[73]	Associated with reduced OS (HR 1.46, 1.13–1.89)	

(CEA: carcinoembryonic antigen; CI: confidence interval; HR: hazard ratio; LT: liver transplantation; OR: odds ratio; OS: overall survival; PVE: portal vein embolization; RR: relative risk)

TABLE 15: Selection criteria for liver transplantation in neuroendocrine tumors.

Criteria	*Milan-NET*	*European Society for Medical Oncology (ESMO)*	*United Network for Organ Sharing (UNOS)/Organ Procurement and Transplantation Network (OPTN)*	*European Neuroendocrine Tumor Society (ENETS)*
Grade	G1–G2	G1/G2 Ki-67 <10%	• G1–G2 • Mitotic rate <20/10 HPF • Ki-67 <20%	G1–G2
Primary tumor site	Drained by the portal system		Drained by the portal system	NA
Tumor involvement	<50% of liver volume	<50% of liver volume	<50% of liver volume	NA
Extrahepatic disease	Ok			No
Primary tumor treatment	Resection of the primary tumor and all extrahepatic tumor deposits	Previous removal of the primary tumor	Resection of primary malignancy and all extrahepatic diseases	Early/refractory to multiple systemic treatments
Interval	Stable disease/good response for ≥6 months	Stable disease for ≥6 months	No recurrence for ≥6 months	NA
Recipient age	<60 years (relative criteria)	<60 years	<60 years	NA
Others	None		• NET limited to the liver, bilobar, not amenable to resection • Negative metastatic workup (PET, somatostatin receptor, DOTA Gallium-68 DOTATATE PET scan)	Low bilirubin Carcinoid syndrome or functional NETs

(HPF: high-power field; NET: neuroendocrine tumor; PET: positron emission tomography)

from primary tumors in the lower rectum, esophagus, lung, adrenal gland, and thyroid are not LT candidates.

The North American Neuroendocrine Tumor Society (NANETS) considers LT controversial but an option for patients meeting Milan-NET and European Neuroendocrine Tumor Society (ENETS) criteria.[75]

Hepatic Epithelioid Hemangioendothelioma

Liver transplantation for HEHE, even with extrahepatic disease, has excellent long-term outcomes and low recurrence rates.[76-79]

Hepatic epithelioid hemangioendothelioma transplant propensity score =
5 × (*pathologic macrovascular invasion*) +
3 × (*waitlist time of 120 days*) +
2 × (*Hilar LN invasion at pathology*)

The score prognosticates post-LT recurrence risk:

- *Low risk (0–2)*: 5-year disease-free survival (DFS) 93.9%
- *Intermediate risk (3–5)*: 5-year DFS 76.9%
- *High -risk (6–10)*: 5-year DFS 38.5%

LIVER TRANSPLANTATION FOR INBORN ERRORS OF METABOLISM

Inborn errors of metabolism often occur due to enzyme deficiencies or dysfunctional pathways and may lead to serious metabolic disturbances, progressive liver disease, neurological impairment, and/or multisystem problems. Medical treatments and dietary restrictions are first-line therapy but may be very challenging for patients and their families. About 10% of pediatric LTs are done for IEMs, the most common indications being α1-antitrypsin deficiency, urea cycle defects, tyrosinemia, cystic fibrosis, and Wilson's disease **(Table 16)**.[80]

CONTRAINDICATIONS FOR LIVER TRANSPLANTATION

Liver transplantation is contraindicated if it poses a prohibitive surgical risk or has a low likelihood of long-term survival or acceptable quality of life after LT. The criteria vary between centers, depending on local facilities and expertise available and the reversibility of the condition. **Table 17** provides a comprehensive list of the contraindications to a liver transplant.

TABLE 16: Inborn errors of metabolism (IEMs) requiring LT.

Disease/Description	*Indications for LT*
Group A: Disorders with enzyme defect only in the liver, and LT is done predominantly for ESLD and its related complications	
Tyrosinemia (HT-1): • The risk of recurrence of HCC after LT surveillance is required • Renal-sparing immunosuppression is preferred	• HCC • Decompensated cirrhosis • Noncompliance with medical therapy • ALF
Alpha 1 antitrypsin deficiency: • Pulmonary function may continue to deteriorate after LT • Higher incidence of hepatic artery thrombosis	• Decompensated cirrhosis • HCC
Galactosemia type 1: • Early recognition with withdrawal of lactose/galactose improves the clinical status and liver function. LT is rarely indicated	• Progressive liver dysfunction despite a galactose-free diet • HCC
Wilson's disease: • LT is not recommended for neurologic-only presentation, as liver disease can be stabilized with medical therapy, and neuropsychiatric symptoms may not improve after LT, but may be considered in the absence of response to chelation therapy • The asymptomatic heterozygous family donor can safely donate their liver	• Decompensated cirrhosis • CLD with failure of response to medical therapy • Acute liver injury with coagulopathy unresponsive to vitamin K, New Wilson's index persistently ≥11, progression to ALF • Acute liver failure (8–20% of patients) • HCC
Hereditary fructosemia: • Prompt recognition and withholding of fructose in the diet reverses symptoms and liver disease	• Synthetic failure • Portal hypertension • Malignancies • Growth retardation
Glycogen storage disease types III and IV: • Type III GSD involves the striated muscles in 85% of cases, and cardiac disease should be ruled out before LT • Type IV GSD may have muscle involvement and infantile presentations such as spinal muscular atrophy	• Synthetic failure • Portal hypertension • Cirrhosis • HCC
Congenital disorder of glycosylation	ESLD
Lysosomal storage disorders: • Enzyme replacement is continued after the LT period to control extrahepatic symptoms and prevent disease recurrence	ESLD
Group B: Disorders with enzyme defects limited to the liver. These patients rarely have ESLD; LT is performed for extrahepatic organ involvement	
Urea cycle disorders: • LT arrests the progression of neurological damage by preventing hyperammonemia and metabolic crisis	Severe metabolic defects • Elevated ammonia >300 μmol/L • Refractoriness to medical therapy
Porphyrias: • Tramadol, ketamine, thiopentone, azole antifungals, cotrimoxazole, and carbapenems should be avoided • Porphyrin levels should be maintained by plasmapheresis or by heme infusion	Timely LT before onset and/or progression of neuronal injury and/or autonomic dysfunction
Glycogen storage disease type 1: • SLKT may be required for coexisting ESRD • Renal-sparing immunosuppression is preferred	• Poor metabolic control despite a complex carbohydrate diet (e.g., uncooked corn starch) • Multiple and growing hepatic adenomas • HCC • Growth retardation

Contd...

Contd…

Disease/Description	*Indications for LT*
Primary hyperoxaluria: • If EF < 40–45%, aggressive dialysis for 4–6 weeks may decrease systemic oxalate load and improve cardiac contractility • Higher risk of bleeding after LT due to platelet dysfunction • Heterozygous donors are screened for urine oxalate levels, even with normal renal function. They can be liver donors but not kidney donors because of the risk of long-term renal failure risk	• eGFR > 50 mL/m^2/min → isolated LT • eGFR > 50 mL/m^2/min/renal stones → SLKT
Familial hypercholesterolemia: • Early childhood atherosclerosis can cause coronary artery disease/myocardial infarction	• LT is curative • Recommended before the development of atherosclerosis
Crigler–Najjar syndrome	LT prevents further neurological injury and may reverse the changes
Group C: Disorders having enzyme defects in the liver and extrahepatic tissue, and LT only partially corrects the underlying metabolic disease and alleviates symptoms of extrahepatic organ involvement	
Methylmalonic aciduria: • 60% can have progressive renal dysfunction • Pancreatitis, cognitive deficits, metabolic strokes • Optic atrophy may not be completely prevented even after a successful LT	Recurrent metabolic crises in early infancy
Propionic academia: • Higher incidence of hepatic artery thrombosis • Injury to the brain and heart is usually irreversible • Annual monitoring with clinical examinations and investigations is required	LT provides good control of the metabolism, decreases the toxic metabolic burden, and improves QoL
Maple syrup urine disease	• Recurrent seizures and cognitive dysfunction • LT prevents metabolic crises and arrests neurological progression
Mitochondrial hepatopathies: • LT only corrects hepatic manifestations • Other problems, such as pulmonary hypertension, progressive neurological dysfunction, and cardiomyopathy, may continue to worsen and may lead to mortality	Primary hepatic involvement without apparent extrahepatic organ involvement

(ALF: acute liver failure; CLD: chronic liver disease; EF: ejection fraction; eGFR: estimated glomerular filtration rate; ESLD: end-stage liver disease; ESRD: end-stage renal disease; GSD: glycogen storage disease; HCC: hepatocellular carcinoma; LT: liver transplantation; SLKT: simultaneous liver-kidney transplant)

TABLE 17: Contraindications for LT.

	Contraindication	*Remarks*
Severe cardiac disease	• Symptomatic coronary artery disease • Advanced coronary artery disease not amenable to revascularization • Severe ventricular dysfunction (EF <45%, cardiac index <3 L/min/m^2) • Advanced cardiomyopathy • Severe valvular heart disease • Aortic stenosis with poor ventricular function	• Patients may be eligible after revascularization (CABG or angioplasty) after myocardial ischemia has resolved and/or correction of valvular dysfunction • Some patients may need simultaneous CABG with LT • Good cardiac medical and surgical backup with ECMO may be required
Pulmonary hypertension	PA systolic >50 mm Hg and/or PVR >240 dynes/s/cm^5 and/or mean pulmonary arterial pressure (PAP) >35 mm Hg	Patients who respond to medical treatment become eligible for LT when PAP is <35 mm Hg

Contd…

Contd...

	Contraindication	***Remarks***
Pulmonary disease	• Severe HPS with arterial hypoxemia (<50 mm Hg PaO_2) • Oxygen-dependent chronic obstructive airway disease (COPD) • Advanced pulmonary fibrosis • Advanced pulmonary disease (FEV1/FVC ratio <0.5 or PO_2 <60 mm Hg in the absence of HPS or on home oxygen)	• Severe HPS patients may need backup with nitric oxide and ECMO • Reactive airway disease, hepatic hydrothorax, and others can/should be controlled before LT
Irreversible cerebral injury	• ALF with cerebral edema and brainstem herniation • CVA with irreversible disabling neurologic deficits	
Infections	• Active uncontrolled infection • Extensively drug-resistant (XDR) infections • Septic shock • AIDS/HIV with low CD4, high viral load	Patients may be eligible for LT after control/ treatment of infection
Malignancy	• Extrahepatic malignancies • Metastatic primary liver tumor	• Localized treated skin cancer patients may be considered for LT • For most other extrahepatic tumors, the patient may be considered for LT 2–5 years after remission of disease-free
Technical	• Extensive portomesenteric thrombosis without collateralization may make transplant technically unfeasible • Extensive adhesions/cocoon abdomen make dissection risky	
Psychosocial problems/ compliance	• Active alcohol abuse • Active illicit substance/drug abuse • Severe, uncontrolled, untreated psychiatric disease • Lack of family/social support, unsatisfactory caregiver plan • Inability or unwillingness to comply with a psychosocial plan • Behavior determined by the multidisciplinary team to pose a risk for noncompliance	LT may be offered at some centers for SAH, depending on certain criteria and the acuity of organ shortage locally
Poor functional status	• Severe sarcopenia, frailty • Severe muscle wasting	
Others		• Elderly patients may be LT candidates if they are functionally well preserved with controlled comorbidities • Patients with BMI <19 kg/m^2 and >50 at the time of transplant • LT during pregnancy is avoided unless life-threatening, such as ALF

(AIDS: acquired immunodeficiency syndrome; ALF: acute liver failure; BMI: body mass index; CABG: coronary artery bypass graft; CVA: cerebrovascular accident; EF: ejection fraction; FEV1/FVC: forced expiratory volume in 1 second/forced vital capacity; HIV: human immunodeficiency virus; HPS: hepatopulmonary syndrome; LT: liver transplantation; SAH: severe alcoholic hepatitis)

CONCLUSION

LT should be offered to patients at an optimum time within the entire spectrum of liver disease. It should be done at an appropriate time where benefits outweigh the expected risk. If too early, patients might miss out on the chance of spontaneous recovery and not be delayed to the point that patients are too sick to tolerate a transplant.

The number of LT has been steadily increasing worldwide. Presently, the most common indication of LT is still from decompensated chronic liver disease.

While, chronic Hepatitis B infection as an indication for transplant is declining worldwide due to universal vaccination, indication for MASLD has been steadily increasing. Appropriate timing for LT on acute liver failure and acute on chronic liver failure is suitable. The indications of LT are continually expanding, especially in tumors. The field of Transplant oncology is promising.

REFERENCES

1. Devarbhavi H, Asrani SK, Arab JP, Nartey YA, Pose E, Kamath PS. Global burden of liver disease: 2023 update. J Hepatol. 2023;79(2):516-37.
2. Paik JM, Golabi P, Younossi Y, Mishra A, Younossi ZM. Changes in the global burden of chronic liver diseases from 2012 to 2017: the growing impact of NAFLD. Hepatology. 2020;72(5):1605.
3. Starzl TE, Marchioro TL, Kaulla KNV, Hermann G, Brittain RS, Waddell WR. Homotransplantation of the liver in humans. Surg Gynecol Obstet. 1963;117:659.
4. Terrault NA, Francoz C, Berenguer M, Charlton M, Heimbach J. Liver Transplantation 2023: status report, current and future challenges. Clin Gastroenterol Hepatol. 2023;21(8):2150-66.
5. Kwong AJ, Kim WR, Lake JR, Schladt DP, Schnellinger EM, Gauntt K, et al. OPTN/SRTR 2022 annual data report: liver. Am J Transplant. 2024;24(2):S176-S265.
6. Anand AC, Nandi B, Acharya SK, Arora A, Babu S, Batra Y, et al. Indian National Association for the Study of the Liver Consensus Statement on Acute Liver Failure (Part 1): epidemiology, pathogenesis, presentation and prognosis. J Clin Exp Hepatol. 2020;10(4):339-76.
7. European Association for the Study of the Liver (EASL) clinical practice guidelines: liver transplantation. J Hepatol. 2016;64(2):433-85.
8. Younossi ZM, Wong G, Anstee QM, Henry L. The global burden of liver disease. Clin Gastroenterol Hepatol. 2023;21(8):1978-91.
9. Tian F, Feld JJ, Feng Z, Sander B, Wong WWL. Feasibility of hepatitis B elimination in high-income countries with ongoing immigration. J Hepatol. 2022;77(4):947-56.
10. Stockdale AJ, Meiring JE, Shawa IT, Thindwa D, Silungwe NM, Mbewe M, et al. Hepatitis B vaccination impact and the unmet need for antiviral treatment in Blantyre, Malawi. J Infect Dis. 2022;226(5):871-80.
11. Battistella S, Grasso M, Catanzaro E, D'Arcangelo F, Corrà G, Germani G, et al. Evolution of liver transplantation indications: expanding horizons. Medicina. 2024;60(3):412.
12. Sarin SK, Kumar M, Eslam M, George J, Mahtab MA, Akbar SMF, et al. Liver diseases in the Asia-Pacific region: a Lancet Gastroenterology & Hepatology Commission. Lancet Gastroenterol Hepatol. 2020;5(2):167-228.
13. Williams I. Epidemiology of hepatitis C in the United States. Am J Med. 1999;107(6):2-9.
14. Klevens RM, Hu DJ, Jiles R, Holmberg SD. Evolving epidemiology of hepatitis C virus in the United States. Clinical infectious diseases. 2012;55(suppl_1):S3-9.
15. Younossi ZM, Kalligeros M, Henry L. Epidemiology of metabolic dysfunction associated steatotic liver disease. Clin Mol Hepatol. 2025;31(Suppl):S32-S50.
16. Paik JM, Henry L, Younossi Y, Ong J, Alqahtani S, Younossi ZM. The burden of nonalcoholic fatty liver disease (NAFLD). Hepatol Commun. 2023;7(10):e0251.
17. Murray CJL, Aravkin AY, Zheng P, Abbafati C, Abbas KM, Abbasi-Kangevari M, et al. Global burden of 87 risk factors in 204 countries and territories, 1990–2019: a systematic analysis for the Global Burden of Disease Study 2019. Lancet. 2020;396(10258):1223-49.
18. Huang DQ, Terrault NA, Tacke F, Gluud LL, Arrese M, Bugianesi E, et al. Global epidemiology of cirrhosis—etiology trends and predictions. Nat Rev Gastroenterol Hepatol. 2023;20:388-98.
19. Wu XN, Xue F, Zhang N, Zhang W, Hou JJ, Lv Y, et al. Global burden of liver cirrhosis and other chronic liver diseases caused by specific etiologies from 1990 to 2019. BMC Public Health. 2024;24:363.
20. Younossi ZM, Stepanova M, Ong J, Trimble G, AlQahtani S, Younossi I, et al. Nonalcoholic steatohepatitis is the most rapidly increasing indication for liver transplantation in the United States. Clin Gastroenterol Hepatol. 2021;19: 580-9.
21. D'Amico G, Garcia-Tsao G, Pagliaro L. Natural history and prognostic indicators of survival in cirrhosis: a systematic review of 118 studies. J Hepatol. 2006;44(1):217-31.
22. Kamath PS, Wiesner RH, Malinchoc M, Kremers W, Therneau TM, Kosberg CL, et al. A model to predict survival in patients with end-stage liver disease. Hepatology. 2001;33(2):464-70.
23. Kim WR, Mannalithara A, Heimbach JK, Kamath PS, Asrani SK, Biggins SW, et al. MELD 3.0: the model for end-stage liver disease updated for the modern era. Gastroenterology. 2021;161(6):1887-95.e4.
24. Merion RM, Schaubel DE, Dykstra DM, Freeman RB, Port FK, Wolfe RA. The survival benefit of liver transplantation. Am J Transplant. 2005;5(2):307-13.
25. Francoz C, Nadim MK, Durand F. Kidney biomarkers in cirrhosis. J Hepatol. 2016;65(4):809-24.
26. Dickson ER, Grambsch PM, Fleming TR, Fisher LD, Langworthy A. Prognosis in primary biliary cirrhosis: model for decision making. Hepatology. 1989;10(1):1-7.
27. Grambsch PM, Dickson ER, Wiesner RH, Langworthy A. Application of the Mayo primary biliary cirrhosis survival model to Mayo liver transplant patients. Mayo Clin Proc. 1989;64(6):699-704.
28. Murtaugh PA, Dickson RE, Van Dam GM, Malinchoc M, Grambsch PM, Langworthy AL, et al. Primary biliary cirrhosis: prediction of short-term survival based on repeated patient visits. Hepatology. 1994;20(1):126.

29. Carbone M, Sharp SJ, Flack S, Paximadas D, Spiess K, Adgey C, et al. The UK-PBC risk scores: derivation and validation of a scoring system for long-term prediction of end-stage liver disease in primary biliary cholangitis. Hepatology. 2016;63(3):930-50.
30. Lammers WJ, Hirschfield GM, Corpechot C, Nevens F, Lindor KD, Janssen HLA, et al. Development and validation of a scoring system to predict outcomes of patients with primary biliary cirrhosis receiving ursodeoxycholic acid therapy. Gastroenterology. 2015;149(7):1804-12.e4.
31. O'Grady JG, Alexander GJM, Hayllar KM, Williams R. Early indicators of prognosis in fulminant hepatic failure. Gastroenterology. 1989;97(2):439-45.
32. Bernuau J, Goudeau A, Poynard T, Dubois F, Lesage G, Yvonnet B, et al. Multivariate analysis of prognostic factors in fulminant hepatitis B. Hepatology. 1986;6(4):648.
33. Bismuth H, Samuel D, Castaing D, Williams R, Pereira SP. Liver transplantation in Europe for patients with acute liver failure. Semin Liver Dis. 2008;16:415-25.
34. Hadem J, Stiefel P, Bahr MJ, Tillmann HL, Rifai K, Klempnauer J, et al. Prognostic implications of lactate, bilirubin, and etiology in German patients with acute liver failure. Clin Gastroenterol Hepatol. 2008;6(3):339-45.
35. Dhiman RK, Jain S, Maheshwari U, Bhalla A, Sharma N, Ahluwalia J, et al. Early indicators of prognosis in fulminant hepatic failure: an assessment of the Model for End-Stage Liver Disease (MELD) and King's College Hospital Criteria. Liver Transpl. 2007;13(6):814-21.
36. Kumar R, Shalimar, Sharma H, Goyal R, Kumar A, Khanal S, et al. Prospective derivation and validation of early dynamic model for predicting outcome in patients with acute liver failure. Gut. 2012;61(7):1068-75.
37. Bechmann LP, Jochum C, Kocabayoglu P, Sowa JP, Kassalik M, Gieseler RK, et al. Cytokeratin 18-based modification of the MELD score improves prediction of spontaneous survival after acute liver injury. J Hepatol. 2010;53(4):639-47.
38. Bernal W, Donaldson N, Wyncoll D, Wendon J. Blood lactate as an early predictor of outcome in paracetamol-induced acute liver failure: a cohort study. Lancet. 2002;359(9306):558-63.
39. Schmidt LE, Dalhoff K. Serum phosphate is an early predictor of outcome in severe acetaminophen-induced hepatotoxicity. Hepatology. 2002;36(3):659-65.
40. Schmidt LE, Larsen FS. MELD score as a predictor of liver failure and death in patients with acetaminophen-induced liver injury. Hepatology. 2007;45(3):789-96.
41. Rutherford A, King LY, Hynan LS, Vedvyas C, Lin W, Lee WM, et al. Development of an accurate index for predicting outcomes of patients with acute liver failure. Gastroenterology. 2012;143(5):1237-43.
42. Taylor RM, Davern T, Munoz S, Han SH, McGuire B, Larson AM, et al. Fulminant hepatitis A virus infection in the United States: incidence, prognosis, and outcomes. Hepatology. 2006;44(6):1589-97.
43. Ganzert M, Felgenhauer N, Zilker T. Indication of liver transplantation following amatoxin intoxication. J Hepatol. 2005;42(2):202-9.
44. Westbrook RH, Yeoman AD, Joshi D, Heaton ND, Quaglia A, O'Grady JG, et al. Outcomes of severe pregnancy-related liver disease: refining the role of transplantation. Am J Transplant. 2010;10(11):2520-6.
45. Ichai P, Legeai C, Francoz C, Boudjema K, Boillot O, Ducerf C, et al. Patients with acute liver failure listed for superurgent liver transplantation in France: reevaluation of the clichy-villejuif criteria. Liver Transpl. 2015;21(4):512.
46. O'Grady JG, Alexander GJM, Hayllar KM, Williams R. Early indicators of prognosis in fulminant hepatic failure. Gastroenterology. 1989;97(2):439-45.
47. Solà E, Fernandez J, Ginès P. Acute-on-chronic liver failure: the role of precipitating illness. Semin Liver Dis. 2016;36:117-22.
48. Mazzaferro V, Regalia E, Doci R, Andreola S, Pulvirenti A, Bozzetti F, et al. Liver transplantation for the treatment of small hepatocellular carcinomas in patients with cirrhosis. N Engl J Med. 1996;334(11):693-700.
49. Yao FY, Ferrell L, Bass NM, Watson JJ, Bacchetti P, Venook A, et al. Liver transplantation for hepatocellular carcinoma: expansion of the tumor size limits does not adversely impact survival. Hepatology. 2001;33(6):1394-403.
50. Yao FY, Ferrell L, Bass NM, Bacchetti P, Ascher NL, Roberts JP. Liver transplantation for hepatocellular carcinoma: comparison of the proposed UCSF criteria with the Milan criteria and the Pittsburgh modified TNM criteria. Liver Transpl. 2002;8(9):765.
51. Silva M, Moya A, Berenguer M, Sanjuan F, López-Andujar R, Pareja E, et al. Expanded criteria for liver transplantation in patients with cirrhosis and hepatocellular carcinoma. Liver Transpl. 2008;14(10):1449-60.
52. Kaido T, Ogawa K, Mori A, Fujimoto Y, Ito T, Tomiyama K, et al. Usefulness of the Kyoto criteria as expanded selection criteria for liver transplantation for hepatocellular carcinoma. Surgery. 2013;154(5):1053-60.
53. Fan J, Yang GS, Fu ZR, Peng ZH, Xia Q, Peng CH, et al. Liver transplantation outcomes in 1,078 hepatocellular carcinoma patients: a multi-center experience in Shanghai, China. J Cancer Res Clin Oncol. 2009;135(10):1403-12.
54. Sugawara Y, Tamura S, Makuuchi M. Living donor liver transplantation for hepatocellular carcinoma: Tokyo University Series. Dig Dis. 2007;25(4):310-2.
55. Toso C, Asthana S, Bigam DL, Shapiro AMJ, Kneteman NM. Reassessing selection criteria prior to liver transplantation for hepatocellular carcinoma utilizing the scientific registry of transplant recipients database. Hepatology. 2009;49(3):832-8.
56. Soejima Y, Taketomi A, Yoshizumi T, Uchiyama H, Aishima S, Terashi T, et al. Extended indication for living donor liver transplantation in patients with hepatocellular carcinoma. Transplantation. 2007;83(7):893.

57. Zheng SS, Xu X, Wu J, Chen J, Wang WL, Zhang M, et al. Liver transplantation for hepatocellular carcinoma: Hangzhou experiences. Transplantation. 2008;85(12):1726.
58. Mazzaferro V, Llovet JM, Miceli R, Bhoori S, Schiavo M, Mariani L, et al. Predicting survival after liver transplantation in patients with hepatocellular carcinoma beyond the Milan criteria: a retrospective, exploratory analysis. Lancet Oncol. 2009;10(1):35-43.
59. Toso C, Meeberg G, Hernandez-Alejandro R, Dufour JF, Marotta P, Majno P, et al. Total tumor volume and alpha-fetoprotein for selection of transplant candidates with hepatocellular carcinoma: a prospective validation. Hepatology. 2015;62(1):158-65.
60. Lee SG, Hwang S, Moon DB, Ahn CS, Kim KH, Sung KB, et al. Expanded indication criteria of living donor liver transplantation for hepatocellular carcinoma at one large-volume center. Liver Transpl. 2008;14(7):935-45.
61. Sapisochin G, Goldaracena N, Laurence JM, Dib M, Barbas A, Ghanekar A, et al. The extended Toronto criteria for liver transplantation in patients with hepatocellular carcinoma: a prospective validation study. Hepatology. 2016;64(6):2077-88.
62. Nordlinger B, Guiguet M, Vaillant JC, Balladur P, Boudjema K, Bachellier P, et al. Surgical resection of colorectal carcinoma metastases to the liver: a prognostic scoring system to improve case selection, based on 1568 patients. Cancer. 1996;77(7):1254-62.
63. Hoti E, Adam R. Liver transplantation for primary and metastatic liver cancers. Transpl Int. 2008;21(12):1107-17.
64. Nagashima I, Takada T, Nagawa H, Muto T, Okinaga K. Proposal of a new and simple staging system of colorectal liver metastasis. World J Gastroenterol. 2006;12(43):6961.
65. Konopke R, Kersting S, Distler M, Dietrich J, Gastmeier J, Heller A, et al. Prognostic factors and evaluation of a clinical score for predicting survival after resection of colorectal liver metastases. Liver Int. 2009;29(1):89-102.
66. Margonis GA, Sasaki K, Gholami S, Kim Y, Andreatos N, Rezaee N, et al. Genetic and morphological evaluation (GAME) score for patients with colorectal liver metastases. Br J Surg. 2018;105(9):1210-20.
67. Whitrock JN, Pratt CG, Shah SA. Expanding MELD exceptions for colorectal liver metastasis: data and policy. Current Opinion in Organ Transplantation. 2024;29(3):195-9
68. Sasaki K, Morioka D, Conci S, Margonis GA, Sawada Y, Ruzzenente A, et al. The Tumor Burden Score: a new "Metro-ticket" prognostic tool for colorectal liver metastases based on tumor size and number of tumors. Ann Surg. 2018;267(1):132.
69. Amygdalos I, Müller-Franzes G, Bednarsch J, Czigany Z, Ulmer TF, Bruners P, et al. Novel machine learning algorithm can identify patients at risk of poor overall survival following curative resection for colorectal liver metastases. J Hepato-Biliary-Pancreat Sci. 2023;30(5):602-14.
70. Viganò L, Capussotti L, Lapointe R, Barroso E, Hubert C, Giuliante F, et al. Early recurrence after liver resection for colorectal metastases: risk factors, prognosis, and treatment. A LiverMetSurvey-based study of 6,025 patients. Ann Surg Oncol. 2014;21(4):1276-86.
71. Mao R, Zhao JJ, Bi XY, Zhang YF, Li ZY, Zhou JG, et al. A postoperative scoring system for post-hepatectomy early recurrence of colorectal liver metastases. Oncotarget. 2017;8(60):102531.
72. Dueland S, Yaqub S, Syversveen T, Carling U, Hagness M, Brudvik KW, et al. Survival outcomes after portal vein embolization and liver resection compared with liver transplant for patients with extensive colorectal cancer liver metastases. JAMA Surg. 2021;156(6):550-7.
73. Imai K, Allard MA, Benitez CC, Vibert E, Sa Cunha A, Cherqui D, et al. Early recurrence after hepatectomy for colorectal liver metastases: what optimal definition and what predictive factors? Oncologist. 2016;21(7):887-94.
74. Jiang LM, Zhang YP, Wang CW, Zhang WD, He W, Qiu JL, et al. More liver metastases detected intraoperatively indicates worse prognosis for colorectal liver metastases patients after resection combined with microwave ablation. J Oncol. 2022;2022(1):3819564.
75. NANETS Guidelines (2022). [online] Available from https://nanets.net/images/guidelines/21513_NANETS_2022_Guidelines_Compendium.pdf. [Last accessed May, 2025].
76. Mihir B, Stacey P, Therese B. Liver transplantation for hepatic epithelioid hemangioendothelioma is facilitated by exception points with acceptable long-term outcomes. Transplant. 2020;104(6):1187-92.
77. Remiszewski P, Szczerba E, Kalinowski P, Gierej B, Dudek K, Grodzicki M, et al. Epithelioid hemangioendothelioma of the liver as a rare indication for liver transplantation. World J Gastroenterol. 2014;20(32):11333-9. doi: 10.3748/wjg.v20.i32.11333. PMID: 25170219; PMCID: PMC4145773.
78. Nudo CG, Yoshida EM, Bain VG, Marleau D, Wong P, Marotta PJ, et al. Liver transplantation for hepatic epithelioid hemangioendothelioma: the Canadian multicentre experience. Can J Gastroenterol. 2008;22(10):821-4.
79. Lai Q, Feys E, Karam V, Adam R, Klempnauer J, Oliverius M, et al. Hepatic Epithelioid Hemangioendothelioma and Adult Liver Transplantation: Proposal for a Prognostic Score Based on the Analysis of the ELTR-ELITA Registry. Transplant. 2017;101(3):555-64.
80. McDiarmid SV, Anand R, Martz K, Millis MJ, Mazariegos G. A multivariate analysis of pre-, peri-, and post-transplant factors affecting outcome after pediatric liver transplantation. Ann Surg. 2011;254(1):145-54.

CHAPTER 2

Surgical Steps in Living Donor and Cadaveric Liver Transplant: What Intensivists Must Know?

Binoj ST, Shweta Mallick, Krishnanunni Nair, Guhan Venkatakrishnan, Sudhindran S

INTRODUCTION

"He bled to death as we worked desperately to stop the haemorrhage. The operation could not be completed. Bennie was only three years old and had not enjoyed a trouble-free day in his life. Now, his wound was closed and he was wrapped in a plain white sheet after being washed off by a weeping nurse. They took him away from this place of sanitised hope to the cold and unhygienic morgue, where an autopsy did not add to the understanding of our failure. The surgeons stayed in the operating room for a long time after, sitting on the low stools around the periphery, looking at the ground saying nothing. The orderlies came and began to mop the floor. It was necessary to prepare for the next case".

This is a poignant excerpt from Thomas Starzl's autobiography on the first-ever liver transplant performed in the world. From this point in history, we have now arrived at a stage where transplants are performed as a routine surgery, often without any transfusion and virtually without any death on table.

Liver transplant surgery can be discussed under the following headings:

- Liver graft procurement from the donor (either deceased or living)
- Preparation of the graft on the back table/bench
- Explantation of the diseased liver from the recipient
- Implantation of the graft liver in the recipient

Graft procurement: Until 1987, deceased donors were the only sources of grafts for transplantation. Today, living donors constitute the bulk of grafts for liver transplant in India and Southeast Asian countries.

DECEASED DONOR ORGAN PROCUREMENT

Deceased donors can be either heart-beating donors (HBDs) or nonheart-beating donors (NHBDs).

- *Heart-beating donors [donation after brain death (DBD)]* where death is diagnosed as defined by the brain stem death criteria first described in 1968.[1] As the heart is beating and the circulation is maintained to the abdominal and thoracic organs, the surgery does not involve extraordinary blood losses. A state of coagulopathy with disseminated intravascular coagulation may occur after brain death needing correction with plasma. During retrieval, the brain-dead donor muscle relaxants are required as spinal reflexes are preserved despite brain death.
- *Nonheart-beating donors [donation after cardiac death (DCD)]* where death is diagnosed by heart criteria. According to the Maastricht criteria, there are four categories of NHBDs based predominantly on the duration of cardiac arrest before retrieval.[2] Most DCD retrievals are type 3, where once the decision to donate is consolidated with the full consent of the family, all necessary life supports are withdrawn under supervision and retrieval is initiated after the cessation of cardiac activity.[2] Nonheart-beating donation is rarely performed in India.

The primary aim of organ retrieval is to keep the warm ischemia as short as possible, which is traditionally defined as the time from aortic cross-clamping in the donor to perfusion of the graft with a preservative solution. Retrieval entails dissection of the liver for perfusion as well as easy removal. Perfusion entails exsanguination of the patients and flushing with preservative solution.

The extent of dissection of the liver before perfusion varies from surgeon to surgeon and the clinical situation. If time and the vital condition of the donor permit, the liver can be mobilized from all its attachments and the HA, portal vein (PV), and inferior vena cava (IVC) are dissected as much as possible (warm dissection phase). However, if the donor is unstable, then the dissection is to be kept minimal and the procedure of organ perfusion should be performed rapidly after placing inflow and outflow perfusion cannulas.

For perfusion of the liver, most surgeons use the common iliac artery and PV for inflow. The outflow chosen would depend upon other organ retrievals planned. If heart retrieval is not planned, then the suprahepatic IVC can be opened and used as the outflow. If cardiac retrieval is to be done, then the cardiac surgeons usually clamp the suprahepatic IVC, and the infrarenal IVC is used as the outflow of the perfusate.

Once the cannulation has been performed, the retrieval team stands prepared for perfusion. In an HBD, perfusion is started while the heart is still beating, consequently resulting in zero warm ischemia time. In NHBDs, since cannulation is done after cessation of cardiac activity, the warm ischemia is likely to last >10 minutes. Quick exposure and cannulation of the iliac vessel followed by supraceliac cross clamping and perfusion are imperative to reduce the warm ischemia time. Subsequent dissection of the liver for retrieval is termed cold dissection phase. This too needs to be kept as short as possible. The liver is retrieved with PV, HA with the celiac axis (in case of accessory right from SMA, combined celiac and SMA patch may be taken), and IVC. The liver is then placed in cold perfusate fluid, which is covered with ice slush. This initiates the cold ischemia phase, which starts from the organ perfusion with cold perfusate to the beginning of implantation in the recipient. Ideal core cooling of the organ occurs at 4°C, and at this temperature, the liver graft can be kept viable for 7–8 hours. There is a short period between the placement of the liver in the body till its perfusion with portal blood during the implantation phase, which is termed secondary warm ischemia time (here, organ is still cold but not as low as 4°C).

PRESERVATION OF ORGAN AFTER EXPLANT: MACHINE PERFUSION

With the increase in NHBD, much interest has been garnered by machine perfusion, either hypothermic (HOPE) or normothermic perfusion (NRP). This is because, unlike cold ischemia, each minute of warm ischemia induces much cellular damage to the hepatocytes and cholangiocytes. Machine perfusion helps by removing the graft from the ischemic toxic environment and restoring the perfusion of normal oxygenated blood through the machine. It also provides ways to assess the function of the graft during perfusion by assessing bile production, bile pH, lactate clearance, and other by-products. Thus, the postoperative primary graft nonfunction (PGNF), which is a relatively common occurrence in DBD, can be predicted and such grafts discarded. Nevertheless, the predominant effect observed so far has been in mitigating the incidence of ischemic cholangiopathy.[3,4]

Another development with regard to improving the quality of NHBD organ has been the technique of NRP. NRP is a method of maintaining the allografts during DCD donation by instituting venoarterial extracorporeal membrane oxygenation (VA-ECMO) to maintain organ perfusion, allowing them time to recover from warm ischemic injury. Normothermic blood is perfused through the iliac/femoral artery while the supraceliac aorta and the suprahepatic IVC are clamped or balloon occluded to prevent escape of blood to the thoracic and cerebral circulation. The perfused blood is drained through the IVC and recirculated through an oxygenated machine pump. At the end of the 60 minutes, if the organs are suitable for transplant, then NRP perfusion is stopped, and the organs are perfused with the University of Wisconsin (UW) solution and are harvested.[5] In essence, NMP converts a DCD to a DBD by re-establishing circulation to extracerebral organs. Following NRP retrieval, machine perfusion can be continued if required.

LIVING DONOR ORGAN PROCUREMENT

Living donor liver transplantation is technically more challenging as the graft is partial and the blood vessels and bile ducts may have complex anatomy. Donor selection and optimal evaluation are probably the keys to a successful living donor liver transplant. Donor evaluation entails relevant blood tests, multiphase CECT (for assessment of degree of fat, anatomy of graft vasculature, and volumetric), MRI (for assessment of donor biliary anatomy and fat quantification), and a thorough multidepartmental systemic evaluation. What graft is taken depends upon the donor's future liver remnant (FLR) and graft-recipient weight ratio (GRWR) which should ideally be >30% and >0.8, respectively. The right lobe usually makes up about 65% of the graft and the left lobe about 35%. Therefore, in adults weighing 65 kg, a 650-g graft is ideal, for which a right lobe graft is almost always required. Right lobe grafts are informally divided into right, modified right, and extended right lobe grafts depending upon the limit of parenchyma transection with respect to the middle hepatic vein (MHV; without MHV and with partial MHV and total MHV, respectively).

Usually, donor surgery is through a right subcostal or midline incision and starts with mobilization of the liver, according to the graft planned. Right lobe mobilization involves the division of the triangular and coronary ligaments, and all the diaphragmatic attachments followed by the division of the caudate branches to the IVC, including the Makuuchi ligament. The next step involves dissection of the hepatic hilum to delineate the branches of the HA and PV and demarcation of the biliary bifurcation. Demarcation for transection planes between the right and left lobes can be achieved by temporary clamping of the vessels of the desired side. Most surgeons pass an umbilical tape through the RHV-MHV groove anterior to IVC behind the mobilized caudate which is brought out at the hilum over the right PV and HA. This is referred to as the hanging maneuver and aids faster transection.

Parenchymal transection is performed mainly by a cavitron ultrasonic suction aspirator (CUSA), which is an ultrasonic shear, the tip of which vibrates at 23 kHz and causes the water molecules in the cells to implode, leading to tissue fragmentation (cavitation). Tissues with high water content like liver parenchyma easily disrupt, but tissues with low water content like connective tissue of the wall of the blood vessels stay intact, and this prevents unwanted bleeding. These vessels can be tackled separately by clipping, ligature, or coagulation. Bleeding during transection is nevertheless a major concern and can be reduced by keeping the central venous pressure (CVP) low and lowering of the head end as most of these bleeds are from hepatic veins. Some centers use Pringle's maneuver either routinely or during bleeds. Another potential advantage of Pringle's maneuver is that it may prepare the liver for prolonged ischemia by ischemic preconditioning.[6]

Bile duct division entails a careful preoperative anatomic assessment by MRCP. Additionally, an intra-operative cholangiogram can be performed before division. Only approximately 40% of the population has "normal" anatomy with a single right hepatic duct. Many have multiple ducts at the bifurcation which can increase the complexities of biliary reconstruction in the graft. The right duct is divided sharply at the bifurcation, and the stump on the donor side is suture closed. This could be one potential area from where postoperative bile leak can occur in the donor.

Retrieval starts after completion of parenchymal transection and duct division with the division of the right HA and PV. This marks the onset of warm ischemia. This is followed by the division of the right hepatic vein and removal of the graft by placing it in cold perfusate fluid in an ice slush. The left lobe graft retrieval is relatively simpler compared to the right. Mobilization is done by the division of the left triangular ligament and division of the caudate veins draining the IVC. Left grafts can be taken with or without the caudate (providing an 8–12% gain in left graft weight). For left lateral segmentectomy (segments 2 and 3), which is without the caudate lobe, the transection plane is just on the right of the falciform ligament and slants toward the ligamentum venosum groove.

Minimally invasive donor hepatectomy (MIDH) has been performed lately which can be either laparoscopic or robotic. This has been widely adopted for the left lateral segmentectomy and is now perhaps the standard of care. However, minimally invasive right or left hepatectomies are restricted to a few centers. Here, the whole transection is performed laparoscopically or robotically, and the graft is removed using a remote small incision, often a Pfannenstiel for its evident cosmetic benefits. The current literature reports lesser morbidity, pain, and hospital stay for MIDH compared to its open counterpart with almost equivalent results in the recipients.[7,8]

Bench Work

In DDLT, bench work involves the removal of unwanted tissue like the diaphragm, adrenal gland, retroperitoneal fat, lymphatics, and the fibromuscular tissue around the blood vessels to give them adequate length for safe anastomosis. In the case of multiple hepatic arteries, appropriate reconstruction may be done to achieve a single anastomosis.

In LDLT, following harvest of the graft and placement in ice, the blood is flushed out with perfusion fluid histidine-tryptophan-ketoglutarate (HTK) or UW solution through the PV, and the organ is core cooled. Most centers do not perfuse through the artery on account of its small size and fear of intimal damage. After optimal perfusion, bench work involves the reconstruction of the anterior sector drainage. A right lobe graft is one where the donor right lobe is taken without any portion of the middle hepatic vein (MHV) whereas a modified right lobe graft is one where a part of the MHV is taken. In a right lobe graft, the segment V & VIII veins are reconstructed to form the neo-MHV whereas in a modified right lobe graft, the partial MHV and segment VIII veins are reconstructed to form the neo-MHV by either using a venous graft prepared from the recipient PV or a cadaveric iliac vein graft or a synthetic graft: Polytetrafluoroethylene fluoroethylene or a Dacron graft.

If the graft portal anatomy is more complex, such as a type II or III PV wherein the graft liver has two portal ostia, a venous graft from the recipient PV is used to reconstruct the multiple openings into a single one. Often, a patch or a cuff placement might be required to augment inferior hepatic veins with significant caliber for implantation **(Fig. 1)**.

In liver transplants in small children, a major concern is the space constraint as a large graft cannot be placed in the abdomen. Besides, larger grafts may not receive adequate perfusion by the child's portal circulation, and these can affect the graft function. The ideal GRWR in children is between 1 and 4. So, if the GRWR of a left lateral graft (segments II and III) is >4, it requires reduction to a monosegment graft which can be performed either in situ or on the bench.[9,10] In the case of deceased donor grafts, a size-matched graft from a pediatric donor or the left lateral segment by splitting the adult whole liver can be used. Split livers increase the donor pool for pediatric transplants in places where living donor transplant is not commonly performed.[11]

EXPLANT HEPATECTOMY OF THE RECIPIENT

The incision for this surgery is either through a reverse L-shaped incision or bilateral subcostal with vertical upper extension (Mercedes Benz), as this provides good access to the recipient. The explant hepatectomy can be challenging if the surgeon encounters adhesions either due to episodes of spontaneous bacterial peritonitis or prior surgeries. Such adhesions are often vascular and result in massive bleeding. The caudate is invariably hypertrophied in cirrhotics and raises concerns when it encircles the IVC. In such cases, early dissection of the PV and doing a PV shunt may help by reducing the bleeding from the liver as well as facilitating ease of mobilization **(Fig. 2)**. However, this is at the expense of a prolonged anhepatic phase. Clamping the IVC, either partially or totally, may also help in dissection by reducing bleeding. Explant starts with the hilar dissection which involves dissection and isolation of the HA, bile duct, and PV in preparation for implant. The artery and bile duct are divided early on while the patient remains "hepatic" on the portal flow to match timing with the graft procurement. One usually encounters multiple collaterals as a consequence of portal hypertension. These collaterals are seen at the liver hilum, splenorenal,

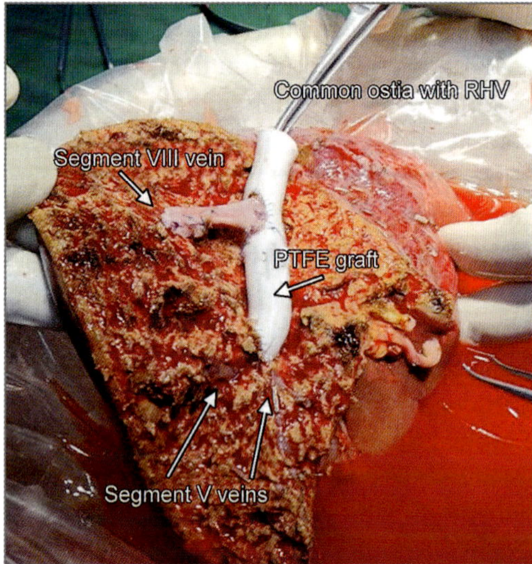

Fig. 1: Bench preparation of the graft- In a right lobe graft, segment V and segment VIII veins are reconstructed to create a neo-MHV. This can be done by using either the native recipient portal vein or any synthetic graft. Neo- MHV can be implanted either as a common ostia with the right hepatic vein or separately onto the left hepatic vein/inferior vena cava. (MHV: middle hepatic vein; RHV: right hepatic vein; PTFE: polytetrafluoroethylene graft)

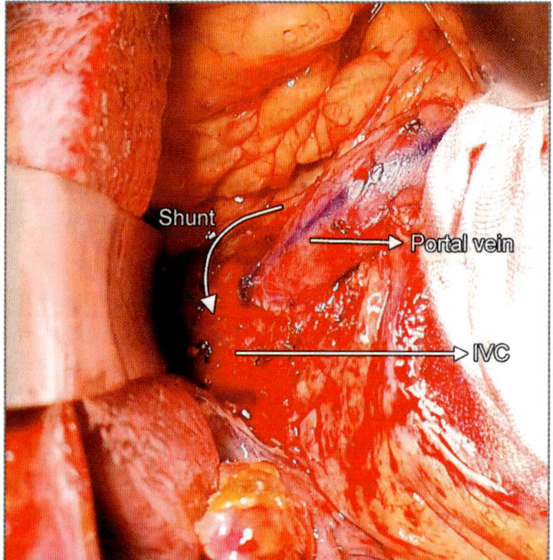

Fig. 2: Demonstrates a porto-caval shunt—During recipient hepatectomy, the portal vein is divided and anastomosed to the inferior vena cava in an end to side fashion, thereby creating a temporary shunt between the mesenteric and systemic circulation during the anhepatic phase. It helps by reducing the bleeding and preventing bowel oedema due to congestion. (PV: portal vein; IVC: Inferior vena cava)

left gastric, and gastroepiploic areas. The tortuous and distended collaterals contribute to significant bleeding during the dissection phase. After the hilar dissection, the liver is mobilized, and the caudate attachment to the IVC is freed by securing caudate branches. Most centers prefer to perform a temporary portocaval shunt. This can reduce portal hypertension and decompress the mesenteric blood to IVC, resulting in less bowel congestion-related edema and bleeding from collaterals. In portocaval shunting, the main PV is divided, and an end-to-side portocaval vascular anastomosis is created. Once mobilization is adequately complete, the right, middle, and left hepatic veins are divided between clamps or by using vascular staplers preferably leaving a long stump for venous implant. For deceased donor whole liver grafts with IVC, recipient hepatectomy can be performed as en bloc removal of the liver with IVC above the renal vein and above the diaphragm, the "classical hepatectomy" with caval resection. This requires clamping of the supra- and infrahepatic IVC and can be done only in patients who tolerate cross-clamping.

If the patient is hemodynamically unstable when portal and caval clamps are applied, a venovenous bypass is required where the portal and caval blood is routed to a machine and pumped back into the heart usually through the internal jugular vein. The problem with venovenous bypass is an attendant risk of clot formation in the circulation, which can lead to pulmonary embolism. To overcome this, anticoagulation is often required, and this may lead to major bleeding in an already coagulopathic and hypothermic patient. Nowadays, venovenous bypass and en bloc resection of the liver with IVC are rarely done. The usual practice in most units is the removal of the liver while preserving the cava in total. Although this dissection is more tedious, the need for a venovenous bypass can be avoided.[12]

An auxiliary partial orthotopic liver transplantation (APOLT)[13,14] is performed in acute liver failure wherein the native liver can regenerate after the acute insult or in metabolic liver disorders where the liver is normal but unable to synthesize the enzyme where only a part of a new liver sufficient to synthesize the enzyme needs to be transplanted. The advantage of APOLT in ALF is that once the acute phase abates, the liver regenerates adequately and the immunosuppression can be withdrawn, leading to rejection of the implanted graft and allowing the recipient to live a normal immunosuppression-free life (Q). In APOLT for metabolic disease, even though the graft needs lifelong immunosuppression, the proposed advantages for the recipient are a less morbid surgery (partial hepatectomy vs. total one) and virtual abolishment of the risk of primary nonfunction even if the transplanted graft does not work.

Familial amyloid polyneuropathy (FAP) occurs due to a mutated transthyretin gene and results in debilitating wheelchair-dependent neuropathy, developing over a period of 15–20 years. The liver is otherwise macroscopically normal. Such livers can be transplanted to patients whose expected survival is to the tune of 10 years, like those with hepatocellular carcinoma. This is called a domino transplant, where the explant liver goes from one individual to another. It could also be subjected to a split and used in two recipients. In maple syrup urine disease (MSUD), too, a domino transplant can be carried out. Here, in affected children, there is a total lack of production of the enzyme branched-chain alpha-keto acid dehydrogenase, resulting in accumulated branched-chain amino acids and leading to their deleterious effects. However, the hepatic production of the enzyme is minor, and hence, MSUD livers can be transplanted to recipients for other indications without subsequent metabolic effects.[15]

IMPLANTATION OF THE GRAFT LIVER

The order of anastomosis of the graft liver is the hepatic veins, followed by the portal vein that marks the graft reperfusion and the end of secondary warm ischaemia. Following this the hepatic artery and then the bile duct. In deceased donor grafts where classical hepatectomy has been performed and the graft comes with a segment of the donor IVC, the upper and lower ends of the caval segments are anastomosed to the supra and infra hepatic portion of the recipient's IVC respectively **(Fig. 3)**. More often than not, nowadays, the recipient IVC is left intact during explant, and the graft IVC is anastomosed in piggyback fashion, where the suprahepatic portion of the graft cava is joined to the suprahepatic cava of the recipient and the lower end is closed or as a side-to-side cavocavostomy.

In LDLT with right lobe grafts, the hepatic venous anastomosis is more complex and can be done either as a single outflow where the common opening of the graft RHV-Neo (reconstructed) MHV is anastomosed to the recipient RHV or given separately as a double outflow. Inferior hepatic veins with significant drainage are drained

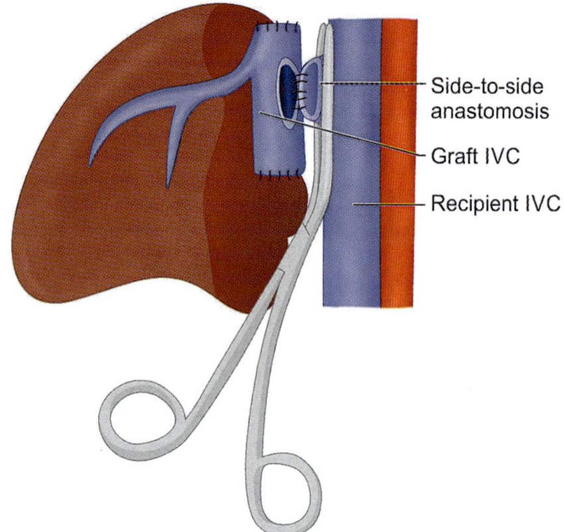

Fig. 3: A side-to-side cavo-caval anastomosis in a deceased donor graft implant. The superior and inferior ends of the graft IVC are closed, and a new opening is created onto which the recipient's cava is anastomosed in a side-to-side fashion. (IVC: inferior vena cava)

to the IVC directly or by using a venous cuff/patch if necessary.[16]

Portal vein anastomosis is carried out in an end-to-end fashion. Just before the reperfusion, most of the centers wash out the remaining perfusion fluid from the graft either by a forward flush using albumin or Ringer's lactate solution or by back bleeding from the IVC. This flushing helps in removing accumulated perfusate and toxic metabolites of organ ischemia and in reducing the extent of reperfusion-related hypotension. Caution should be used while using UW solution as the perfusate solution, as it has high potassium content and may lead to hyperkalemic cardiac arrest.[17]

When the native portal veins are atretic, as in biliary atresia, venoplasties or venous grafts may be required. It is critical to assess the portal flow before reperfusion, and this is where inflow modulation techniques are employed, depending upon the flow velocity. It is now routine to measure the portal pressures after implantation, and the ideal portal pressure is below 20 mm Hg. High portal flows for small-sized grafts require modulation to reduce the flow like splenic artery ligation, splenectomy, mesocaval shunt, or hemiportocaval shunts. This is to prevent sinusoidal damage from the heavy flow, which can cause graft dysfunction and small-for-size syndrome. If the portal flow is low, coexisting large portocaval shunts need to be ligated. If there are multiple shunts, ligation of the renal vein and other retroperitoneal veins needs to be performed to reroute the mesenteric flow to the liver.[18]

Reconstructions on atretic PVs may result in a thrombus that poses a major surgical challenge. When that happens, an endovenous thrombectomy is attempted. If this does not restore the blood flow, a jump graft from the patent part of the portal or superior mesenteric vein to the graft PV can be attempted. In desperate cases where the portal flow cannot be restored, options like renoportal anastomosis or hemi-cavoportal transposition (where the suprarenal cava is transected and anastomosed to graft PV as the inflow supply) should be sought.[19]

Hepatic artery anastomosis is the most technically challenging vascular anastomosis in liver transplant, especially in LDLT, as the caliber of the HA is very small (2–4 mm). Fine suture materials and the use of a microscope or a magnifying loupe make the task easier. Sometimes, when the recipient arteries are not structurally good such as in post-transarterial chemoembolization for hepatocellular carcinoma, or when the flow is less (coeliac stenosis), one might need to do extra-anatomic anastomosis using recipient splenic, gastroduodenal, and gastroepiploic arteries or conduit from the aorta.

Biliary anastomosis is often called the "Achilles' heel" in liver transplantation as complications like biliary leak and stricture make the patient a biliary cripple. The graft bile duct is usually anastomosed to the recipient bile duct in an end-to-end fashion using absorbable fine sutures. But when the recipient duct is not usable [as in primary sclerosing cholangitis (PSC) or biliary atresia] or there are multiple ducts in the graft (due to variant donor biliary anatomy), a bilioenteric anastomosis is unavoidable (usually a Roux-En-Y choledochojejunostomy). The advantages of duct-to-duct anastomose are that they are easy to create, are easy for future biliary interventions (like ERCP and stenting), and allow faster recovery of bowel functions (E, F, G).

Liver transplantation is a complex surgical procedure, which needs careful planning, meticulous surgical techniques, and comprehensive postoperative care. A knowledge of the steps and procedures involved allows the intensivist to anticipate and manage problems in the intensive care unit (ICU).

A multispecialty team is the key for every successful transplant. With the vast amount of experience gained over the years and advancements in anesthesia, surgical techniques, and critical care, the outcomes of liver transplantation have improved significantly, and a 1-year survival of >85–90% is not unusual in most high-volume centers.[20]

REFERENCES

1. Spears W, Mian A, Greer D. Brain death: a clinical overview. J Intensive Care. 2022;10(1):16.
2. Potts JT Jr, Herdman R. Non-heart-beating organ transplantation: medical and ethical issues in procurement. Washington (DC): National Academies Press (US); 1997. p. 4, The Modern Non-Heart-Beating Donor.
3. Hessheimer AJ, Billault C, Barrou B, Fondevilla C. Hypothermic or normo-thermic abdominal regional perfusion in high risk donors with extended warm ischemic times: impact on outcomes? Transpl Int. 2014;28:700e707.
4. Weeder PD, van Rijn R, Porte RJ. Machine perfusion in liver transplantation as a tool to prevent non-anastomotic biliary strictures: rationale, current evidence and future directions. J Hepatol. 2015;63:265e275.
5. Meinders AM, Hobeika MJ, Currie I. Normothermic regional perfusion in donation after circulatory death for liver transplantation: a narrative review. Curr Surg Rep. 2024;12:15-25.
6. Clavien PA, Yadav S, Sindram D, Bentley RC. Protective effects of ischemic preconditioning for liver resection performed under inflow occlusion in humans. Ann Surg. 2000;232(2):155-62.
7. Soubrane O, Eguchi S, Uemoto S, Kwon CHD, Wakabayashi G, Han HS, et al. Minimally Invasive Donor Hepatectomy for Adult Living Donor Liver Transplantation: An International, Multi-institutional Evaluation of Safety, Efficacy and Early Outcomes. Ann Surg. 2022;275(1):166-74.
8. Varghese CT, Chandran B, Sudhindran S. Approach to minimally invasive donor hepatectomy: Laparoscopic, robotic, or bit of both! Ann Gastroenterol Surg. 2023;7:696-7.
9. Enne M, Pacheco-Moreira L, Balbi E, Cerqueira A, Santalucia G, Martinho JM. Liver transplantation with monosegments. Technical aspects and outcome: a meta-analysis. Liver Transpl. 2005;11(5):564-9.
10. Kasahara M, Kaihara S, Oike F, Ito T, Fujimoto Y, Ogura Y, et al. Living-donor liver transplantation with monosegments. Transplantation. 2003;76(4):694-6.
11. Hackl C, Schmidt KM, Süsal C, Döhler B, Zidek M, Schlitt HJ. Split liver transplantation: current developments. World J Gastroenterol. 2018;24(47):5312-21.
12. Khajeh E, Ramouz A, Aminizadeh E, Sabetkish N, Golriz M, Mehrabi A, et al. Comparison of the modified piggyback with standard piggyback and conventional orthotopic liver transplantation techniques: a network meta-analysis. HPB (Oxford). 2023;25(7):732-46.
13. Shrivastav M, Rammohan A, Reddy MS, Rela M. Auxiliary partial orthotopic liver transplantation for acute liver failure. Ann R Coll Surg Engl. 2019;101(3):e71-2.
14. Shanmugam NP, Valamparampil JJ, Reddy MS, Al Said KJ, Al-Thihli K, Al-Hashmi N, et al. Auxiliary partial orthotopic liver transplantation for monogenic metabolic liver diseases: single-centre experience. JIMD Rep. 2019;45: 29-36.
15. Marques HP, Barros I, Li J, Murad SD, di Benedetto F. Current update in domino liver transplantation. Int J Surg. 2020;82:163-8.
16. Jeng LB, Thorat A, Yang HR, Li PC. Venous outflow reconstruction in living donor liver transplantation: dealing with venous anomalies. World J Transplant. 2015;5(4): 145-53.
17. Stoll WD, Hand WR, Chavin KD, Felton DH, Wolf BO, Davis GP, et al. Post-reperfusion syndrome in liver transplantation: does a caval blood flush vent help? Ann Transplant. 2019;24:631-8.
18. Bharathy KG, Shenvi S. Portal hemodynamics after living-donor liver transplantation: management for optimal graft and patient outcomes—a narrative review. Transplantology. 2023;4(2):38-58.
19. Bhangui P, Fernandes ESM, Di Benedetto F, Joo DJ, Nadalin S. Current management of portal vein thrombosis in liver transplantation. Int J Surg. 2020;82S:122-7.
20. Ghelichi-Ghojogh M, Rajabi A, Mohammadizadeh F, Shojaie L, Vali M, Afrashteh S, et al. Survival rate of liver transplantation in Asia: a systematic review and meta-analysis. Iran J Public Health. 2022;51(10):2207-20.

CHAPTER 3

Preoperative Cardiac Evaluation of Liver Transplant Recipients

Sunaina Tejpal Karna, Kelika Prakash, Bhushan Shah

INTRODUCTION

Major adverse cardiac events (MACE), such as heart failure (HF), acute coronary syndrome (ACS), and myocardial infarction (MI), are the third most important cause of mortality after infection and rejection in liver transplant candidates.[1] The transplant candidate demographics are expanding with the inclusion of older patients with comorbidities like diabetes, tobacco addiction, hypertension, and ventricular hypertrophy.[2,3] The hemodynamic changes secondary to bleeding, vena cava clamping, and postreperfusion syndrome impose significant stress on the heart during transplant surgery. Patients with end-stage liver disease (ESLD) may have a varied spectrum of cardiac involvement, which may be pre-existing or may be associated with cirrhosis **(Flowchart 1)**. Hence, the main goal of preoperative cardiac workup in these patients before transplant surgery is to:

- Identify the cardiac involvement with appropriate evaluation.
- Plan appropriate optimization where possible.
- Stratify risk, prognosticate, and exclude candidates too fragile to tolerate perioperative stress.

Flowchart 1: Spectrum of cardiovascular involvement in patients with end-stage liver diseases (ESLDs).

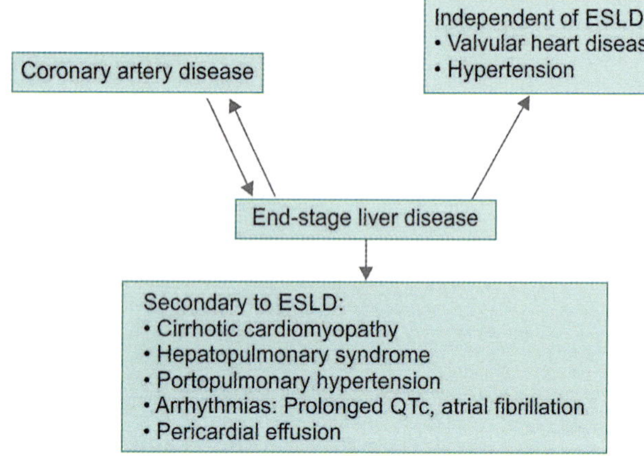

- Preoperative cardiac evaluation starts with assessing age, gender, comorbidities (renal disease, diabetes), and meticulous physical examination focusing on the cardiovascular system [coronary artery disease (CAD), systolic or diastolic dysfunction, or pulmonary hypertension].

SPECTRUM OF CARDIOVASCULAR INVOLVEMENT IN LIVER DISEASE

Coronary Artery Disease

Evidence indicates that the patient age considered high risk for CAD has decreased from 60 to 40 years in the past decade, from 2012 to 2023.[4,5] Though CAD is equally prevalent in patients with ESLD as in the general population, it is masked because of the low systemic vascular resistance (SVR).[6] Chronic inflammation along with hyperdynamic circulation in liver disease predisposes to plaque rupture and ACS, the majority unmasked in the first month after surgery.[7]

The most recent scientific statement on screening for CAD in transplant candidates from the American College of Cardiology (ACC) and the American Heart Association (ACC/AHA), released in 2023, recognizes that patients with nonalcohol-related steatohepatitis (NASH) have a high risk of CAD.[5] It is associated with critical coronary stenosis, diastolic dysfunction, and increased left atrial volume, which in turn are predictors of morbidity and mortality.

Cardiomyopathy

Cardiomyopathy typically has structural and functional changes in the heart, and even in the absence of primary cardiac disease, the stress response is impaired. This condition may be present in about 40–50% of cirrhotic patients.[8] The 2005 definition of cirrhotic cardiomyopathy (CCM) included echocardiographic and biochemical criteria. The American Society of Echocardiography and the European Association of Cardiovascular have redefined cardiomyopathy to include tissue Doppler and strain patterns.[9] Similar to CAD, the CCM may also get unmasked by the strain placed on an already compromised cardiovascular system by transfusion, fluid, anesthesia, and mechanical ventilation. Periods of stress, like surgery, exercise, and infections, may precipitate cardiac failure.[10,11]

Besides CCM and CAD, several systemic diseases like hemochromatosis, secondary iron overload, and amyloidosis may affect the heart along with the liver and need to be evaluated with echocardiography and cardiac magnetic resonance imaging. In iron overload cardiomyopathy, which may occur in ESLD patients, profound left ventricular (LV) diastolic dysfunction preceding LV systolic dysfunction is typical, with a reduction in the ejection fraction as a relatively late-stage finding.[12]

In alcoholic liver disease, cardiac involvement may start even before significant liver damage.[6] Further autonomic dysfunction, if present in ESLD, is associated with a high (30%) 4-year mortality in comparison to those without dysautonomia (6%). With the presence of ascites, the diastolic dysfunction may be more severe, which may precede the systolic dysfunction.[13]

Portopulmonary Hypertension

Portopulmonary hypertension (PoPH) is an uncommon condition occurring in 2–10% of patients with underlying portal hypertension, which may or may not be associated with the presence of cirrhosis. It is a cause of precapillary pulmonary hypertension. PoPH increases morbidity and mortality, as severe PoPH can lead to right HF.[14]

Until recently, PoPH was defined as the presence of both portal and pulmonary hypertension. Pulmonary arterial hypertension (PAH) was defined by the following criteria:

- Mean pulmonary arterial pressure (mPAP) >25 mm Hg on right heart catheterization (RHC)
- Pulmonary vascular resistance (PVR) >3 Woods units (240 dynes s cm^{-5})
- Pulmonary capillary wedge pressure (PCWP) <15 mm Hg

However, the recent 2022 European Society of Cardiology (ESC)/European Respiratory Society (ERS) guidelines have "lowered the mPAP limit from ≥25 to >20 mm Hg and the PVR threshold from >3 to >2 Wood units (WU) to diagnose PAH".[15]

The severity of PoPH is based on the mPAP (mild 20–35 mm Hg, moderate 36–45 mm Hg, and severe >45 mm Hg). A liver transplant is considered in PoPH only if the baseline mPAP is <35 mm Hg. Values above this cut-off need medical optimization. Patients with mPAP ≥35 can also be considered for liver transplantation (LT) if the PVR is <240 dynes s cm^{-5} with normal RV function. However, mPAP >45 mm Hg is usually considered an absolute contraindication to transplant.

Hepatopulmonary Syndrome

Hepatopulmonary syndrome (HPS), defined by the "presence of hypoxemia and intrapulmonary shunts in a patient with ESLD and this has a prevalence of 5–32%".[14]

INVESTIGATIVE APPROACH FOR PREOPERATIVE ASSESSMENT OF LIVER TRANSPLANT RECIPIENTS

Electrocardiography

Preoperative 12-lead electrocardiogram is done, as a routine in all LT candidates as a basic investigation. Corrected QT interval (QTc) should be determined in all LT patients. QTc prolongation is defined as >0.47 seconds in women and >0.45 seconds in men. Prolonged QTc is associated with a risk of torsade de pointes. QT interval (QTc) of >440 ms, an electrophysiologic hallmark of CCM, is present in 30–60% of ESLD patients.[16] Though hypokalemia and hypomagnesemia lead to prolonged QTc, it may also occur in the absence of dyselectrolytemia. If present, potassium levels should be corrected prior to surgery. Almost 1–6% of LT candidates are seen to have atrial fibrillation (AF), and any underlying cardiac pathology should be thoroughly investigated. Preexisting AF increases the risk of post-LT complications by sixfold.[17] The AHA guidelines, in 2012, emphasized that "baseline 12-lead electrocardiography and transthoracic echocardiography are necessary for preoperative evaluation of liver and kidney transplant recipients".[4]

2D-Transthoracic Echocardiography

Transthoracic echocardiography (TTE) is routinely done to assess cardiac chambers, biventricular and valvular function, pericardial involvement, and estimation of pulmonary hypertension. In the presence of left ventricular systolic dysfunction [left ventricular ejection fraction (LVEF) <40%] or regional wall motion abnormalities, it is prudent to rule out ischemic etiology with coronary angiography (CA).

Evaluation of potential LT recipients must include a two-dimensional-TTE (2D-TTE) as well as a tissue Doppler to detect CCM. The Cirrhotic Cardiomyopathy Consortium redefined CCM in 2020.[16] with the new criteria of:

- *Systolic dysfunction* ***(Fig. 1)****:* Either LVEF <50% or absolute global longitudinal strain (GLS) <18%, as is seen in the abnormal polar plot strain map with left ventricle GLS of 14.5%, suggestive of CCM.
- *Diastolic dysfunction* ***(Figs. 2A and B)****:* Presence of three or more of the following:
  - Septal mitral annular early diastolic velocity (e′) by tissue Doppler <7 cm/s
  - Mitral inflow early diastolic velocity (E) to e′ ratio >15
  - Left atrial (LA) volume index (LAVI) >34 mL/m^2
  - Tricuspid regurgitation (TR) velocity >2.8 m/s in the absence of PoPH

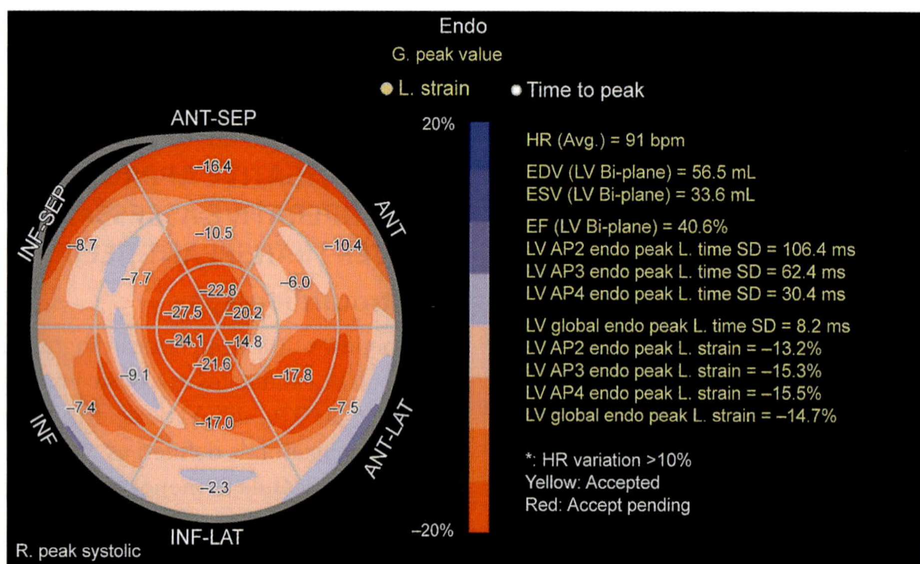

Fig. 1: Polar map of strain for the left ventricle on echocardiography showing reduced LV systolic function, LVEF 40.6%, and LV GLS—14.7%. Abnormal polar plot strain map (LV GLS—14.5%) suggestive of cirrhotic cardiomyopathy. (ANT-SEP: AnteroSeptal; ANT-LAT: AnteroLateral; GLS: global longitudinal strain; INF-SEP: InferoSeptal; INF-LAT: InferoLateral; LV: left ventricular; LVEF: left ventricular ejection fraction)

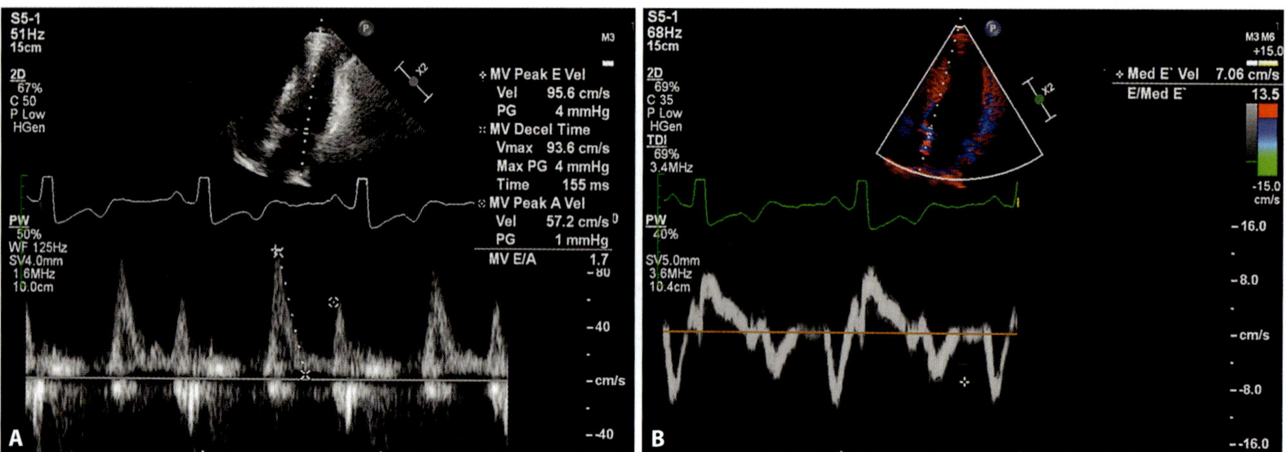

Figs. 2A and B: Pulse wave and tissue Doppler evidence of diastolic dysfunction in ESLD. (A) Transmitral pulse wave Doppler inflow; (B) tissue Doppler annular velocity in a patient with ESLD documenting abnormal mitral inflow and annular tissue velocities consistent with diastolic dysfunction. (ESLD: end-stage liver disease)

Heart failure in ESLD patients may manifest with either reduced (HFrEF) or preserved (HFpEF) LVEF. The presence of preoperative LV dysfunction is a risk factor for perioperative MACE. There is no established LVEF cut-off to preclude LT, although an ejection fraction of <40% is considered an absolute contraindication.[18]

Valvular regurgitation (mitral MR, tricuspid TR, or both) has been reported in approximately 28% of LT recipients.[19] Mild-to-moderate valvular regurgitation is usually tolerated in the perioperative period and does not preclude LT. Poor post-LT outcomes are observed with the presence of moderate to severe TR. In moderate to severe MR, bradycardia and dehydration should be avoided. Asymptomatic mild to moderate aortic stenosis (AS) is not a contraindication to LT.[20] Severe AS is associated with hemodynamic instability as well as reduced myocardial perfusion. Patients with severe symptomatic AS should be considered for valvular correction. Surgical or percutaneous balloon valvuloplasty or transcatheter aortic valve implantation. For stenotic lesions, especially AS, noninvasive approaches like transcatheter aortic valve replacement may be attempted in patients with a life expectancy >1 year orthotopic liver transplant (OLT).[21]

Bubble contrast-enhanced TTE (BCE-TTE) is used to detect intrapulmonary shunts **(Figs. 3A to D)**. Microbubbles that appear late in the left side of the heart after injection of bubbles in the venous system (four to eight cardiac cycles) are seen in the presence of pulmonary shunts. The appearance of microbubbles in one to four cardiac cycles is seen in the presence of an intracardiac defect.[22]

The initial screening test for PoPH in LT candidates is transthoracic Doppler echocardiography, which is used to estimate the right ventricular systolic pressure (RVSP)

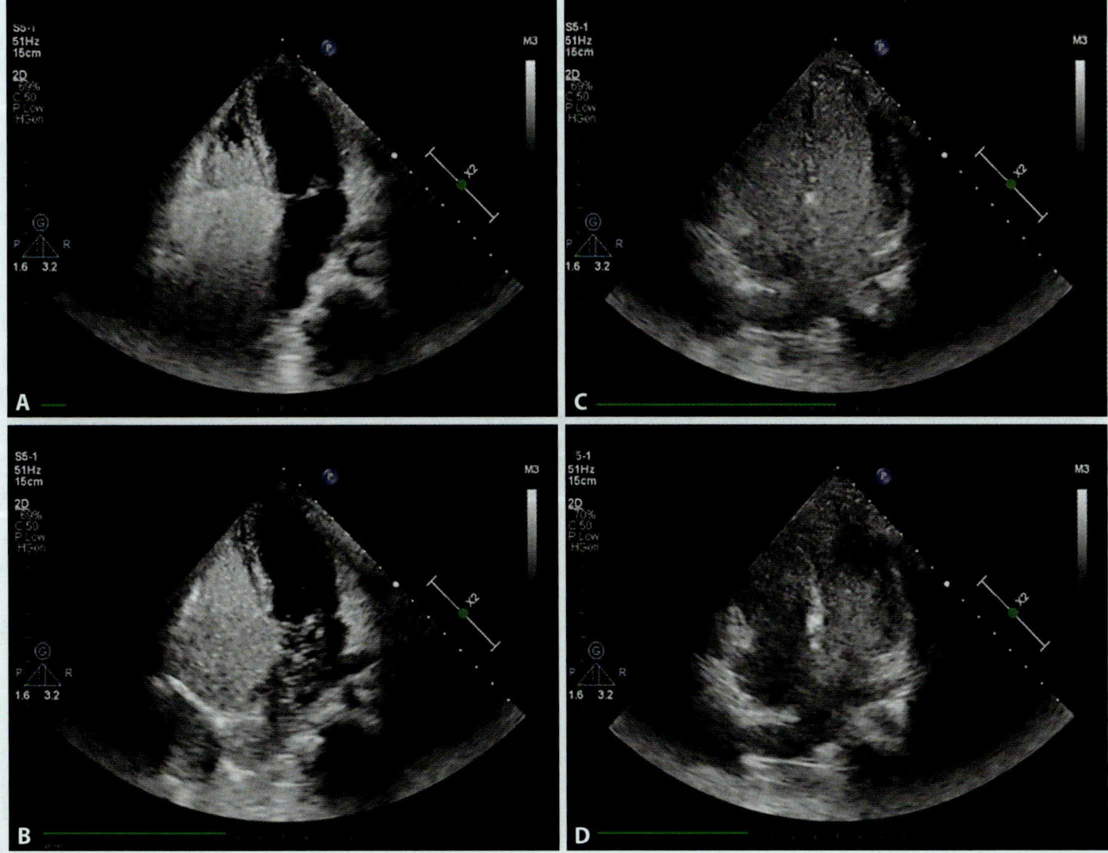

Figs. 3A to D: Bubble contrast transthoracic echocardiography performed in a patient with ESLD revealing marked right-to-left shunt through intrapulmonary AVM. (A) Immediately after the appearance of saline bubble contrast in right-sided heart chambers; (B) appearance of bubble contrast on left-sided heart chambers after six beats; (C) approximately 12 seconds after injection of saline bubble contrast reveals equal contrast in both the right and left ventricles; (D) recorded approximately 18 seconds following injection of saline bubble contrast reveals continued appearance of contrast into the left heart chambers while contrast is diminishing in the right heart chambers. (AVM: arteriovenous malformation; ESLD: end-stage liver disease)

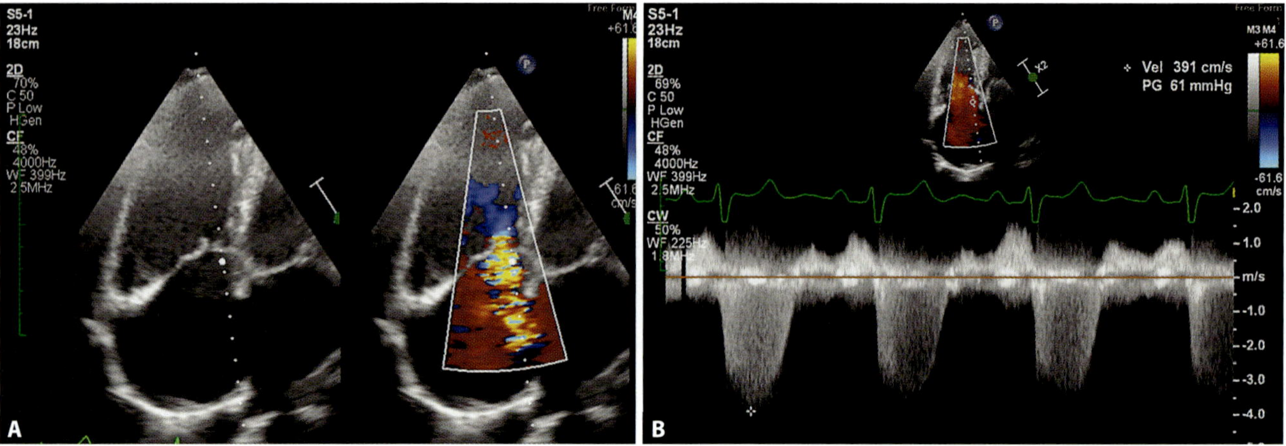

Figs. 4A and B: Portopulmonary hypertension (PoPH) related to end-stage liver disease (ESLD). (A) Right ventricular focused view reveals a dilated right atrium and right ventricle, and moderate tricuspid regurgitation; (B) continuous wave Doppler documents a 61 mm Hg gradient with severe pulmonary hypertension.

(Figs. 4A and B). Abnormalities like TR, right ventricular dilatation, right ventricular dysfunction, and pulmonary artery dilation are other features seen in patients with PoPH. An estimated RVSP >40–50 mm Hg is an indication of RHC.[22] Only an RHC can adequately determine accurate pulmonary pressures, as an echocardiogram only offers estimates based on the TR velocity. Adequate RV function, a surrogate of cardiac output, is the best predictor of operative survival. The American Association for the Study of Liver Diseases (AASLD) recommends that RHC should be performed in patients who either have an RSVP ≥45 mm Hg and/or other evidence suggestive of increased mPAP.[2] However, the ERS and the Mayo Clinic recommend that RHC be performed in patients with RSVP ≥50 mm Hg.[22]

Pericardial effusion is seen in almost 22% of ESLD patients, especially in the presence of ascites, and requires no treatment. However, cardiac tamponade should be treated with pericardiocentesis or pericardial window before LT.

Dobutamine Stress Echocardiography

Ischemic evaluation with exercise stress testing has poor predictive value in LT candidates due to deconditioning and limited ability to exercise to achieve a target heart rate; thus, pharmacologic stress testing is frequently required. It is widely used for the identification of significant CAD and risk stratification of patients with ESLD who are scheduled to undergo LT. However, dobutamine stress echo (DSE) in LT candidates has poor sensitivity (13–37%), high specificity (85%), low positive predictive value (PPV) (22%), and intermediate negative predictive value (75%) for obstructive CAD.[23] This can be explained by various reasons like splanchnic and systemic vasodilatation in ESLD patients, leading to low SVR and a hypercontractile left ventricle , which causes difficulty in identification of small ischemic regions, owing to the tethering by adjacent segments which become hyperkinetic with stress; wide use of beta-blockers as prophylaxis against esophageal variceal bleeding results in impaired chronotropic response; presence of ascites may limit the acquisition of high-quality images. Positive stress in ESLD patients without significant coronary stenosis may be because of microvascular dysfunction, which is more prevalent in patients with nonalcoholic fatty liver disease (NAFLD). With an intermediate negative predictive value, a normal DSE test may be useful in identifying patients at low risk of perioperative MACE.

Various cardiac risk factors have been identified in cirrhotic patients **(Table 1)**. For LT recipients, AHA in 2012 recommended that noninvasive stress testing be considered for patients with three or more risk factors. In 2014, joint guidelines by the AASLD and the American Society of Transplantation (AST) recommended that "stress echocardiography should be performed in all potential LT candidates".[2] In the same year, the ESC and European Society of Anaesthesiology (ESA) issued a consensus recommendation for stress testing in LT candidates as patients with >2 traditional risk factors or diabetes mellitus (high pre-test probability of having

TABLE 1: Summary of risk factors identified in various guidelines.

Guideline	*Risk factors*
AHA/ACC scientific statement, 2012[4]	Diabetes mellitus, prior cardiovascular disease, left ventricular hypertrophy, age >60 years, smoking, hypertension and dyslipidemia
AASLD clinical practice guideline, 2014[2]	Hyperlipidemia, hypertension, diabetes, cigarette consumption, age >60 years
EASL clinical practice guidelines, 2015[3]	Age >50 years, male sex, hypertension, and diabetes mellitus
AST consensus recommendations, 2018[18]	• Age (Men >45 years Women >55 years), hypercholesterolemia, hypertension, tobacco use, family history of early CAD (first degree male relative <55 years or female <65 years) • Independent risk factor: DM (two-fold risk of sudden cardiac death)
AHA scientific statement, 2022[5]	>2 traditional risk factors (male sex, hypertension, hyperlipidemia, smoking, age >60 years, left ventricular hypertrophy, prior cardiovascular disease, or diabetes), or NASH, DM

(AASLD: American Association for the Study of Liver Diseases; AHA/ACC: American Heart Association/American College of Cardiology; AST: American Society of Transplantation; CAD: coronary artery disease; DM: diabetes mellitus; EASL: European Association for the Study of the Liver; NASH: nonalcoholic steatohepatitis)

CAD) and poor functional capacity [<4 metabolic equivalents (METs)] **(Flowchart 2)**.[18,24] In 2015, the European Association for the Study of the Liver (EASL) recommended that cardiopulmonary exercise testing (CPET) should be performed in high-risk patients and stress testing should be considered only in those patients who failed to achieve the target heart rate.[3] The difference in recommendations reflects the low sensitivity of stress testing in detecting CAD in cirrhotic patients.

Myocardial Perfusion Imaging

Single-photon emission computed tomography (SPECT) myocardial perfusion imaging (MPI) for preoperative cardiac risk stratification is a widely used noninvasive imaging modality. However, the evaluation of CAD by SPECT MPI in LT candidates has yielded conflicting results due to the heterogeneity of studies. SPECT MPI has low sensitivity (37%) and specificity (61%) but high negative predictive values (NPVs) for diagnosing severe CAD (95%) in LT candidates.[25] Based on the various studies, SPECT imaging is an inaccurate initial screening test with poor diagnostic ability to detect significant CAD. Nevertheless, a study by Baker et al. demonstrated that SPECT imaging was more effective with PPV and NPV of 67% and 97%, respectively, when it was applied only to patients at high risk for CAD.[26] The preexisting vasodilated state in ESLD patients and underlying coronary microvascular dysfunction mitigate the effects of pharmacologic vasodilatory agents (adenosine, regadenoson, and dipyridamole). Thus, both false positive and false negative findings are seen. Two studies comparing DSE with SPECT MPI did not show any advantage over DSE.[26,27] Positron emission tomography (PET) provides high-resolution images and is a promising tool to evaluate CAD. PET has been validated against dobutamine stress echocardiography, though studies in LT candidates are lacking.[28]

Cardiovascular Magnetic Resonance Imaging

Cardiovascular magnetic resonance imaging (CMR) is an operator-independent integrated modality with high reproducibility. CMR provides a turnkey approach to evaluate cardiac structure, function, ischemia, and viability. It also helps in the assessment of liver anatomy and thoracoabdominal vasculature in LT candidates.[29] It can detect regional wall motion abnormalities during pharmacologic stress (dobutamine) tests, improving the sensitivity and specificity than DSE. Moreover, myocardial perfusion abnormalities can be detected using a gadolinium contrast. Myocardial scars can also be identified using CMR. The spatial resolution of CMR myocardial perfusion is superior to other nuclear imaging modalities (SPECT/PET), and thus subendocardial ischemia can be more reliably identified.[30] In LT candidates, a negative CMR stress test is associated with an almost 100%, 12-month CAD event-free survival.[29] If there is a high index of suspicion that hemochromatosis is a cause of ESLD or myocardial iron overload, CMR may be useful. CMR imaging with a T2*-based sequence diagnoses the severity of myocardial iron overload, if indicated.

Coronary Artery Calcium Score and Coronary Computed Tomography Angiography

Coronary Artery Calcium Score (CACS) with coronary computed tomography angiography (CCTA) identifies subclinical CAD by determining the amount of coronary artery calcium, evaluating the degree of coronary artery

Flowchart 2: Preoperative cardiovascular evaluation and investigative approach strategies in patients scheduled for liver transplant surgery.

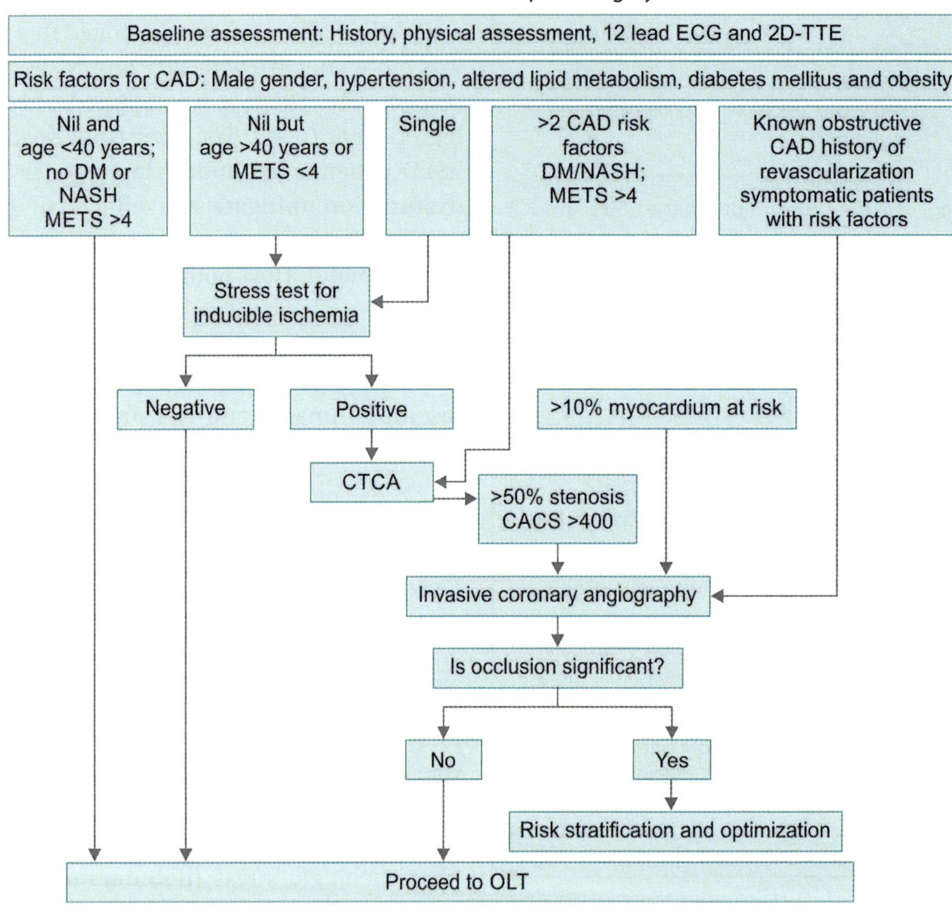

(2D-TTE: two-dimensional transthoracic echocardiogram; CAD: coronary artery disease; CACS: coronary artery calcium score; CTCA: computed tomography coronary angiography; DM: diabetes mellitus; ECG: electrocardiogram; METS: metabolic equivalents; NASH: nonalcoholic steatohepatitis; OLT: orthotopic liver transplant)

stenosis, composition of the atherosclerotic plaque, and measuring the fractional flow reserve-computed tomography (FFR-CT).

Coronary Artery Calcium Score identifies and quantifies the calcification of the coronary plaques CACS [defined in hounsfield units (HUs)] which is graded as absent (0), minimal (1–10), mild (11–100), moderate (101–400), or extensive (>400). A CACS of <10 HU correlates with the absence of significant coronary obstructive lesion, whereas CACS >400 HU is associated with the presence of significant (50%) or critical (70%) coronary artery stenosis on invasive CA Patients with CACS >400 HU also have higher rates of post-LT cardiovascular complications at 1 month. It has been seen that 30% of LT candidates have at least moderate (stenosis of 50%) asymptomatic CAD on CACS.[31]

Noninvasive CCTA, with its high sensitivity (nearly 90%) and negative predictive value (above 95%), may be considered an acceptable alternative to invasive CA for excluding significant CAD in "low-risk" patients with regular, nontachycardic rhythm, able to lie flat and to perform required breath-holding maneuvers.[32] Patients with left ventricular systolic dysfunction (LVEF 40%), angina, or stress testing that shows mild ischemia, or equivocal results can undergo confirmatory CCTA. The presence of severe coronary artery calcification or prior coronary stent placement may preclude accurate assessment for the presence of obstructive CAD. Significant limitations to CT coronary angiography (CTCA) in ESLD patients are renal failure, severe ascites, orthopnea, need for relative bradycardia, and hepatic encephalopathy. Nevertheless, due to the poor predictive value of stress imaging and improvements in noninvasive CCTA, it is the ideal test for screening obstructive CAD in LT candidates, reserving invasive CA as the gold standard in case of doubt. In LT candidates with coronary artery stenosis 50% or greater on CCTA or in cases of CACS 400, CA is mandatory to quantify the stenosis and to define the need for interventional procedures.[18]

Computed tomography-based testing has been gaining prominence in screening and diagnosing CAD. Though the majority of the studies have been conducted in noncirrhotic populations, there is growing evidence that CT-based testing is a good screening test for CAD, given that these tests are not affected by the underlying vasodilated state and hyperdynamic circulation seen in cirrhosis. Recent guidelines for screening for CAD have now included CT-based tests. The AST stated in 2018 that "Coronary angiography, invasive or noninvasive, remains the standard criterion for detection of CAD".[18] They recommend that invasive or noninvasive angiography should be considered in patients with known CAD, abnormal noninvasive test, or a high pretest probability of CAD (e.g., diabetes or ≥2 traditional risk factors; 2C). CACS >400 is associated with significant CAD requiring revascularization, and patients with CACS >400 are advised to undergo invasive CA. ACC/AHA recommends that CCTA should be performed in all high-risk patients (≥2 risk factors) and those with diabetes mellitus (DM) or NASH. Their approach limits the use of stress tests to only those patients who have one risk factor or patients with no risk factors who are >40 years of age or unable to achieve METs >4. Patients <40 years of age and with no risk factors for CAD, DM, or metabolic dysfunction-associated steatohepatitis (MASH) can proceed for LT directly if they can achieve METS >4.[30,33] Computed tomography-fractional flow reserve (CT-FFR) for intermediate lesions is yet to be validated in ESLD patients.

Invasive Coronary Angiography

Invasive CA remains the gold standard for the diagnosis of CAD. The prevalence of CAD in asymptomatic LT candidates varies from 13 to 26% and is related to traditional cardiovascular risk factors.[34] Routine CA as the initial diagnostic modality for the evaluation of CAD is controversial. Indications for CA include the presence of positive noninvasive stress testing, evidence of obstructive CAD on CCTA (50% stenosis), and evaluation of certain patients with a history of revascularization or known obstructive CAD to assess graph patency when indicated. Assessment of LT candidates who had undergone coronary artery bypass grafting (CABG) should be based on their pretransplant LV ejection fraction and ischemic testing. ESLD patients who are LT candidates are susceptible to thrombocytopenia, anemia, and renal failure, making them prone to increased risk of femoral artery vascular complications; however, CA can be safely performed in LT candidates via a transradial approach compared to the femoral approach, thereby reducing bleeding complications.[35] Radial artery occlusion (RAO) incidence in the first week after intervention is 5.5%. Maintenance of the patency of the radial artery should be an integral part of all procedures undertaken through the radial approach. High-dose heparin, along with shorter compression times and patent hemostasis, is recommended in reducing RAO.[36]

Risk Scores Using Combination of Tests

Coronary artery disease in liver transplant (CAD-LT): Rachwan et al., in their retrospective study of 1771 LT candidates over 10 years, proposed the use of CAD-LT score, which has risk factors (age, male gender, diabetes, hypertension, tobacco use, family history of CAD, and personal history of CAD). The score and the derived algorithm independently predicted significant CAD, defined as stenosis ≥50% in a major vessel or ≥70% in a moderate-size vessel branch. Preoperative screening with CAD-LT score was able to identify 89% of patients with significant CAD, reducing unnecessary testing with stress tests (57%) or invasive angiography (44%).[37]

Cardiovascular risk in orthotopic liver transplantation: This score, formulated in 2017, uses a point-based system to find the 1-year risk for mortality or hospital admission secondary to a MACE after LT. The risk factors included in this scoring system are age, gender, race, diabetes, hypertension, obesity, chronic kidney disease, end-stage kidney disease, smoking, and dyslipidemias.[38] The 1-year mortality due to cardiovascular causes estimated by this score may range from optimal (<5%) to high (>45%).

CONCLUSION

Preoperative cardiovascular assessment needs multidisciplinary collaboration and an investigative approach. Electrocardiogram (ECG), 2D-TTE with Doppler, and BCE-TTE are to be performed in all LT candidates, with

TABLE 2: Noninvasive and invasive diagnostic modalities for evaluation of CAD in liver transplant candidates.

Screening test	*Sensitivity*	*Specificity*	*Positive predictive value*	*Negative predictive value*	*Disadvantages in ESLD*
Dobutamine stress echocardiography (DSE)	13–32%	78–85%	0–33%	75–100%	Limited accuracy of DSE to detect CAD due to: • ESLD patients typically have hypercontractile left ventricle • Use of beta-blockers results in failure to achieve target heart rates during the test • Presence of ascites may result in pseudo dyskinesis of the posterior wall • Microcirculatory dysfunction
• Myocardial perfusion imaging (MPI) • Single photon emission computed tomography (SPECT)	37–100%	50–88%	15–28%	77–100%	Limited accuracy of MPI due to: • Impaired vasodilatory reserve in ESLD patients may reduce the effectiveness of a vasodilatory stress test • Image artifacts secondary to splenomegaly and ascites
CT coronary angiography (CTCA)	95–99%	83–91%	64%	83–99%	• False-positive results in case of diffuse coronary calcification or prior implanted stent • Major limitations: – Nephrotoxicity – Need for relative bradycardia
Coronary angiography	NA	NA	NA	NA	Complications: • Bleeding • Blood transfusions

(CAD: coronary artery disease; CT: computed tomography; ESLD: end-stage liver disease; NA: not applicable)

further investigations individualized according to the patient-specific cardiac assessment **(Table 2)**. A negative stress test helps in ruling out the presence of CAD. For initial CAD evaluation in cirrhotic patients with more than two risk factors, CACS and CCTA are acceptable screening noninvasive modalities of choice. If the CACS is >400 or >50% stenosis is present, then the risk-benefit of the investigative approach must be individualized. Invasive CA is the ultimate investigative tool in the armamentarium **(Fig. 1)**. Though there is a risk of inappropriate and unnecessary coronary revascularization and its complications, the benefits need to be weighed against them.

REFERENCES

1. Kim WR, Lake JR, Smith JM, Schladt DP, Skeans MA, Harper AM, et al. OPTN/SRTR 2016 annual data report: liver. Am J Transplant. 2018;18 Suppl 1:172-253.
2. Martin P, DiMartini A, Feng S, Brown R Jr, Fallon M. Evaluation for liver transplantation in adults: 2013 practice guideline by the American Association for the Study of Liver Diseases and the American Society of Transplantation. Hepatology. 2014;59(3):1144-65.
3. European Association for the Study of the Liver. Electronic address: easloffice@easloffice.eu. EASL clinical practice guidelines: liver transplantation. J Hepatol. 2016;64(2):433-85.
4. Lentine KL, Costa SP, Weir MR, Robb JF, Fleisher LA, Kasiske BL, et al. Cardiac disease evaluation and management among kidney and liver transplantation candidates: a scientific statement from the American Heart Association and the American College of Cardiology Foundation. J Am Coll Cardiol. 2012;60(5):434-80.
5. Cheng XS, VanWagner LB, Costa SP, Axelrod DA, Bangalore S, Norman SP, et al. Emerging evidence on coronary heart disease screening in kidney and liver transplantation candidates: a scientific statement rom the American Heart Association: endorsed by the American Society of Transplantation. Circulation. 2022;146(21):e299-324.
6. Jha AK, Lata S. Liver transplantation and cardiac illness: current evidences and future directions. J Hepatobiliary Pancreat Sci. 2020;27(5):225-41.

7. Nicolau-Raducu R, Gitman M, Ganier D, Loss GE, Cohen AJ, Patel H, et al. Adverse cardiac events after orthotopic liver transplantation: a cross-sectional study in 389 consecutive patients. Liver Transpl. 2015;21(1):13-21.
8. Shahvaran SA, Menyhárt O, Csedrik L, Patai ÁV. Diagnosis and prevalence of cirrhotic cardiomyopathy: a systematic review and meta-analysis. Curr Probl Cardiol. 2021;46(10):100821.
9. Nagueh SF, Smiseth OA, Appleton CP, Byrd BF, Dokainish H, Edvardsen T, et al. Recommendations for the evaluation of left ventricular diastolic function by echocardiography: an update from the American Society of Echocardiography and the European Association of Cardiovascular Imaging. J Am Soc Echocardiogr. 2016;29(4):277-314.
10. Yoon KT, Liu H, Lee SS. Cirrhotic cardiomyopathy. Curr Gastroenterol Rep. 2020;22(9):45.
11. Liu H, Lee SS. Diagnostic criteria of cirrhotic cardiomyopathy: out with the old, in with the new? Hepatology. 2021;74(6):3523-5.
12. Kremastinos DT, Farmakis D. Iron overload cardiomyopathy in clinical practice. Circulation. 2011;124(20):2253-63.
13. Hendrickse MT, Thuluvath PJ, Triger DR. Natural history of autonomic neuropathy in chronic liver disease. Lancet. 1992;339(8807):1462-4.
14. Soulaidopoulos S, Goulis I, Cholongitas E. Pulmonary manifestations of chronic liver disease: a comprehensive review. Ann Gastroenterol. 2020;33(3):237-49.
15. Humbert M, Kovacs G, Hoeper MM, Badagliacca R, Berger RMF, Brida M, et al. 2022 ESC/ERS Guidelines for the diagnosis and treatment of pulmonary hypertension [published correction appears in Eur Heart J. 2023; 44(15):1312]. Eur Heart J. 2022;43(38):3618-731.
16. Bernardi M, Calandra S, Colantoni A, Trevisani F, Raimondo ML, Sica G, et al. Q-T interval prolongation in cirrhosis: prevalence, relationship with severity, and etiology of the disease and possible pathogenetic factors. Hepatology. 1998;27(1):28-34.
17. Bargehr J, Trejo-Gutierrez JF, Patel T, Rosser B, Aranda-Michel J, Yataco ML, et al. Preexisting atrial fibrillation and cardiac complications after liver transplantation. Liver Transpl. 2015;21(3):314-20.
18. VanWagner LB, Harinstein ME, Runo JR, Darling C, Serper M, Hall S, et al. Multidisciplinary approach to cardiac and pulmonary vascular disease risk assessment in liver transplantation: an evaluation of the evidence and consensus recommendations. Am J Transplant. 2018;18(1):30-42.
19. Alper I, Ulukaya S, Demir F, Kilic M. Effects of cardiac valve dysfunction on perioperative management of liver transplantation. Transplant Proc. 2009;41(5):1722-6.
20. Zinoviev R, Aksoy O. Aortic valve hemodynamics in liver cirrhosis. Circulation. 2024;150(Suppl_1):A4145296-.
21. Khan MZ, Khan MU, Munir MB, Khan SU, Osman M, Balla S. Contemporary trends and outcomes in aortic valve replacement in patients with end-stage liver disease. Catheter Cardiovasc Interv. 2020;96(4):947-55.
22. Krowka MJ, Fallon MB, Kawut SM, Fuhrmann V, Heimbach JK, Ramsay MA, et al. International Liver Transplant Society practice guidelines: diagnosis and management of hepatopulmonary syndrome and portopulmonary hypertension. Transplantation. 2016;100(7):1440-52.
23. Harinstein ME, Flaherty JD, Ansari AH, Robin J, Davidson CJ, Rossi JS, et al. Predictive value of dobutamine stress echocardiography for coronary artery disease detection in liver transplant candidates. Am J Transplant. 2008;8(7):1523-8.
24. Kristensen SD, Knuuti J, Saraste A, Anker S, Bøtker HE, Hert SD, et al. 2014 ESC/ESA Guidelines on non-cardiac surgery: cardiovascular assessment and management: the Joint Task Force on non-cardiac surgery: cardiovascular assessment and management of the European Society of Cardiology (ESC) and the European Society of Anaesthesiology (ESA). Eur Heart J. 2014;35(35):2383-431.
25. Bhutani S, Tobis J, Gevorgyan R, Sinha A, Suh W, Honda HM, et al. Accuracy of stress myocardial perfusion imaging to diagnose coronary artery disease in end stage liver disease patients. Am J Cardiol. 2013;111(7):1057-61.
26. Baker S, Chambers C, McQuillan P, Janicki P, Kadry Z, Bowen D, et al. Myocardial perfusion imaging is an effective screening test for coronary artery disease in liver transplant candidates. Clin Transplant. 2015;29(4):319-26.
27. Snipelisky D, Ray J, Vallabhajosyula S, Matcha G, Squier S, Lewis J, et al. Usefulness for predicting cardiac events after orthotopic liver transplantation of myocardial perfusion imaging and dobutamine stress echocardiography preoperatively. Am J Cardiol. 2017;119(7):1008-11.
28. Tincopa MA, Weinberg RL, Sengupta S, Slivnick J, Corbett J, Sonnenday CJ, et al. The utility of noninvasive PET/CT myocardial perfusion imaging in adult liver transplant candidates. Transplant Direct. 2022;8(4):e1311.
29. Reddy ST, Thai NL, Oliva J, Tom KB, Dishart MK, Doyle M, et al. Cardio-hepatic risk assessment by CMR imaging in liver transplant candidates. Clin Transplant. 2018;32(5): e13229.
30. Greenwood JP, Maredia N, Younger JF, Brown JM, Nixon J, Everett CC, et al. Cardiovascular magnetic resonance and single-photon emission computed tomography for diagnosis of coronary heart disease (CE-MARC): a prospective trial. Lancet. 2012;379(9814):453-60.
31. Su A, Almazan E, Sakulsaengprapha V, Shay J, Wittstein I, Hammami M, et al. High coronary artery calcium score is associated with increased major adverse cardiac events after liver transplantation. Transplant Direct. 2023;9(2):e1426.
32. Moon YJ, Kwon HM, Jung KW, Jeong HW, Park YS, Jun IG, et al. Risk stratification of myocardial injury after liver

transplantation in patients with computed tomographic coronary angiography-diagnosed coronary artery disease. Am J Transplant. 2019;19(7):2053-66.

33. VanWagner LB, Harinstein ME, Runo JR, Darling C, Serper M, Hall S, et al. Multidisciplinary approach to cardiac and pulmonary vascular disease risk assessment in liver transplantation: an evaluation of the evidence and consensus recommendations. Am J Transplant. 2018;18(1):30-42.
34. Xia VW, Taniguchi M, Steadman RH. The changing face of patients presenting for liver transplantation. Curr Opin Organ Transplant. 2008;13(3):280-4.
35. Feng K, Gupta V, Terrazas E, Yeghiazarians Y, Ports T, Gregoratos G, et al. Trans-radial versus trans-femoral access in patients with end-stage liver disease undergoing cardiac catheterization. Am J Cardiovasc Dis. 2014;4(3):133-9.
36. Rashid M, Kwok CS, Pancholy S, Chugh S, Kedev SA, Bernat I, et al. Radial artery occlusion after transradial interventions: a systematic review and meta-analysis. J Am Heart Assoc. 2016;5(1):e002686.
37. Rachwan RJ, Kutkut I, Timsina LR, Bou Chaaya RG, El-Am EA, Sabra M, et al. CAD-LT score effectively predicts risk of significant coronary artery disease in liver transplant candidates. J Hepatol. 2021;75(1):142-9.
38. VanWagner LB, Ning H, Whitsett M, Levitsky J, Uttal S, Wilkins JT, et al. A point-based prediction model for cardiovascular risk in orthotopic liver transplantation: the CAR-OLT score. Hepatology. 2017;66(6):1968-79.

CHAPTER 4

Selection and Evaluation of Donors in Living Donor Liver Transplantation

Rohan J Chaudhary, Ketul Shah, Makrand Karpe, Kalpana Tathe

INTRODUCTION

Living donor liver transplantation (LDLT) has emerged as a highly effective treatment option for end-stage liver disease, comparable to deceased donor liver transplantation (DDLT). Surgical protocols across various centers have focused on ensuring donor safety while refining biliary and vascular techniques. However, criteria for donor selection vary significantly between centers, influenced by factors such as the proportion of DDLT versus LDLT performed, the availability of living donors, regional disease patterns, and the timeline of development for both DDLT and LDLT.

Experienced centers are increasingly accepting donors with more complex anatomical features, posterior sector grafts (PSGs), and lower graft-to-recipient weight ratios (GRWR). Nevertheless, the concept of double equipoise remains crucial in evaluating the balance between donor risk and recipient benefit. LDLT should only be considered when the potential risk to the donor is justified by an acceptable outcome for the recipient.[1]

The primary focus of donor evaluation is safety. Key objectives include ensuring that there is adequate parenchymal volume, vascular inflow, venous outflow, and biliary drainage for both the partial allograft and the donor remnant. Additionally, it is critical to assess that the donor faces no systemic risks during the partial hepatectomy and that the donor fully understands the process and potential psychological effects.

Definitions

A *modified right lobe graft (MRLG)* refers to a graft that includes separate segment 5 and 8 hepatic veins, with the middle hepatic vein (MHV) retained in the donor's remnant liver.

An *RL with partial or subtotal MHV* involves retrieving half or nearly the entire MHV along with the RL.

A *standard RLG* does not involve any reconstruction of the anterior sector venous outflow.

Mild mental subnormality describes someone who has a slower cognitive process but is still capable of providing informed consent.

Upper-extremity disability refers to an individual who is independent but cannot fully use one or both arms due to amputation, injury, previous illness, or neurological weakness.

Lower-extremity disability refers to an individual who is independent but cannot fully use one or both legs due to amputation, injury, previous illness, or neurological weakness.

DONOR SELECTION CRITERIA

The key aspects in donor selection are given in the following text.

Donor Age

The acceptable lower and upper age limits among donors are 18 and 55 years, respectively. Donor candidates over the age of 45 years should be considered with stricter criteria, i.e., GRWR >0.8 and remnant volume >35%. In a recent study by Macshut et al.,[2] it was found that a donor age above 45 years independently contributed to the risk of small-for-size syndrome (SFSS), early graft loss, and increased 1-year mortality rates in recipients.

Donor Body Mass Index

The ideal donor body mass index (BMI) should be between 18 and 28 kg/m^2. However, the majority of centers accept donor candidates up to a BMI of 33 kg/m^2. Donors with a BMI above 30 kg/m^2, or those with a BMI of 28 kg/m^2 and >2 metabolic syndrome (MS) parameters [such as waist circumference >102 cm in men or >88 cm in women, fasting blood glucose >100 mg/dL, blood pressure >130/85 mm Hg, high-density lipoprotein (HDL) cholesterol <40 mg/dL in men or <50 mg/dL in women, and serum triglycerides >150 mg/dL], should undergo a liver biopsy to exclude fatty liver or steatohepatitis and can be selected if they have <20% macrosteatosis with no fibrosis on biopsy. To ensure an extra margin of safety, we subtract the percentage of macrosteatosis from the estimated graft and remnant volumes while calculating the GRWR or remnant percentage. Donors with higher BMI can have higher postoperative complications (pulmonary infections, decreased mobility, and increased surgical site infections).[3] The lower limit of BMI can be lowered to 16 kg/m^2 in selected cases after ruling out physical illness or chronic disease and mental illness such as anorexia nervosa or other eating disorders.

ABO Compatibility

The ideal donor should be ABO compatible with the recipient. However, in Asia, where there is a shortage or absence of deceased donors, protocols for ABO-incompatible adult-to-adult LDLT have been developed and have yielded acceptable results.[4,5] Additionally, paired exchange donation offers another option for utilizing medically suitable ABO-incompatible donors. In liver transplantation, swap transplants can be for blood group or volume incompatibility. These innovations have helped to increase the live donor pool and reduce recipient waiting list mortality.

Least Acceptable Donor Liver Remnant

For RLG, most centers consider a minimum of 30% remnant as the cutoff for donor selection. Few centers have age-specific criteria for remnant selection, like 28% for donors below the age of 35 years, 30% for those above 35 years, and >35% for donors aged >45 years. This is owing to perhaps lower regeneration potential in older donors.[1]

Lower Cutoff of Graft to Recipient Weight Ratio

Graft to recipient weight ratio (GRWR) is calculated as graft volume in kilogram by recipient weight in kilogram. The previously accepted lower limit of GRWR in RL LDLT is 0.8%. The majority of the centers currently accept a GRWR of 0.7% or even lower in selected cases, with similar cutoffs in right and left lobe (RL and LL) LDLT.[7]

Donors with Comorbidity

Candidates with well-controlled diabetes mellitus, hypo/hyperthyroidism, hypertension, and asthma can be considered for liver donation. History of coronary artery disease or cerebrovascular accidents is a contraindication for liver donation.

Procoagulant Workup

It is advisable to screen high-risk donors (BMI >28 kg/m^2, age >50 years) for procoagulant disorders. Nondonor hepatectomy data suggest a higher incidence of thrombotic complications among those older than 50 years, with surgery longer than 4 hours, and a BMI >28 kg/m^2.[2,8]

Acceptable Transaminases

Few centers accept "the normal range" of their laboratory, but majority consider an upper limit between 40 and 50 IU/mL. While mild elevation of transaminases (>2–3 × normal) is acceptable in a deceased donor liver where the volume of the liver graft is more than sufficient graft volume, this is not the case in adult LDLT where both the remnant and the graft are partial livers. In LDLT, even mild and self-limiting donor liver pathology at the time of donation/transplantation may lead to remnant liver or graft dysfunction, respectively. While the actual value of elevated transaminases is less important, the presence of inflammation and/or necrosis must be ruled out on a liver biopsy. As per the American Gastroenterological Association (AGA)[9] recommendations, a liver biopsy seems logical prior to rejecting a donor with an unexplained mild elevation of serum transaminases.[10]

Assessment of Donor Liver Steatosis

The acceptable steatosis in adult LDLT is <20% macrovesicular fat. It is <30% in pediatric LDLT with a larger graft (GRWR >2). Hepatic steatosis is the most common cause of rejection of otherwise medically fit donors. Ultrasound, noncontrast computed tomography (NCCT) scan, and magnetic resonance imaging (MRI) scan are the commonly used noninvasive tests to assess steatosis.[11,12] Frequently used methods include the ratio of liver to splenic attenuation (L/S) or the difference between the two (liver attenuation index or LAI) in Hounsefield units (HU) on NCCT scan and spectrophotometry or 3-point Dixon on MRI **(Table 1)**. If LAI is >5, the liver is accepted; biopsy is considered if LAI is between 0 and 5;

TABLE 1: Liver attenuation index.

NCCT for liver fat assessment	
LAI	***Estimation of liver steatosis***
<–10	>30%
–10 to +5	6%–30%
>5	0–5%

(LAI: liver attenuation index; NCCT: noncontrast computed tomography)

if LAI is <0, the donor is either rejected or subjected to weight-reduction treatment.[13]

Limitations of computed tomography (CT)/LAI: (1) Hemosiderin deposition can cause falsely elevated liver attenuation and (2) radiologically occult diffuse liver disease may be missed.

Histologically, microsteatosis consists of fat droplets measuring 1–2 μm that do not displace the nucleus, commonly seen in alcoholic or drug-induced liver disease or as a nonspecific finding. Macrosteatosis, on the other hand, involves droplets larger than 20 μm that displace the nucleus. This can occur due to the coalescence of microsteatotic droplets in alcoholic liver disease or develop independently in nonalcoholic fatty liver disease. While macrovesicular steatosis is generally agreed to impact graft function, microsteatosis in a healthy liver graft with sufficient volume is typically not a concern.

In the largest study of donor steatosis, which analyzed 9,677 deceased donors using the United Network for Organ Sharing (UNOS) and the European Liver Transplant Registry (ELTR) databases,[14,15] microsteatosis did not negatively affect survival across any categories of balance of risk (BAR) scores. However, when macrosteatosis exceeded 30%, survival rates were adversely impacted, especially with higher BAR scores. Donor liver steatosis may be reversible, depending on factors such as age, severity, and cold ischemia time. The functional capacity of steatotic hepatocytes compared to nonsteatotic ones remains a subject of debate. Cho et al.[16] found that mild steatosis does not hinder hepatic regeneration in grafts. However, other studies suggest that steatotic hepatocytes contribute to an ischemic environment, compromising the functional quality of those cells.[17]

Consensus recommendations are as follows: (1) The upper acceptable limit of macrovesicular steatosis for RL and LL grafts should be 10–20%, (2) the presence of steatosis on noninvasive imaging should trigger a predonation liver biopsy to assess the extent of steatosis and check for hepatitis, and (3) potential steatotic donors can undergo preoperative treatment with a carefully monitored diet and exercise regimen for 4–8 weeks to reduce weight, thereby improving their suitability as donors.[18,19] The donor with steatosis, along with any other adverse pathological findings like inflammation, fibrosis, or hepatocyte ballooning, is not acceptable for liver donation.

BOX 1: Indications for donor liver biopsy.

- Body mass index (BMI) >30 kg/m^2
- Dyslipidemia
- Presence of risk factors for metabolic syndrome
- Liver attenuation index (LAI) ≤5
- Low graft recipient weight ratio <0.7% (graft-side biopsy)
- Liver remnant: <30–32% (remnant side liver biopsy)

Donor Liver Biopsy

A selective donor liver biopsy is performed in the presence of one or more of the following: Age >50 years, BMI >30 kg/m^2, low GRWR <0.7%, low remnant <30–32%, any component of MS, steatosis on imaging, and elevated liver enzymes **(Box 1)**. While a selective predonation liver biopsy is usual, its criteria remain controversial and vary between centers.[18,19] Steatosis detected on noninvasive imaging, abnormal transaminases, and two or more components of MS are the most common indications for predonation liver biopsy. Thresholds for biopsy are lower among older donors and those with borderline remnant and graft volumes. Elevated triglycerides and/or MS have been linked to steatosis and steatohepatitis. Regeneration potential reduces with age; therefore, donor age, metabolic parameters, and remnant and graft volumes must all be factored in when deciding on performing a biopsy and the acceptable degree of steatosis.

Histopathologic evidence of significant inflammation and/or fibrosis (F1 or higher) is clearly not acceptable. The significance of nonspecific granulomas (not associated with tuberculosis/other infections/sarcoidosis) on donor biopsy is controversial.

Protocol for Liver Biopsy in Liver Donor

To evaluate liver fat

- Body mass index >30 kg/m^2
- Liver attenuation index ≤5

Liver biopsy in the presence of normal LAI:

- In case of borderline residual liver volume (<30%)

- In case of anticipated small-for-size graft volume (GRWR <0.7)
  (In both of these situations, even a small amount of fat, 5–10%, will compromise the liver volumes.)
- To evaluate for suspected liver pathology when transaminases are elevated

Exclusion Criteria Based on Donor Comorbidity and Abnormal Laboratory Tests

Hepatitis B core antibody (HBcAb)-positive donors are universally acceptable. In such cases, the long-term risk to recipients of transmission of hepatitis B seropositivity is 20–30%, and conversion to hepatitis B virus deoxyribonucleic acid (DNA) positive status is 10–30%. Currently, post-transplant therapy with nucleotide and nucleoside analogs (entecavir or tenofovir) is recommended for such recipients for at least 5 years.

Donors with transient *elevation of serum transaminases* can be accepted provided they normalize before donation and the biopsy is normal.

The minimal *acceptable Hb* is 9.5 g/dL, although some accept less. Potential donors with beta thalassemia minor and those with correctable anemia can be eligible for liver donation after correction.

Donors with a previous *psychiatric illness* in remission can be accepted carefully; caution is prudent in such donors since living donation is a significant psychological stress, and there are reports of depression and even suicide among donors.

Physical disability among donors that would not interfere with recovery to preoperative functional status is acceptable. Again, evidence that physical composite scores after donation normalize over 6 months lends support to this policy.

There is a clear consensus to exclude those with a previous history of coronary artery disease, stroke, nonskin extracranial malignancy, and previous drug abuse. However, accepting reformed alcoholics as donors, even if they had a normal liver biopsy, is controversial.

A history of upper abdominal surgeries and laparoscopic cholecystectomy should not be considered a barrier to donation,[20] as such procedures do not increase donor morbidity. Asymptomatic first-degree relatives of recipients with hereditary or autoimmune liver diseases, like Wilson disease, hemochromatosis, hemophilia, and maple syrup urine disease, can still be considered as donors, though they may require predonation liver biopsy, enzyme tests, or genetic studies.

CT Volumetry

A triple-phase contrast-enhanced CT scan (CECT) of the abdomen is done in all donors. The gold standard method for preoperative liver volumetry is manual CT volumetry. Transverse images of the portal-venous phase are used because hepatic veins are depicted with maximum contrast in this phase. Semiautomated interactive commercial software called AW Volume Share 6 (GE Healthcare, Chicago, Illinois, USA) is used. All major vessels, such as the extrahepatic portal vein in the area of the porta hepatis and inferior vena cava, as well as larger fissures, the gallbladder, and the hepatic ligamentum teres are manually excluded from the total liver volume analysis because they have no metabolic function and therefore cannot be added to the volume of the graft. The liver outline is determined by either the pencil trace or the paintbrush method in a craniocaudal direction.

The radiological plane of transection is drawn along the MHV to delineate the RL and the LL of the liver **(Figs. 1A and B)**. The volume of the caudate lobe is calculated separately. The following volumes are calculated: Total liver volume, RL including MHV, RL excluding MHV, LL including MHV, and LL excluding MHV. While calculating the GRWR for the RL graft, RL excluding MHV is taken as the graft weight, whereas for the LL graft, LL including MHV is taken as the graft weight. For the left lateral segment graft, the radiological plane of transection is drawn just to the right of the falciform ligament caudally and close to the ostia of the left hepatic vein (LHV) cranially, and the volume of the left lateral segment is calculated.

The vascular inflow and outflow, as well as the volumetric analysis of the liver lobes or segments, can also be done with 3D modeling on MeVis, Merion, or Synapse Vincent software. These afford high-resolution depiction of the hepatic arterial, portal venous, and hepatic venous systems, which can be superimposed.[21]

Donor Vascular and Biliary Anatomy

The anatomy of the liver should be delineated clearly preoperatively by a triple-phase contrast imaging, with or without three-dimensional reconstruction, which remains invaluable in planning the operative approach to preserving arterial and venous inflow and venous outflow of the graft, without compromising the remnant inflow and outflow, especially in RLGs. An ideal graft anatomy is a single long hepatic artery, a single portal vein, and a single hepatic duct, which is seen in 40–50%

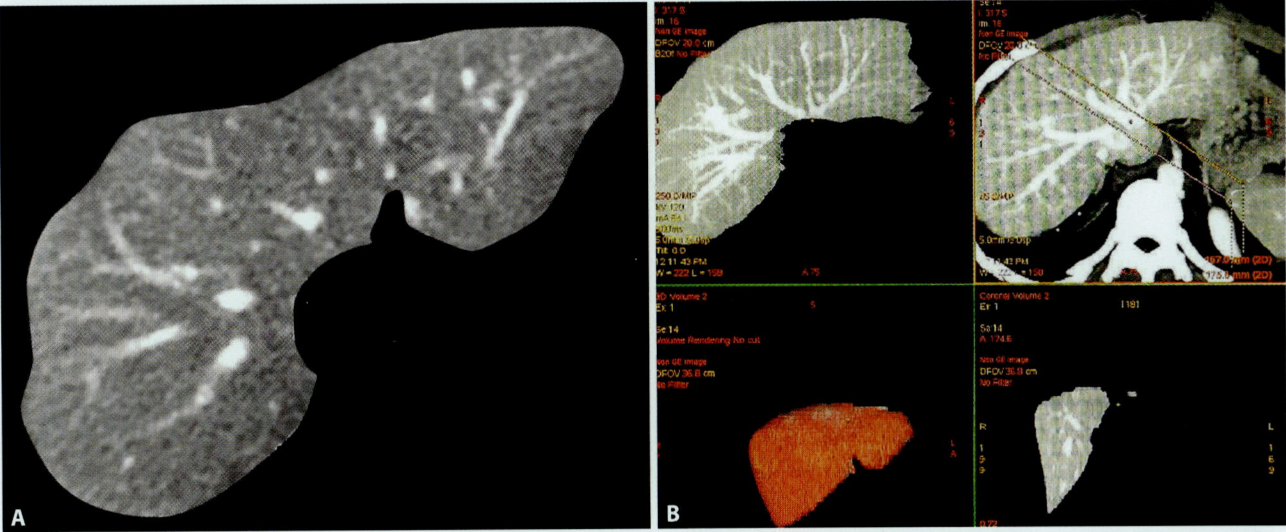

Figs. 1A and B: CT volumetry image: Liver border is outlined by the pencil trace method (A); Radiological plane of transection (B).[21]

of cases in high-volume centers. The rest of the cases have anatomical variations, and selection in such cases is based on institutional experience.[22]

The more experienced LDLT centers would accept grafts with three or more arteries, especially if there are common areas of supply between arteries, and eventually, up to two arterial anastomoses are expected. As for portal vein anomalies **(Table 2)**, the majority of centers would reject Nakamura types D and E or high takeoff of the right anterior portal vein from the left portal vein (LPV) for RLGs.[23,24] Left-sided gallbladders are frequently accompanied by type E portal vein anatomy and can be suitable only for left lateral sector donation in a few cases.

Biliary complications are more common in LDLT compared to DDLT, with an incidence of 11–38% due to the presence of multiple, small graft ducts requiring reconstruction. Magnetic resonance pancreaticography (MRCP) and/or intraoperative cholangiogram (IOC) is performed to assess duct anatomy, and it is not uncommon to reject donors with three or more graft ducts **(Fig. 2)**.

Type of Graft

The selection of the graft is primarily influenced by the recipient's preoperative condition, GRWR, the donor's remnant liver volume, and the vascular anatomy. Three variations of RLGs are used depending on the extent of the MHV retrieved from the donor: Modified extended right lobe graft (MERLG) or subtotal MHV graft, which preserves the cranial segment 4a vein; the partial right lobe graft (PRLG), which includes a partial MHV; and the MRLG, where the segment 5 and 8 veins are reconstructed on the bench, with no MHV involved.[26]

TABLE 2: Nakamura' classification of portal vein anatomy.[23,24]

Classifications		***Anatomical variants***
Nakamura et al. Type A Normal classical	Cheng et al. Type I	Right PV, Left PV
Nakamura et al. Type B Trifurcation	Cheng et al. Type II	RAS, Left PV, RPS
Nakamura et al. Type C	Cheng et al. Type III	RAS, Left PV, RPS
Nakamura et al. Type D	Cheng et al. Type IV	RAS, Left PV, RPS
Nakamura et al. Type E	Cheng et al. Type IV (Others)	S4, S8, S5, Left PV, RPS

(LV: left ventricle; RAS: right anterior sectoral; RPS: right posterior sectoral)

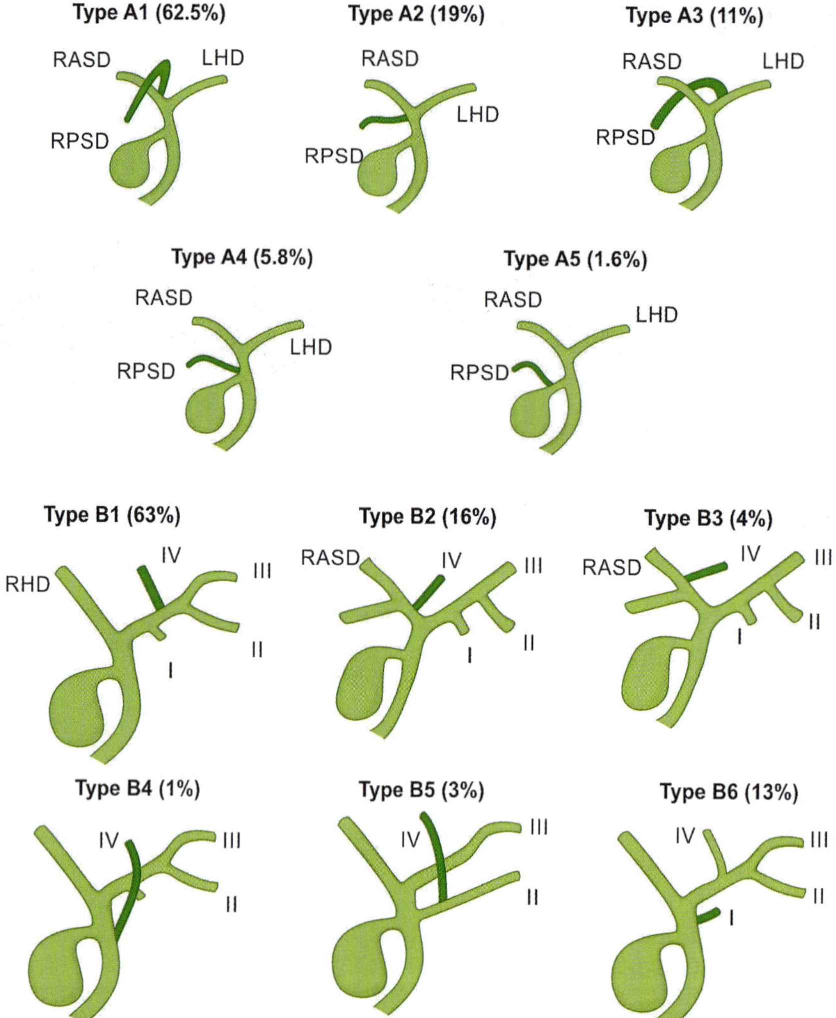

Fig. 2: Huang's classification of hepatic duct anatomy.[25] (A) For right lobe grafts; (B) For left lobe grafts. (LHD: left hepatic duct; RASD: right anterior sectoral duct; RHD: right hepatic duct; RPSD: right posterior sectoral duct).

The actual surgical plane of parenchymal transection is defined by intraoperative inflow occlusion of the lobe to be removed and may differ from the preoperative radiological plane. In a left lateral sector graft, the surgical plane of transection is 1 cm right to the falciform ligament.

Selection of Right/Left Lobe Graft[27,28]

- RL GRWR ≥0.8 (preferred), up to 0.70 acceptable in low MELD recipients
- LL GRWR ≥1 preferable
- The remnant volume should be >32% preferably (acceptable up to 30%).

The most commonly used grafts in adult liver transplantation are RLGs, with modified RLGs being the preferred choice. Some centers have reported successful outcomes using left lobe grafts (LLGs) for adults. Any viable approach must ensure adequate remnant volume, as well as proper vascular inflow and outflow.

Posterior sector grafts are considered when the donor's anatomy is favorable, with the posterior sector having a larger volume than the LL, and when the remnant volume is insufficient with an RLG. The ideal anatomical conditions for PSG include a long extrahepatic right posterior hepatic artery, a type C portal vein, and Huang A4 hepatic ducts. Kokudo et al.[29] reported on 28 PSG grafts from 437 LDLTs, with a 90% graft survival rate, 10% vascular complications, and 33% biliary complications. To reduce the incidence of biliary complications in PSG, microscopic arterial reconstruction and the avoidance of multiple hepatic ducts, along with Huang A4 biliary anatomy, may be beneficial.

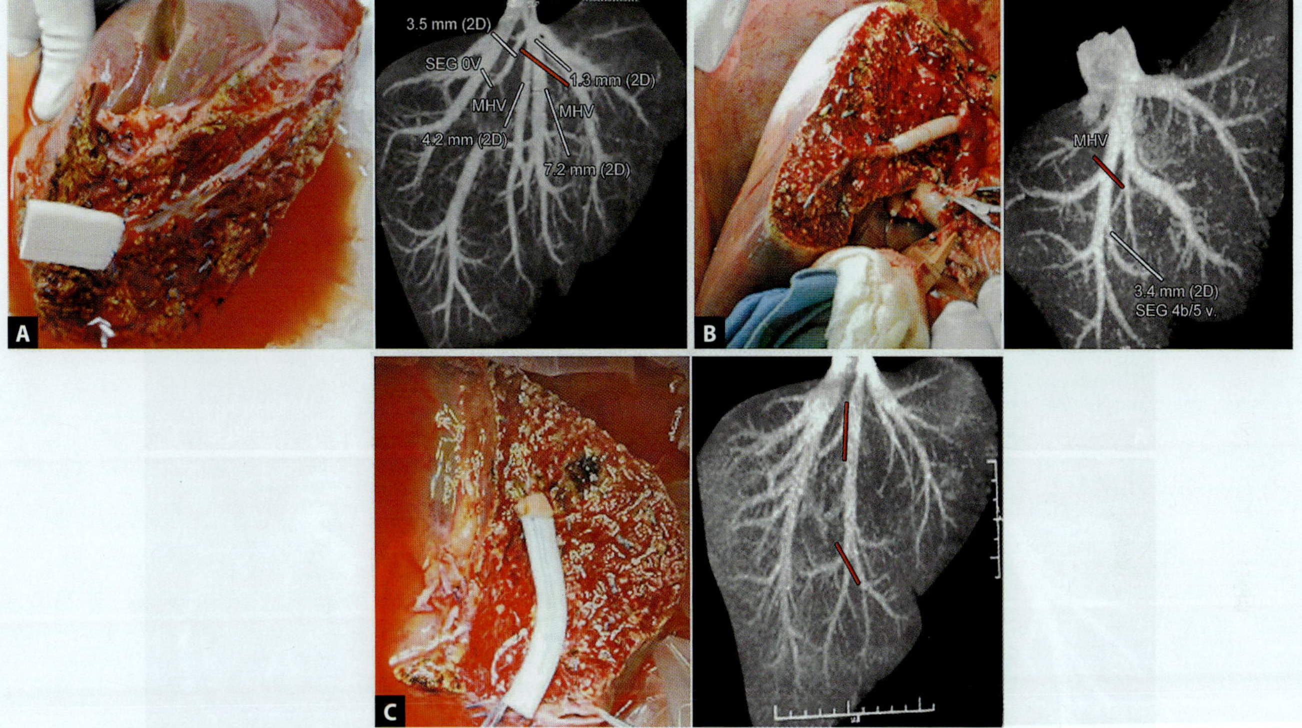

Figs. 3A to C: Type of RLG. (A) Subtotal MHV RLG; (B) Partial MHV RLG; (C) Modified MHV RLG.[26] (MHV: middle hepatic vein; RLG: right lobe graft)

- *MHV controversy:* The MHV anatomy is categorized into four types by modifying the original Neumann classification, rather than the traditional three types **(Figs. 3A to C)**. The fourth type is essentially a mirror image of type 3, also referred to as a double or bifid MHV **(Figs. 4A to D)**. Type 1 is typically suitable for a MRLG, type 2 for a PRLG, and types 3 and 4 for a MERLG.

Segment 4 venous drainage is classified as either favorable or unfavorable, depending on whether it predominantly drains into the LHV or the proximal MHV, which aligns with the Nakamura classification. The LHV-dominant (Nakamura type 1) anatomy is considered favorable for a MERLG, while Nakamura type 3 is suitable for an MRLG, and partially favorable (Nakamura type 2) venous anatomy is best suited for a PRLG **(Figs. 5A to C)**.

The factors favoring an RLG with partial MHV or a modified RLG are as follows:

- Remnant liver volume: 30–35%
- Donor age >40 years
- Steatosis in liver biopsy >10%
- MHV type 1 (modified RLG)
- MHV type 2 (partial RLG)
- V4 unfavorable (modified RLG)
- V4 Partially favorable (partial RLG)
- GRWR >0.8
- Low MELD recipient <25

These factors are known to affect liver regeneration and have the potential to tip the balance away from donor safety. So, our policy is to leave the MHV with the donor when these factors are encountered in any combination to avoid the segment 4 congestion and inadequate liver regeneration.

Donor Consent

The structured process of donor informed consent is summarized by Gordon[33] and includes: (1) Assessment of donor competence to make decisions; (2) disclosure of information; (3) donor comprehension of the information; (4) a voluntary decision by the donor to donate, free from coercion; and finally (5) donor agreement to undergo the procedure. Donor privacy should always be protected. It must be ensured that the decision to donate is voluntary and without coercion, either self-imposed or the result

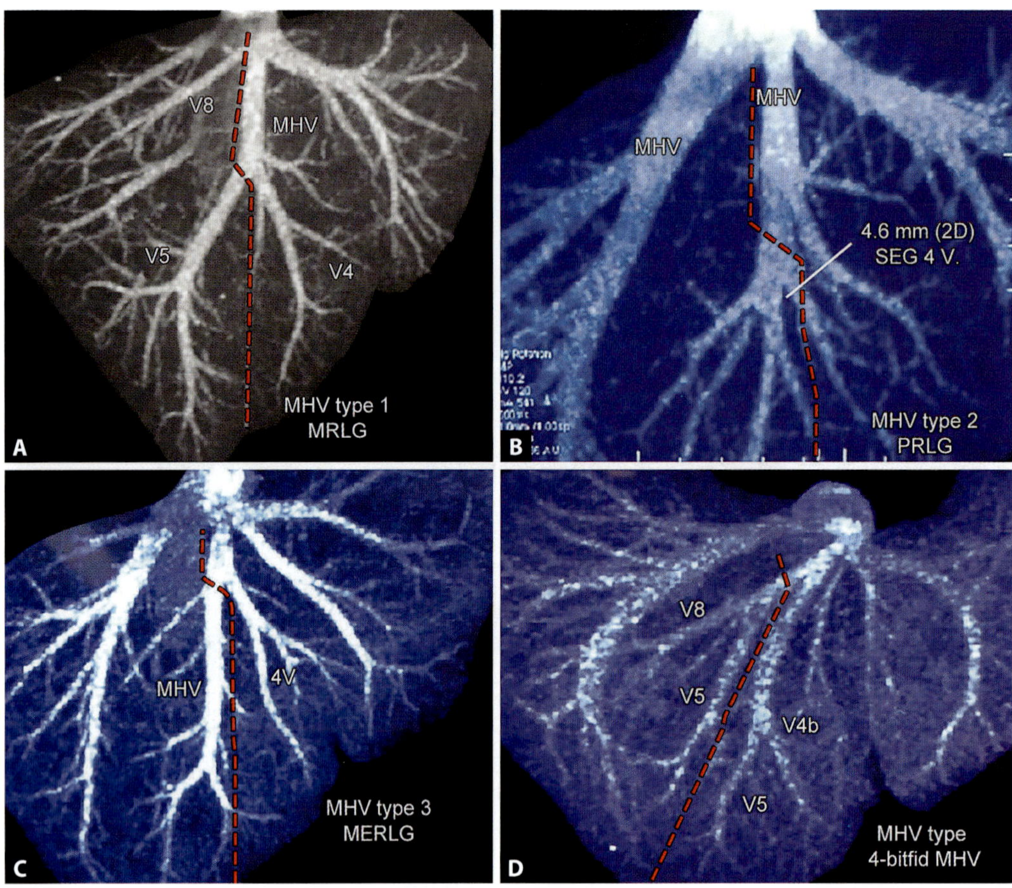

Figs. 4A to D: (A) Neumann type 1 MHV; (B) Neumann type 2 MHV; (C) Neumann type 3 MHV; (D) Neumann type 4 MHV.[30] (MHV: middle hepatic vein)

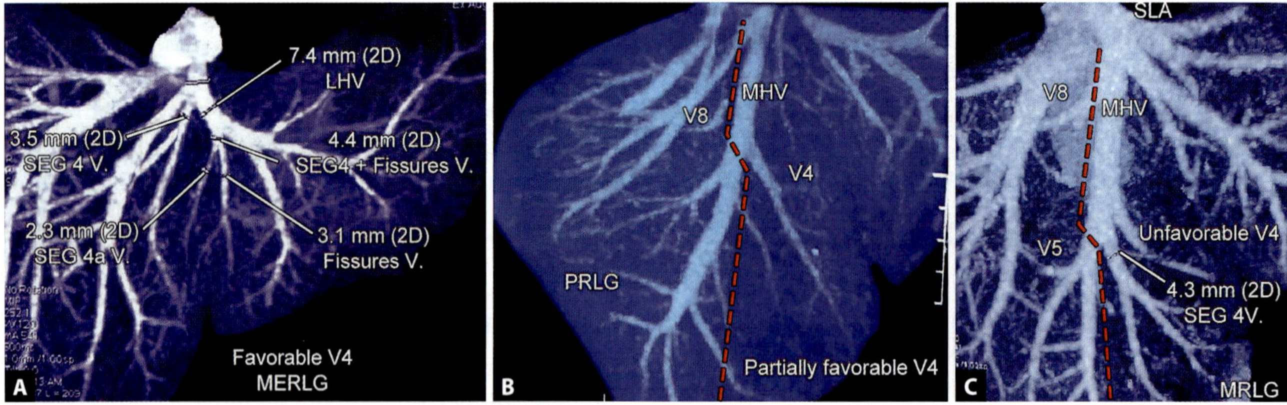

Figs. 5A to C: (A) Nakamura type 1: Favorable V4; (B) Nakamura type 2: Partially favorable V4; (C) Nakamura type 3: Unfavorable V4.[31,32]

of external pressures or manipulation. Informed consent must include full information on the potential surgical, medical, financial, and psychological risks (including death) of a hepatectomy. Potential outcomes for the recipient must be disclosed to the donor.

Aftercare and Follow-up of Donors

Living donor liver transplantation carries a significant estimated donor mortality at 0.1% and 0.5% for left and right liver donors, respectively. A morbidity rate of 20–35%[34-36] is also expected. Immediately after surgery,

TABLE 3: Donor evaluation protocol.

Phase 1	Blood group, complete blood count, differential leukocyte count, liver function test, renal function test, prothrombin time, internationalized ratio, activated partial prothrombin time, lipid profile, thyroid profile, viral marker—anti-HCV/HbsAg/HBcAb/HIV I and II, cytomegalovirus IgG and IgM, venereal disease of research laboratory, random blood sugar, urine routine and microscopic examination, urine culture and sensitivity, urine pregnancy test (for female), dengue profile, hepatitis A virus (HAV IgM), hepatitis E virus (HEV IgM), Epstein-Barr virus (EBV IgM for donor of pediatric recipient only)
	Noncontrast computed tomography for liver attenuation Index
	Magnetic resonance fat estimation
Phase II	Triphasic CT of abdomen for liver volumetry and vascular anatomy
Phase III	Pulmonary function test (PFT)
	Electrocardiogram (ECG) Stress echocardiography (for donor's age >35 years) Echocardiography and treadmill test (TMT) (for donor's age <35 years)
	Chest X-ray (PA view)
	Bilateral mammography (for female donor's age >35 years)
	Transvaginal ultrasonography (TVS) (for married females) Ultrasound pelvis (for unmarried females)
	Magnetic resonance pancreaticography (MRCP)
	Computed tomography calcium scoring (for donor's age >50 years)
	Bilateral carotid vessels Doppler (for donor's age >50 years)
Phase IV	Hepatology/gynecology and breasts (for female)/psychiatry/anesthesia/cardiology: Clearance
	Further investigations are conducted if there is a notable medical history, such as a family history of primary biliary cirrhosis or autoimmune diseases, or any history of addiction, including smoking, alcohol, or substance abuse. Throughout the evaluation process, multiple professionals explain the risks associated with donor hepatectomy, as well as address any questions regarding recovery, return to normal activities, and follow-up care Informed consent is obtained from the donor, and approval from a legal authorization committee is required by the state health authority

(CT: computed tomography; HBcAb: hepatitis B core antibody; HBsAg: hepatitis B surface antigen; HCV: hepatitis C virus; IgG: immunoglobulin G; IgM: immunoglobulin M; PA: posteroanterior)

all donors should receive effective prophylaxis against deep vein thrombosis and stress peptic ulceration **(Table 3)**. Upon discharge from the hospital, all donors should have regular clinical monitoring and follow-up for at least 2 years and preferably for life. Laboratory tests for liver function and platelet counts should be checked at follow-up for at least 1 year. All donors should be advised to have lifetime annual primary care examinations for health maintenance.

Donor Death in Living Donation

Living donor liver transplantation is associated with a well-documented risk of donor morbidity and mortality. No institution engaged in this high-risk clinical activity is immune to this risk. Studies in the field of crisis management show that preparing for a catastrophic event is imperative, both to respond appropriately and for prevention. The key phrase is "when, not if". The International Liver Transplantation Society (ILTS) recommends that hospitals and teams involved in LDLT should create a framework on how to respond to a potential living donor crisis.[37]

REFERENCES

1. Soin AS, Chaudhary RJ, Pahari H, Pomfret EA. A worldwide survey of liver donor selection policies at 24 centers with a combined experience of 19 009 adult living donor liver transplants. Transplantation. 2019;103(2): e39-47.
2. Macshut M, Kaido T, Yao S, Yagi S, Ito T, Kamo N, et al. Older donor age is a risk factor for negative outcomes after adult living donor liver transplantation using small-for-size grafts. Liver Transpl. 2019;25:1524-32.

3. Moss J, Lapointe-Rudow D, Renz JF, Kinkhabwala M, Dove LM, Gaglio PJ, et al. Select utilization of obese donors in living donor liver transplantation: implications for the donor pool. Am J Transplant. 2005;5(12):2974-81.
4. Soin AS, Raut V, Mohanka R, Rastogi A, Goja S, Balachandran M, et al. Use of ABO-incompatible grafts in living donor liver transplantation—first report from India. Indian J Gastroenterol. 2014;33(1):72-6.
5. Tiwari AK, Pandey P, Aggarwal G, Dara RC, Rawat G, Raina V, et al. Cascade plasmapheresis (CP) as a preconditioning regime in ABO-incompatible live related donor liver transplants (ABOi-LDLT). Transplant Res. 2014;3:17.
6. Lee S-G. A complete treatment of adult living donor liver transplantation: a review of surgical technique and current challenges to expand indication of patients. Am J Transplant. 2015;15:17-38.
7. Selzner M, Kashfi A, Cattral MS, Selzner N, Greig PD, Lilly L, et al. A graft to body weight ratio less than 0.8 does not exclude adult-to-adult right-lobe living donor liver transplantation. Liver Transpl. 2009;15:1776-82.
8. Bustelos R, Ayala R, Martinez J, Martin MA, Toledo T, Grande S, et al. Living donor liver transplantation: usefulness of haemostatic and prothrombotic screening in potential donors. Transplant Proc. 2009;41:3791-5.
9. American Gastroenterological Association. American Gastroenterological Association medical position statement: evaluation of liver chemistry tests, this document presents the official recommendations of the American Gastroenterological Association (AGA) on the evaluation of liver chemistry tests. It was approved by the Clinical Practice Committee on March 3, 2002 and by the AGA Governing Board on May 19, 2002. Gastroenterology. 2002;123(4):1364-6.
10. Patel S, Orloff M, Tsoulfas G, Kashyap R, Jain A, Bozorgzadeh A, et al. Living-donor liver transplantation in the United States: identifying donors at risk for perioperative complications. Am J Transplant. 2007; 7:2344-9.
11. Vohra S, Goyal N, Gupta S. Preoperative CT evaluation of potential donors in living donor liver transplantation. Indian J Radiol Imaging. 2014; 24:350-9.
12. Krishan S, Baijal SS, Saraf N, Gautam D, Saigal S, Soin AS. Accuracy of MR based calculation of hepatic fat fraction. J Clin Exp Hepatol. 2014;4:S83.
13. Bhangui P, Sah J, Choudhary N, Gautam D, Gupta V, Srinivasan T, et al. Safe use of right lobe live donor livers with up to 20% macrovesicular steatosis without compromising donor safety and recipient outcome. Transplantation. 2020;104(2):308-16.
14. Dutkowski P, Schlegel A, Slankamenac K, Oberkofler CE, Adam R, Burroughs AK, et al. The use of fatty liver grafts in modern allocation systems risk assessment by the balance of risk (BAR) score. Ann Surg. 2012;256(5):861-9.
15. Dutkowski P, Oberkofler CE, Slankamenac K, Puhan MA, Schadde E, Müllhaupt B, et al. Are there better guidelines for allocation in liver transplantation? A novel score targeting justice and utility in the model for end-stage liver disease era. Ann Surg. 2011; 254:745-53.
16. Cho JY, Suh KS, Kwon CH, Yi NJ, Lee KU. Mild hepatic steatosis is not a major risk factor for hepatectomy and regenerative power is not impaired. Surgery. 2006;139(4): 508-15.
17. Peralta C, Jiménez-Castro MB, Gracia-Sancho J. Hepatic ischemia and reperfusion injury: effects on the liver sinusoidal milieu. J Hepatol. 2013;59(5):1094-106.
18. Choudhary NS, Saraf N, Saigal S, Gautam D, Lipi L, Soin AS. Estimation of normal values of serum transaminases based on liver histology in healthy Asian Indians. J Gastroenterol Hepatol. 2015;30(4):763-6.
19. Choudhary NS, Saraf N, Saigal S, Gautam D, Lipi L, Rastogi A, et al. Rapid reversal of liver steatosis with lifestyle modification in highly motivated liver donors. J Clin Exp Hepatol. 2015;5(2):123-6.
20. Lo CM. Complications and long-term outcome of living liver donors: a survey of 1,508 cases in five Asian centers. Transplantation. 2003;75(suppl):S12-5.
21. Goja S, Yadav SK, Yadav A, Piplani T, Rastogi A, Bhangui P, et al. Accuracy of preoperative CT liver volumetry in living donor hepatectomy and its clinical implications. Hepatobiliary Surg Nutr. 2018;7(3):167-74.
22. Marcos A, Ham JM, Fisher RA, Olzinski AT, Posner MP. Surgical management of anatomical variations of the right lobe in living donor liver transplantation. Ann Surg. 2000;231(6):824-31.
23. Nakamura T, Tanaka K, Kiuchi T, Kasahara M, Uemoto S, et al. Anatomical variations and surgical strategies in right lobe living donor liver transplantation: lessons from 120 cases. Transplantation. 2002;73:1896-903.
24. Cheng YF, Huang TL, Lee TY, Chen TY, Chen CL. Variation of the intrahepatic portal vein; angiographic demonstration and application in living-related hepatic transplantation. Transplant Proc. 1996;28:1667.
25. Huang TL, Cheng YF, Chen CL, Chen TY, Lee TY. Variants of the bile duct: clinical application in the potential donor of living-related hepatic transplantation. Transplant Proc 1996;28:1669.
26. Goja S, Kumar Yadav S, Singh Soin A. Readdressing the middle hepatic vein in right lobe liver donation: triangle of safety. Liver Transpl. 2018;24(10):1363-76.
27. Soin AS, Yadav SK, Saha SK, Rastogi A, Bhangui P, Vohra V, et al. Is portal inflow modulation always necessary for successful utilization of small volume living donor liver grafts? Liver Transpl. 2019;25(12):1811-21.
28. de Villa VH, Chen CL, Chen YS, Wang CC, Lin CC, Cheng YF, et al. Right lobe living donor liver transplantation-addressing the middle hepatic vein controversy. Ann Surg. 2003;238(2):275-82.
29. Kokudo T, Hasegawa K, Arita J, Yamamoto S, Kaneko J, Akamatsu N, et al. Use of a right lateral sector graft in living donor liver transplantation is feasible, but special caution

is needed with respect to liver anatomy. Am J Transplant. 2016;16:1258-65.

30. Neumann JO, Thorn M, Fischer L, Schöbinger M, Schemmer P, et al. Branching patterns and drainage territories of the middle hepatic vein in computer-simulated right living-donor hepatectomies. Am J Transplant. 2006;6(6):1407-15.
31. Nakamura S, Tsuzuki T. Surgical anatomy of the hepatic veins and the inferior vena cava. Surg Gynecol Obstet. 1981;152(1):43-50.
32. Hwang S, Lee SG, Choi ST, Moon DB, Ha TY, Lee YJ, et al. Hepatic vein anatomy of the medial segment for living donor liver transplantation using extended right lobe graft. Liver Transpl. 2005;11(4):449-55.
33. Gordon EJ, Rodde J, Skaro A, Baker T. Informed consent for live liver donors: a qualitative, prospective study. J Hepatol. 2015;63(4):838-47.
34. Goja S, Yadav SK, Saigal S, Soin AS. Right lobe donor hepatectomy: is it safe? A retrospective study. Transpl Int. 2018;31(6):600-9.
35. Goja S, Yadav SK, Roy R, Soin AS. A retrospective comparative study of venous vs nonringed expanded polytetrafluoroethylene extension graft for anterior sector outflow reconstruction in right lobe living donor liver transplantation. Clin Transplant. 2018;32(8):e13344.
36. Yadav SK, Saraf N, Saigal S, Choudhary NS, Goja S, Rastogi A, et al. High MELD score does not adversely affect outcome of living donor liver transplantation: experience in 1000 recipients. Clin Transplant. 2017;31(8).
37. Miller CM, Durand F, Heimbach JK, Kim-Schluger L, Lee SG, Lerut J, et al. The International Liver Transplant Society guideline on living liver donation. Transplantation. 2016;100(6):1238-43.

CHAPTER 5

Liver Transplant in Acute Liver Failure: Preoperative Evaluation and Optimization of Patients

Suvadeep Sen, Aklesh Tandekar

INTRODUCTION

Acute liver failure (ALF) is a catastrophic life-threatening condition, arising from acute dysfunction of the liver leading to a multisystem organ involvement within a short period in a patient who does not have pre-existing liver disease. All patients with ALF must be distinguished from acute-on-chronic liver failure (ACLF) as they are heterogeneous in their clinical course, require different sets of management plans, and have differences in prognostic outcome characteristics. The condition is unique in its presentation in terms of the development of sudden and severe cerebral edema in the absence of any intracranial (IC) cause, normal and sometimes hypercoagulable state even in the presence of deranged biochemical coagulation parameters, development of multiple organ involvement within a short period, and requirement of substantial healthcare resource in the overall management of the condition, delivering tremendous economic and psychological pressure to the family member of the affected. The prognosis of ALF depends on its etiology, the rapidity of development of full-blown encephalopathy, the degree of organ involvement, and the effectiveness of clinical management strategies. The condition is often fatal as there is no artificial system that can support the entire synthetic, metabolic, and excretory function of the liver. The lack of randomized controlled trials on this "orphan disease" makes guidelines about its management mostly based on expert consensus with lower grades of recommendation. A liver transplant (LT) is a potentially curative option in the treatment plan when spontaneous regeneration of the liver is no longer expected. However, intensive care management in both the pretransplant and post-transplant periods to provide organ support plays a dominating role in determining the outcome of most of the cases.

ACUTE LIVER FAILURE DEFINITION AND CLASSIFICATION

Acute liver failure is defined as an acute deterioration of the function of the liver characterized by raised bilirubin, prolonged international normalized ratio (INR) of prothrombin time (>1.5), and encephalopathy in the absence of pre-existing liver dysfunction. There is inconsistency in the duration of liver failure that defines ALF. The American Association for the Study of Liver Diseases (AASLD) accepts a period of illness <26 weeks to define ALF.[1] The Indian National Association for Study of the Liver (INASL) accepts 4 weeks from jaundice to encephalopathy as the cutoff to define ALF.[2] The spectrum of disease is further subdivided based on jaundice to encephalopathy duration into (1) hyperacute (<7 days), (2) acute (7–28 days), and (3) subacute (5–12 weeks) presentation. The duration of illness is important as it provides clues to etiology and sometimes has a prognostic relation in patients with ALF.

ROLE OF LIVER TRANSPLANTATION IN PATIENTS WITH ACUTE LIVER FAILURE

The management of ALF is mainly supportive. An LT is the only treatment that significantly modifies the course and outcome of ALF in patients not responding to medical supportive care. Forty years back in the pretransplant era, ALF used to carry a mortality of 80–85%.[3] With the evolution of LTs and improvement in practices in the intensive care unit (ICU), the overall mortality from ALF over the next 30 years has come down to around 33% and around a quarter of patients with ALF require LTs.[4,5] The survival benefit of patients with ALF requiring LT at 1-year post-LT in patients with ALF is around 80%.[6] The Acute Liver Failure Study Group (ALFSG) registry[7] collecting data from various centers in the UK on the outcome of all patients admitted with ALF and ALI in the time duration from 1998 to 2019 has shown that 22% of patients required liver transplantation while 51% had complete spontaneous recovery from the condition.

ASSESSMENT AND MANAGEMENT OF PATIENTS WITH ACUTE LIVER FAILURE

The assessment of ALF patients includes (1) identification of etiology, (2) confirming of diagnosis of ALF and excluding chronic liver disease, (3) clinical and laboratory investigations to understand etiology and assess severity and complications of the disease, (4) stabilization and support of extrahepatic organs, and (5) determining the need for LT and preparing for the patient for prospective LT.

Identification of Etiology

The identification of etiology is important as this has prognostic implications. Etiology workup may be conducted as per **Table 1**. ALF due to paracetamol overdose, ischemic hepatitis, hepatitis A and E, and pregnancy-related ALF usually recovers spontaneously in >50% of patients without the need for LT, whereas hepatitis B ALF, drug-induced ALF, acute Budd–Chiari or autoimmune hepatitis or ALF of indeterminate etiologies tends to have a more subacute course and have transplant-free survival of <25%.[8] LT is not indicated for secondary causes of ALF like malignant infiltration of the liver, acute ischemic injury, systemic diseases like dengue, malaria, Rickettsial diseases, and hemophagocytic lymphohistiocytosis (HLH) precipitated by viral or fungal infections or hematological malignancies. The etiology of the disease may not be identifiable in around 10–15% of adults and 50% of the pediatric population with ALF, and they have a comparatively poorer course of disease.[9]

Rule Out Cirrhosis and Other Liver Pathologies

It is important to rule out evidence of chronic liver disease in any patients with suspected ALF, irrespective of age bracket. This not only alters the management of the patients but also modifies the whole outcome characteristics. However, there are certain conditions like Budd–Chiari syndrome, reactivation of hepatitis B, Wilson's disease, and autoimmune hepatitis where the diagnosis of ALF may still be acceptable despite having underlying chronic liver pathology.[4] Clinical signs of cirrhosis with portal hypertension like ascites, splenomegaly, caput medusae, rectal hemorrhoids, and palmer erythema should be sought in any patient with deranged liver function. Ultrasonography should be done to assess the liver size, nodularity, and echotexture; splenic size with evidence of ascites; and portal venous Doppler for portal flow, portal vein diameter, and pressure. UGI endoscopy may reveal esophageal varices. Liver biopsy is sometimes required to exclude any infiltrative disorders, Wilson's disease, autoimmune hepatitis, or malignancy before transplant. Routine use of biopsy is not recommended and is potentially dangerous in the presence of coagulopathy. The transjugular approach is safer and more effective, and it is currently the most frequently used route for biopsy compared to the percutaneous route.

Understanding the Severity of Illness in Patients with Acute Liver Failure

All patients with ALF should be closely observed clinically and with periodic laboratory assessments to understand the dynamicity of illness **(Table 2)**. Mental status examination to grade encephalopathy as per West Haven grading needs to be done frequently. The hemodynamic status, oxygenation, breathing, and urine output are the basic parameters that should be observed in all patients. Careful observation for any evidence of bleeding is required in the presence of coagulopathy. Periodic testing of arterial blood gas, lactate level, ammonia level, prothrombin time, and INR and blood sugar measurement is required for understanding the course of illness. The frequency of laboratory evaluation depends on the institutional protocol. This evaluation is extremely important to determine the timing of escalation of management, listing for transplantation, and understanding futility in case the patient becomes too sick. The ALFSG has suggested to use of a checklist at admission for diagnosis and daily evaluation of patients with ALF in the ICU.[10] A web version of the checklist may be accessed from https://alfchecklist.com.

Organ Support and Preparation of Transplant if Required

The following are the usual indications to shift patients with ALF to the ICU:

- Encephalopathy grade 2 and higher
- Hypotension mean arterial pressure (MAP) <60 mm Hg after adequate fluid resuscitation

TABLE 1: *Acute liver failure (ALF):* Etiologies and their salient characteristics.

Etiology	*Cause*	*Salient Characteristics*
Infection	• Hepatotrophic viral infections • Hepatitis B, A, E	• Leading cause of ALF worldwide • Hepatitis A and E is predominant in countries with poor sanitation and hygiene. Hyperacute presentation; higher transplant-free survival • *HBV:* Only 25% recover without transplant • *HEV:* Pregnancy is a categorical risk factor; usually self-limited
	Herpes simplex (HSV), cytomegalovirus (CMV), Epstein–Barr virus (EBV), adenovirus	• Common in immunocompromised patients • Treat with acyclovir or ganciclovir
Drugs	Acetaminophen	Hyperacute presentation with very high aminotransferase level and initial mild elevation of bilirubin
	Complementary and alternative medicines (CAM), antitubercular drugs, immune checkpoint inhibitors, minocycline, nitrofurantoin, azole antifungals, sulfa drugs, antiretrovirals	Around 10% of drug-induced liver injury develop ALF usually, a subacute presentation with high bilirubin at presentation and lower aminotransferase levels; poorer transplant-free survival
Toxins	• Mushroom poisoning • Rat killing pesticides	• Hyperacute and acute presentation • Good transplant-free survival with intensive care support
Genetic/ Metabolic	Acute Wilson's disease, galactosemia, tyrosinemia, α1-antitrypsin deficiency, hemochromatosis	• Usually refractory to medical treatment • Liver transplant is the definitive treatment
Pregnancy	Acute fatty liver of pregnancy (AFLP), hemolysis, elevated liver enzymes, low platelet (HELLP) syndrome	• Present in third trimester or early postpartum • Associated with preeclampsia; early delivery if fetus is crucial • Disseminated intravascular coagulation is common
Autoimmune	Acute severe autoimmune hepatitis	• Acute or subacute presentation • Usually requires autoimmune markers and histopathology for diagnosis • Poor transplant-free survival
Vascular	Acute Budd–Chiari syndrome, veno-occlusive disease, acute hepatic artery thrombosis post-transplant	• Obstruction of the hepatic venous outflow tract • Underlying hypercoagulable disorder
Malignancy	Lymphoma, leukemia, metastatic or primary liver cancer	Liver transplant is not recommended; poor outcome
Secondary causes	• Ischemic liver injury (hypotension, congestive cardiac failure, trauma) • Dengue, malaria, leptospira, and hemophagocytic lymphohistiocytosis (HLH), Reye's syndrome, heat stroke	• Correct the underlying cause • Liver transplant is usually not recommended

- Oliguria despite fluid resuscitation
- Requirement of oxygen to maintain SpO_2 >95

Organ support is vital in the management of patients with ALF. Transplantation is the only curative option. Patients must be stabilized before an emergency or semielective transplant.

Neurological Evaluation

All patients with ALF should be monitored for mental status examination frequently. Any change in mentation or increasing irritability may be an early sign of hepatic encephalopathy (HE). Encephalopathy in ALF is associated with cerebral edema and raised intracranial pressure (ICP). Progression to grade 2 HE warrants a shift to ICU and more frequent neurological monitoring. Worsening of HE is usually correlated with the worsening of the clinical course of ALF. However, the coexistence of infection or extrahepatic organ failure (OF) also worsens the neurological status. All patients should be nursed in a 30° propped-up position with the neck in

TABLE 2: Laboratory evaluation in patients with acute liver failure.

Etiological workup	***Evaluation of organ function***
Virus etiology: Hepatitis A, B, C, E serology	Liver function test, bilirubin, liver enzymes
Serology for herpes, varicella, cytomegalovirus, Epstein–Barr virus (in selected cases)	Blood sugar
Autoimmune markers: Antinuclear antibody, serum IgG level, anti-smooth muscle antibody (ASMA)	Creatinine, electrolytes, phosphorus
Other infective workup: Smear for malaria, dengue and leptospira serology, and PCR	Complete hemogram with differential count
Imaging: Ultrasonography of liver with portal vein Doppler	*Coagulation parameters:* PT, aPTT, fibrinogen, TEG
In selected cases: Paracetamol level, urine toxicology screen, blood ethanol level, urine ethyl glucuronide, β-hCG, serum ceruloplasmin	• ABG with arterial lactate • Arterial ammonia
	• *Infective workup:* Blood and urine cultures
	• ECG, echocardiography
	• X-ray chest

(aPTT: activated partial thromboplastin time; PCR: polymerase chain reaction; PT: prothrombin time; TEG: thromboelastography)

the neutral position in a noise-free quiet environment, avoiding unnecessary stimulation and lights. We usually start 3% saline in patients with encephalopathy with target sodium 145–150 mmol/L and serum osmolality 310–320 mOsm/kg. Mannitol is kept in reserve to control sudden surges in ICP and neurodeterioration. Glasgow Coma Scale (GCS) charting is done 2nd hourly. Grades 3–4 encephalopathy requires elective intubation. All mechanically ventilated patients should receive adequate analgesia with shorter-acting opioids, and sedation with propofol as a cerebroprotective agent and sometimes neuromuscular blockade. EEG may be done to document seizures. Anticonvulsants are not used prophylactically. In case of seizures, levetiracetam, lacosamide, or phenytoin may be used. The American College of Gastroenterology (ACG) guideline recommends starting continuous renal replacement therapy (CRRT) as ammonia-lowering treatment in patients with grade 2 or higher encephalopathy even in the absence of conventional indications of RRT.[11] In patients who are mechanically ventilated and sedated, we routinely monitor optic nerve sheath diameter (ONSD) as a surrogate for raised ICP. The presence of bradycardia with hypertension is an ominous sign of acutely raised ICP and is a poor prognostic sign. Invasive ICP monitoring is not routine in the presence of coagulopathy and associated complexity. The INASL consortium does not recommend invasive ICP monitoring as a routine in all patients. Other surrogate markers of raised ICP are jugular venous oxygen saturation ($SjvO_2$) <50%, increased pulsatility index, and absent diastolic flow in the middle cerebral artery (MCA) as measured in transcranial Doppler (TCD). More often, the arterial ammonia value >150 µmol/L predicts raised ICP and warrants treatment. The presence of encephalopathy warrants consideration of extracorporeal therapies like plasma exchange and continuous veno-venous hemofiltration/hemodiafiltration (CVVHDF). Rifaximin does not have much role in ALF, and lactulose is preferentially avoided as it increases the risk of bowel dilation and ileus. The use of hypothermia in intubated patients in the presence of raised ICP is not evidence-based in current times.

Other causes of altered mentation should also be actively sought. IC bleeding is not uncommon in the presence of coagulopathy. Electrolyte abnormality, hypoglycemia, hypercapnia, and administration of sedation sometimes become contributory factors and should always be ruled out. Hyponatremia worsens cerebral edema as it promotes water entry inside astrocytes. For any patient with grade 4 encephalopathy, or intubated, it is better to do a CT brain to document irreversible IC bleed before taking up for transplant.

Management of Volume and Hemodynamics

Patients with ALF remain at risk of hypovolemia due to multiple episodes of vomiting and poor oral intake. Along with that, the systemic vasodilation from cytokine storm associated with ALF renders them to potential relative hypovolemia. Balanced crystalloids are used for bolus and maintenance fluid. The role of albumin has not been studied in ALF. The assessment of the volume status is difficult. Lactate does not serve as a perfusion parameter in ALF patients, especially in an advanced stage. Central venous oxygen saturation ($ScvO_2$) is also not reliable due to hyperdynamic circulation. Dynamic ultrasound (US)-based bedside assessment of fluid status and checking B lines in lungs at periodic intervals are important. Bedside US to document whether the patient is fluid responsive (i.e., whether stroke volume is increasing with fluid loading) is crucial in the fluid management. The left ventricular outflow tract velocity–time integral (LVOT-VTI) assessment with bedside echocardiography and pulse contour-based cardiac output monitoring (pulse pressure variation) with Flowtraq or PiCCO monitor with information of extravascular lung water (EVLW) in a patient with ventilator are helpful in this context. Often simple methods like end-expiratory occlusion test (EEOT) in ventilated patients to document an increase in cardiac output provide a reliable assessment without expensive gadgets. Passive leg raising (PLR) should generally be avoided in patients with HE with raised ICP. Volume overload is always to be avoided as elevated venous pressure has always been found to be associated with adverse clinical outcomes in any setting. Inferior vena cava (IVC) collapsibility is reliable in understanding elevated right-sided filling pressure.

Systemic vasopressors should be used in case of persistent hypotension despite initial volume loading. Noradrenaline followed by vasopressin are vasopressors of choice. The target MAP is 60–65 mm Hg. In case of persistent hypotension requiring vasopressors, systemic steroids may be considered, as relative adrenal deficiency has been reported in patients with ALF.[4]

Ventilation

The most common indication to put a patient on mechanical ventilation in ALF is grade 3 and 4 HE. Hypoxic respiratory failure due to any cause is another indication of invasive mechanical ventilation. Noninvasive ventilation (NIV) is generally avoided in encephalopathic patients. Elective control of the airway is always superior to emergency intubation. Endotracheal intubation should always be done under a deep plane of anesthesia. Post intubation, a continuous infusion of sedative is required to avoid any agitation or restlessness in the presence of raised ICP. Benzodiazepine is avoided as sedative agents. Propofol and shorter-acting opioids are generally used. Low tidal volume ventilation is the standard of care for all patients. Ventilator-associated pneumonia is a problem in any patient on mechanical ventilation, and preventive measures need to be in place with a bundle care approach. Clinical, microbiological, and radiological surveillance needs to be there for early identification and treatment. It is important to maintain normocarbia. Anyone on mechanical ventilation should have the head end of the bed elevated 30–45°, with the neck in a neutral position as a measure of the raised ICP protocol.

Renal Dysfunction

Renal dysfunction occurs in >50% of patients with ALF and carries higher mortality and need for hospital stay. Hourly urine output is required for the earlier identification of renal dysfunction. Blood urea nitrogen (BUN) is an unreliable parameter in the presence of liver dysfunction. Hypovolemia, sepsis, severe systemic inflammatory response syndrome (SIRS), and nephrotoxic medications, including contrast, are risk factors for acute kidney injury (AKI) in ALF. ACG and European Association for the Study of the Liver (EASL) guidelines suggest early CRRT for managing high ammonia levels, even in the absence of traditional indications of renal replacement therapy (RRT). CRRT is the modality of choice in ALF over intermittent hemodialysis (IHD) to avoid hemodynamic fluctuation and shift of metabolic profiles. CRRT is often conducted without any anticoagulation with the risk of a filter clot. Citrate is generally avoided, and if at all used, it should be used with tight monitoring of the systemic total to ionized calcium ratio. Temperature control and drug dosing need to be optimized in patients undergoing CRRT.

Coagulation in Acute Liver Failure

Coagulopathy in the form of raised INR is an integral component in patients with ALF. However, raised prothrombin time is not a predictor for bleeding in ALF, and bleeding is uncommon unless associated with low fibrinogen, platelet, and elevated activated partial thromboplastin time (APTT).[12] A recent cohort trial suggested that there is a "rebalanced state of hemostasis" in ALF, and bleeding is related to VWF/ADAMTS13 imbalance, which is influenced by the degree of systemic inflammation.[13] A dynamic assessment of coagulation parameters like rotational thromboelastography (TEG) or rotational thromboelastometry (ROTEM) is better to understand the risk of bleeding.[14] However, one drawback of TEG is that it does not adequately assess the activity of Von Willebrand factor (vWF) and protein C, both of which play a critical role in determining the balance of hemostasis in ALF. Prophylactic correction of INR with fresh frozen plasma (FFP) is not recommended as it affects prognostication, delays listing criteria, and increases the risk of transfusion-related acute lung injury (TRALI), volume overload, and other transfusion-associated complications. Regular monitoring of INR helps to understand the dynamicity of the disease and is required for determining the timing of listing for transplantation. TEG-guided correction is required if any invasive procedure is planned like the insertion of an ICP monitor or if there is any evidence of bleeding. The hemoglobin target as a trigger of transfusion is 7 g/dL. All patients should be considered for venous thromboembolism (VTE) prophylaxis, at least with mechanical devices.

Metabolic and Electrolyte Correction

Hypoglycemia is a frequent association in patients with ALF. Blood sugar monitoring needs to be done regularly, and if required, dextrose infusion should be started to prevent hypoglycemia. However, a large volume of hypotonic dextrose solution may exacerbate cerebral edema and should be avoided. We need to maintain serum potassium 4–4.5 mmol/L and prevent hypokalemia as it worsens encephalopathy. Hyponatremia is common in paracetamol-induced ALF and should be corrected. 3% saline is administered in the presence of encephalopathy with serum sodium target 145–150 mEq/L. However, serum sodium levels >150 mEq/L should be avoided.[12] In patients with CRRT, potassium, magnesium, phosphorous, and systemic and ionized calcium should be routinely monitored and replaced as needed. Hypophosphatemia is a sign of liver regeneration and thus acts as a favorable prognostic factor. Hyperlactatemia results from decreased hepatic clearance, and both high lactate and low pH are unfavorable outcome predictors in ALF.

Infection

Patients with ALF develop functional immunoparesis and therefore are at higher risk of infection. Sepsis is often the cause of final death nail in patients with ALF with or without transplantation. The multiple invasive lines, endotracheal tubes, ventilators, and extracorporeal therapies increase the risk of nosocomial infection. Standard infection control practices like hand hygiene, contact precaution, invasive lines, and tube care in a bundle approach should be followed rigorously. Prophylactic antibiotics are frequently used as institutional practice in ALF patients; however, a recent large retrospective cohort study by ALFSG has shown that the use of antimicrobial prophylaxis does not reduce the rate of development of subsequent bloodstream infection (BSI) and has no effect on 21-day mortality.[15] Rather, active surveillance is required to detect any early signs of infection. Identification of sepsis is difficult in this patient group as SIRS response can be due to ALF itself. Biomarkers like C-reactive protein (CRP) and procalcitonin (PCT) are often unreliable in an ALF setting. Regular microbiological surveillance is helpful. However, the frequency of sending surveillance culture depends on institutional infection control practices and management protocol. Monitoring of clinical parameters like new-onset fever, leukocytosis, change in the Sequential Organ Failure Assessment (SOFA) score, hemodynamic parameters, and mental status often provides clues to new-onset sepsis. It is important to adjust the dose of antibiotics when CRRT, plasma exchange, or other extracorporeal devices are used. Severe untreated infection with multidrug-resistant bugs may preclude transplantation. Bacterial infection is the most common form of infection, and among them, gram-negative sepsis is more common than gram-positive sepsis. Fungal infection should be suspected in patients with prolonged ICU stay with ALF. Reactivation of herpes and cytomegalovirus (CMV) may also happen. Strict hand hygiene measures, care of devices and lines with bundle care protocol, and regular tracheobronchial toileting are required to prevent infection. Routine use of prophylactic antimicrobials is discouraged as per the standard guidelines.[11,12] Empiric antibiotics and antifungals should be started in the presence of any clinical deterioration and high-risk patients waiting for liver transplantation and in patients with clinical deterioration like developing renal failure, worsening encephalopathy and hypotension, or fulfilling King's College Criteria (KCC) during their course of illness.[4]

Invasive Line Cannulations

All invasive lines should be cannulated under US guidance by an experienced person. A subclavian line is usually avoided in patients with coagulopathy. A femoral puncture should be done below the inguinal ligament.

Management of Specific Etiologies

N-acetylcysteine (NAC) has proven benefit in paracetamol-induced ALF. Early administration of NAC is better. The intravenous (IV) route is to be chosen in patients having excessive vomiting or abdominal pain. NAC has shown some benefit in nonacetaminophen ALF as well, to improve transplant-free survival when started in sicker patients with a lower grade of HE.[16,17] It has additional antioxidant, anti-inflammatory, and vasodilatory properties that improve microcirculatory flow. The EASL guideline advises to limit NAC infusion for a maximum period of 5 days.

In ALF due to hepatitis B virus (HBV) reactivation, entecavir- or tenofovir-based antivirals need to be started early. For a new hepatitis B infection, starting antiviral might be less relevant in the presence of low viral load, but the usual practice is to start antiviral at the time of diagnosis.

Intravenous Silibinin or Penicillin G is recommended in > ALF from mushroom (*Amanita phalloides*) poisoning.

In acute Wilson's disease, medical therapy like chelators (D-penicillamine and trientine) is usually not effective. These patients should be evaluated and offered LTs early, which is the key to a successful outcome.

In acute severe autoimmune hepatitis, the majority of patients respond well to corticosteroid therapy, but patients progressing to ALF usually require an LT as the definitive treatment.

In pregnancy-specific ALF, supportive care is the mainstay, and it is imperative to deliver the baby at the earliest.

In acute Budd–Chiari syndrome, therapeutic anticoagulation with heparin is considered. Transjugular intrahepatic portosystemic shunt (TIPSS) is done in patients who fail anticoagulation. Once medical and radiological interventions fail. LT needs to be considered.

Acute liver failure may happen rarely post donor nephrectomy in a living donation setting. They should be listed early and considered for transplantation with the best supportive intensive care treatment.

Nutrition

Patients are encouraged to maintain oral intake as much as possible with systemic antiemetics if required unless there is higher-grade encephalopathy. It is better to place a nasogastric (NG) tube after securing the airway to prevent regurgitation and aspiration in an encephalopathic patient. Sometimes, the orogastric tube is preferred over a NG tube in the presence of severe coagulopathy. Patients should receive stress ulcer prophylaxis. These patients usually have higher resting energy expenditure. In the hyperacute form of ALF, the role of nutritional support becomes less crucial due to the shorter duration of the disease. The focus remains largely on maintaining sugar levels and electrolytes. In patients with high-grade encephalopathy and ammonia level >150 mMol/L, sometimes *protein restriction* is contemplated for a shorter duration. However, this is not very much evidence-based practice, especially when the patient is on CRRT or other forms of extracorporeal therapies. In the subacute form of ALF, oral intake is not sufficient after 5–7 days; it is better to start enteral nutritional support to meet calorie and protein requirements. There is a limited role of medical nutritional therapy in the hyperacute form of ALF unless the patient has pre-existing malnutrition. Although there are few pieces of literature suggesting the use of L-leucine, other branched-chain amino acids (BCAA), and hydroxy-beta-methyl butyrate (HMB)-based formulations in patients with ALF,[18] the European Society for Clinical Nutrition and Metabolism (ESPEN) guideline discourages the use of disease-specific formulations over standard enteral formula in ALF.[19]

Extracorporeal Liver-assist Devices

Extracorporeal liver-assist devices are extracorporeal systems to conduct the excretory function of the liver and maintain some homeostasis in the presence of severe SIRS and coagulopathy in ALF. They act either as a bridge to transplant or as a bridge to recovery of native liver function. They mostly use techniques like hemodialysis and charcoal adsorption to remove toxins. Although there are case series and reports of successful management of ALF with this device, well-designed randomized controlled trials (RCTs) failed to prove any mortality benefit of these methods in patients with ALF. Currently, these devices are not US-FDA approved, and their uses are restricted to investigational and compassionate grounds only.[11]

Among all extracorporeal therapies, plasma exchange is proven to be the most successful in terms of mortality benefit. As per the American Society for Apheresis (ASFA) guidelines, high-volume plasma exchange is the class 1 indication for ALF.[20] This recommendation is largely based on a multicentric RCT showing transplant-free survival benefit with high-volume plasmapheresis (8–12

L or 15% of ideal body weight) in patients with ALF.[21] The benefit of plasma exchange is attributed not only to removing ammonia and improving coagulopathy but also to dampening the inflammatory cascade to prevent multiorgan dysfunction. Therapeutic plasma exchange (TPE) can help eliminate both albumin-bound and unbound toxins, including aromatic amino acids, ammonia, endotoxins, indoles, mercaptans, phenols, and other factors that contribute to hepatic coma, hyperkinetic syndrome, decreased systemic vascular resistance, and reduced cerebral blood flow. Multiple studies have shown that TPE improves several clinical parameters, such as cerebral blood flow, MAP, cerebral perfusion pressure, cerebral metabolic rate, hepatic blood flow, and laboratory markers like cholinesterase activity and galactose elimination capacity.

Since plasma contains citrate as an anticoagulant and the liver is already dysfunctional, the whole blood:ACD-A ratio may need to be adjusted to avoid severe hypocalcemia. Alternatively, calcium supplementation during TPE can help to mitigate this risk. Close monitoring is required for metabolic alkalosis, and in some cases, simultaneous hemodialysis has been employed to manage this complication. Plasma is preferred as a replacement fluid due to moderate to severe coagulopathy, but albumin may also be used when necessary.

In ALF, TPE is typically performed daily until liver transplantation or liver regeneration occurs. The biochemical response to TPE should be assessed using laboratory values obtained at least 12 hours after the procedure, as samples collected immediately after TPE are likely to show improvement compared to pre-TPE levels. TPE-HV is often performed over 3 consecutive days for optimal results. The dosing schedule of antibiotics and sedatives needs to be modified with all forms of extracorporeal devices, including plasma exchange.

LIVER TRANSPLANTATION IN A PATIENT WITH ACUTE LIVER FAILURE

Indications

Liver transplantation is indicated in ALF when the regenerative capacity of the liver is exhausted and regeneration is not expected anymore. Three critical parameters are important to understand while evaluating the need for a transplant: (1) Identifying patients who may have spontaneous recovery of liver failure with intensive critical care support and do not need transplant, (2) where the possibility of liver regeneration is low and the patient will have a survival benefit from transplant, and (3) where even after transplant, prognosis may be futile.

Timing is another important factor to understand; too soon consideration opens up the possibility of LT where it might be unnecessary and expose the patient to the risk of lifelong immunosuppression post-transplant complications. Too late decision may render the patient unfit for transplant from a multiorgan failure state (too sick to transplant).

Early identification of factors predicting the need for transplant in patients with ALF is essential. The etiology is important for determining the outcome, as described in the previous section. Duration is also an important prognostic factor. Subacute presentation in nonparacetamol-related liver failure has a poorer prognosis, whereas the hyperacute presentation has a more dramatic course with the early development of high-grade encephalopathy and requirement of organ support but is associated with an overall favorable prognosis. In sub-ALF, even a lower-grade encephalopathy points toward a poorer prognosis and often has a lower chance of survival, especially when liver volume shrinks or ascites develop. Transplant-free survival in this category of patients is less. In general, ALF with grade 3 or 4 encephalopathy, extrahepatic OF, and extreme coagulopathy has a poorer prognosis and is more likely to require LT.[22]

There are conditions where a transplant may be futile. A persistent bilateral dilated, nonreactive pupil with no spontaneous respiration, absent flow in the MCA, uncal herniation, and major intracerebral hemorrhage precludes transplant. Progressive vasoplegic shock, uncontrolled minimal residual disease (MRD) infection, severe acute respiratory distress syndrome (ARDS), and hemorrhagic pancreatitis also preclude transplant in most patients. The United Network for Organ Sharing (UNOS) suggests priority 1A listing for patients with ALF. Similarly, in India, ALF is categorized as hyperacute status for listing for emergency liver transplantation.

All patients with severe acute liver injury should be considered to transfer to a tertiary care center with a facility for liver transplantation. Management in a dedicated liver unit has been shown to improve outcomes even without the need for a transplant in many cases. In case of transfer when higher-grade encephalopathy has already set in, it is important to secure the airway before initiating the shifting process with a deep plane

TABLE 3: Criteria to transfer patients with acute liver failure in a liver transplant unit.

Due to paracetamol or hyperacute causes	*Due to nonparacetamol causes*
Arterial pH <7.3 or HCO_3 <18	Arterial pH <7.3 or HCO_3 <18
INR >3.0 on day 2 or >4 following that	INR >1.8
Oliguria and/or elevated creatinine	Oliguria/renal failure or Na <130 mmol/L
Altered level of consciousness	Encephalopathy, hypoglycemia, or metabolic acidosis
Hypoglycemia	Bilirubin >300 µmol/L (17.6 mg/dL)
Elevated lactate unresponsive to fluid resuscitation	Shrinking liver size

(INR: international normalized ratio)

of anesthesia maintained throughout the transfer. The EASL has published recommendations for early transfer to transplant centers in ALF patients. Along with that, involvement of extrahepatic organs warrants transfer to the ICU in a tertiary center **(Table 3)**.

PROGNOSTIC METHODS IN PATIENTS WITH ACUTE LIVER FAILURE

The ACG guideline recommends the KCC or MELD score for standard prognostic criteria in patients with ALF.[11]

King's College Hospital criteria, published in 1989, were based on cohort studies on cases of ALF at that time. The criteria are highly specific (92–95%) for paracetamol-related etiologies and 82% for etiologies other than paracetamol[23] for predicting mortality without a transplant in patients with ALF in the absence of transplant. This is thus a standard criterion still used worldwide for determining the need and listing for transplant. A dynamic application of KCC with temporal evolution increases its specificity. However, KCC has poorer sensitivity in predicting mortality in ALF even in cases that do not meet the criteria.

The MELD score is the traditional model to predict mortality in patients with cirrhosis and is accepted by the UNOS and Organ Procurement and Transplantation Network (OPTN) for organ allocation in end-stage liver disease (ESLD) patients. A retrospective analysis has shown that MELD has a predictive value in ALF-related mortality as well. A meta-analysis published in 2016 showed that the predictive ability of MELD is superior to KCC in nonparacetamol-induced ALF.[24] Patients presenting with MELD >25 are associated with poor outcome.

The ALFSG index is a novel prognostic score developed by the ALFSG. This model not only includes liver-specific parameters like HE, bilirubin level, and INR but also takes etiology-specific parameters and systemic parameters like the use of vasopressor as determining criteria. This model has been found to have a better prediction for transplant-free survival in ALF in one retrospective analysis of the ALFSG dataset. However, external validation of the model is lacking.[25]

Other prognostic models include Clichy Criteria (used widely in French LT centers), Escudie Criteria for mushroom poisoning, and Swansea Criteria for acute fatty liver of pregnancy (AFLP). They are used for the diagnosis and evaluation of the need for transplant in some centers. New Wilson's criteria are used for Wilson's disease for the evaluation of the need for transplant. The ALF early dynamic (ALFED) model has been found to be superior to other prognostic scores in viral hepatitis-related ALF.[26] The INASL consensus guidelines suggest using dynamic criteria like ALFED score or MELD to decide the need for transplant in ALF.[2] In acute severe autoimmune hepatitis, the SURFASA score based on the evolution of bilirubin and INR can identify steroid nonresponders and the need for urgent LT.[27] Among other infrequently used prognostic scoring systems used in different literatures is the BILE scoring system in ALF of indeterminate etiology, clinical prognostic indicator (CPI) score, ALFA score in hepatitis A, prognostic nomogram for hepatitis E, scoring model of severe viral hepatitis (SMSVH) score, ALF-OF score, etc.[28]

OUTCOME OF ACUTE LIVER FAILURE FOLLOWING LIVER TRANSPLANT

As per the European Liver Transplant Registry (ELTR), ALF constitutes 7–8% of all indications of LT. The 1-year survival is around 75–80% as per the ELTR. As per the UK and Scottish look-back studies, around 25% of patients with ALF required an LT and had a 1-year survival of 80–86%.[5,29] The higher rate of mortality post-transplant in ALF patients is majorly due to neurological and infection-related complications. All these studies revealed better post-transplant outcomes over the last decade, which has been attributed to improvement in the intensive care management of patients in pre- and post-transplant periods. The type of graft also plays an important role in determining the outcome. Usually, an ABO-compatible, nonsteatotic cadaver liver with shorter ischemia times and an uneventful surgical course provides a better post-transplant outcome. ABO-incompatible grafts have been tried in desperate settings but have been found to have a higher rate of rejection, vascular and biliary complications, and inferior graft survival.[30] In Asian countries, living donor liver transplantation is the most common form of LT and is associated with acceptable post-transplant outcomes as in cadaveric transplantation.[31,32] Auxiliary orthotopic liver transplantation (APPOLT) is an interesting option in cases of ALF where there is a potential for liver regeneration. However, this strategy is technically more challenging and is associated with complications like bleeding and frequent post-transplant infection and hence, is not a routine practice.

Improvement in organ procurement, use of extra-corporeal devices such as liver-assist devices, and use of LDLT without waiting for the cadaver pool are also important factors in improving overall outcomes. It is important to identify patients who are too sick to transplant based on their poor prognostic factors.

Evaluation for transplant in patients with ALF requires multidisciplinary efforts. Apart from the clinician's effort in medical stabilization, it also requires psychosocial support to the patients and family, financial support especially in countries like India where penetration and eligibility of insurance schemes are low, medicolegal counseling and support in terms of evaluation of potential living donation, and support of logistics and administrative authorities for conduction of emergency transplantation.

CONCLUSION

Acute liver failure is a condition with a medical emergency. Time is synonymous with "life" here, and a delay in recognition of the condition and its progression and failure to institute timely intervention is universally fatal. Clinicians should have a thorough understanding of the etiologies, pathophysiology, and prognostic characteristics of this condition for prompt escalation of treatment and/or transfer to a dedicated LT center. A multidisciplinary approach collaborating with hepatologists, intensivists, transplant surgeons, and social and administration teams is important for the successful management of this intractable condition. Finally, peritransplant organ support by the intensive care physician plays the most important factor in determining the overall outcome.

REFERENCES

1. Polson J, Lee WM. American Association for the Study of Liver Disease. AASLD position paper: the management of acute liver failure. Hepatology. 2005;41:1179-97.
2. Anand AC, Nandi B, Acharya SK, Arora A, Babu S, Batra Y, et al. Indian National Association for the Study of the Liver Consensus Statement on Acute Liver Failure (Part 1): Epidemiology, Pathogenesis, Presentation and Prognosis. J Clin Exp Hepatol. 2020;10:339-76.
3. Bernuau J, Rueff B, Benhamou JP. Fulminant and sub-fulminant liver failure: definitions and causes. Semin Liver Dis. 1986;6:97-106.
4. Stravitz RT, Lee WM. Acute liver failure. Lancet. 2019;394:869-81.
5. Donnelly MC, Davidson JS, Martin K, Baird A, Hayes PC, Simpson KJ. Acute liver failure in Scotland: changes in aetiology and outcomes over time (the Scottish Look-Back Study). Aliment Pharmacol Ther. 2017;45:833-43.
6. Germani G, Theocharidou E, Adam R, Karam V, Wendon J, O'Grady J, et al. Liver transplantation for acute liver failure in Europe: outcomes over 20 years from the ELTR database. J Hepatol. 2012;57:288-96.
7. Lee W. NIDDK Central Repository. Acute Liver Failure Study Group: Adult Acute Liver Failure Study (AALF). DOI: https://doi.org/10.58020/9n48-q075.
8. Castaldo ET, Chari RS. Liver transplantation for acute hepatic failure. HPB. 2006;8:29-34.
9. Martínez-Martínez LM, Rosales-Sotomayor G, Jasso-Baltazar EA, Torres-Díaz JA, Aguirre-Villarreal D, de León IH, et al. Acute liver failure: management update and prognosis. Rev Gastroenterol México. 2024;89(3):404-17.
10. Fix OK, Liou I, Karvellas CJ, Ganger DR, Forde KA, Subramanian RM, et al. Development and pilot of a checklist for management of acute liver failure in the intensive care unit. PLoS One. 2016;11(5):e0155500.
11. Shingina A, Mukhtar N, Wakim-Fleming J, Alqahtani S, Wong RJ, Limketkai BN, et al. Acute Liver Failure Guidelines. Am J Gastroenterol. 2023;118:1128-53.
12. Wendon J, Cordoba J, Dhawan A, Larsen FS, Manns M, Samuel D, et al. EASL Clinical Practical Guidelines on the management of acute (fulminant) liver failure. J Hepatol. 2017;66:1047-81.
13. Driever EG, Stravitz RT, Zhang J, Adelmeijer J, Durkalski V, Lee WM, et al. VWF/ADAMTS13 imbalance, but not global coagulation or fibrinolysis, is associated with outcome and bleeding in acute liver failure. Hepatology. 2021;73:1882-91.
14. Nanchal R, Subramanian R, Alhazzani W, Dionne JC, Peppard WJ, Singbartl K, et al. Guidelines for the Management of Adult Acute and Acute-on-Chronic Liver Failure in the ICU: Neurology, Peri-Transplant Medicine, Infectious Disease, and Gastroenterology Considerations. Crit Care Med. 2023;51:657-76.

15. Karvellas CJ, Cavazos J, Battenhouse H, Durkalski V, Balko J, Sanders C, et al. Effects of antimicrobial prophylaxis and blood stream infections in patients with acute liver failure: a retrospective cohort study. Clin Gastroenterol Hepatol. 2014;12:1942-9.e1.
16. Lee WM, Hynan LS, Rossaro L, Fontana RJ, Stravitz RT, Larson AM, et al. Intravenous N-acetylcysteine improves transplant-free survival in early stage non-acetaminophen acute liver failure. Gastroenterology. 2009;137:856-64.e1.
17. Walayat S, Shoaib H, Asghar M, Kim M, Dhillon S. Role of N-acetylcysteine in non-acetaminophen-related acute liver failure: an updated meta-analysis and systematic review. Ann Gastroenterol. 2021;34:235.
18. Abenavoli L, Maurizi V, Boccuto L, Di Berardino A, Giostra N, Santori P, et al. Nutritional support in acute liver failure. Diseases. 2022;10(4):108.
19. Bischoff SC, Bernal W, Dasarathy S, Merli M, Plank LD, Schütz T, et al. ESPEN practical guideline: clinical nutrition in liver disease. Clin Nutr. 2020;39:3533-62.
20. Connelly-Smith L, Alquist CR, Aqui NA, Hofmann JC, Klingel R, Onwuemene OA, et al. Guidelines on the Use of Therapeutic Apheresis in Clinical Practice - Evidence-Based Approach from the Writing Committee of the American Society for Apheresis: the Ninth Special Issue. J Clin Apher. 2023;38:77-278.
21. Larsen FS, Schmidt LE, Bernsmeier C, Rasmussen A, Isoniemi H, Patel VC, et al. High-volume plasma exchange in patients with acute liver failure: an open randomised controlled trial. J Hepatol. 2016;64:69-78.
22. Grande RG, Pérez MJ. Liver transplantation in acute liver failure: indications and outcome. In: Liver Research and Clinical Management. IntechOpen; 2017. DOI: 10.5772/intechopen.72664.
23. McPhail MJW, Wendon JA, Bernal W. Meta-analysis of performance of Kings's College Hospital Criteria in prediction of outcome in non-paracetamol-induced acute liver failure. J Hepatol. 2010;53:492-9.
24. McPhail MJW, Farne H, Senvar N, Wendon JA, Bernal W. Ability of King's College Criteria and model for end-stage liver disease scores to predict mortality of patients with acute liver failure: a meta-analysis. Clin Gastroenterol Hepatol. 2016;14:516-25.e5.
25. Koch DG, Tillman H, Durkalski V, Lee WM, Reuben A. Development of a model to predict transplant-free survival of patients with acute liver failure. Clin Gastroenterol Hepatol. 2016;14:1199-206.e2.
26. Shalimar, Sonika U, Kedia S, Mahapatra SJ, Nayak B, Yadav DP, et al. Comparison of dynamic changes among various prognostic scores in viral hepatitis-related acute liver failure. Ann Hepatol. 2018;17:403-12.
27. De Martin E, Coilly A, Chazouillères O, Roux O, Peron JM, Houssel-Debry P, et al. Early liver transplantation for corticosteroid non-responders with acute severe autoimmune hepatitis: the SURFASA score. J Hepatol. 2021;74:1325-34.
28. Biswas S, Kumar R, Acharya SK, Shalimar. Prognostic scores in acute liver failure due to viral hepatitis. Diagnostics. 2023;13(6):1035.
29. Bernal W, Hyyrylainen A, Gera A, Audimoolam VK, McPhail MJW, Auzinger G, et al. Lessons from look-back in acute liver failure? A single centre experience of 3300 patients. J Hepatol. 2013;59:74-80.
30. Thorsen T, Dahlgren US, Aandahl EM, Grzyb K, Karlsen TH, Boberg KM, et al. Liver transplantation with deceased ABO-incompatible donors is life-saving but associated with increased risk of rejection and post-transplant complications. Transpl Int. 2015;28:800-12.
31. Pamecha V, Vagadiya A, Sinha PK, Sandhyav R, Parthasarathy K, Sasturkar S, et al. Living donor liver transplantation for acute liver failure: donor safety and recipient outcome. Liver Transpl. 2019;25:1408-21.
32. Shingina A, Ziogas IA, Vutien P, Uleryk E, Shah PS, Renner E, et al. Adult-to-adult living donor liver transplantation in acute liver failure. Transplant Rev. 2022;36:100691.

CHAPTER 6

Pretransplant Optimization of Patients Admitted with Acute-on-Chronic Liver Failure in ICU

Suvadeep Sen, Amey Sonavane

INTRODUCTION

Acute-on-chronic liver failure (ACLF) is a life-threatening clinical condition in patients with decompensated cirrhosis. This has a heterogeneous presentation and often takes a dynamic course with multiple hepatic and extrahepatic organ involvement and is associated with very high short-term mortality. Liver transplantation (LT) is the only treatment that improves survival in this condition. In high-volume transplant centers, LT is being performed routinely for sick ACLF patients. However, LT is not easy to perform in patients with multiorgan involvement and is associated with higher rates of posttransplant complications and mortality compared to non-ACLF patients. Support of different organ systems is required both pre- and posttransplantation. Intensive care unit (ICU) management plays a crucial role in the overall survival of patients. It is important to identify conditions of futility even after offering transplantation. In this current text, we will discuss how to identify this condition early, how to prognosticate, and how we can optimize a patient's condition medically before semielective liver transplantation.

ACUTE-ON-CHRONIC LIVER FAILURE: DEFINITION AND PROGNOSIS

The American Association for the Study of Liver Diseases (AASLD) working definition of ACLF is: "acute deterioration of preexisting chronic liver disease (CLD) usually related to a precipitating event, usually associated with increased mortality at 3 months due to multisystem organ failure".

Acute-on-chronic liver failure is a common but difficult-to-treat medical condition. There is heterogeneity in the definition of the condition in various societies' guidelines. This makes characterization of its prognosis and treatment-related outcome also extremely variable.

The diagnostic criteria as per the European Association for the Study of the Liver–Chronic Liver Failure-Consortium (EASL-CLIF-C) are widely acceptable in current times for identifying patients with ACLF and have stemmed from the CANONIC study published in 2013.[1] This definition combines liver-related decompensation factors along with the sepsis organ failure assessment (SOFA) score, commonly used in patients requiring intensive care treatment for assessment of organ dysfunction in the setting of sepsis.[2] In the SOFA-CLIF score, organ function status is evaluated based on six parameters denoting the function of six organs—(1) bilirubin, (2) creatinine, (3) encephalopathy, (4) international normalized ratio (INR), (5) blood pressure, and (6) P/F ratio **(Table 1)**. The presence or absence of organ failure was determined by predefined criteria. Based on the patient population and outcome characteristics, patients with cirrhosis with decompensation are subdivided into four subgroups **(Table 2)**. CLIF-SOFA score was later simplified by Jalan, et al. using data from the same patient population after following them up for a subsequent year.[3] In this validation model, CLIF consortium organ failure score (CLIF-C OFs) was developed to diagnose and grade ACLF in a simpler format, and CLIF-C OFs and two other independent clinical and biochemical variables (age and white blood cell count) were combined to design CLIF consortium ACLF score (CLIF-C ACLFs), which is an ACLF-specific prognostication score (score range from 0 to 100 points) for mortality in patients with ACLF depending on its grade. The concordance index analysis of the derivation cohort revealed that the discriminative ability of CLIF-C ACLF score is better than the prognostic accuracy of the model for end-stage liver disease (MELD), MELD-Na, and Child-Turcotte-Pugh (CTP) scores to predict 1-year mortality in ACLF patients in the absence of liver transplant. The online application for the calculation of CLIF-C ACLF score is available online at

TABLE 1: CLIF-SOFA scoring system.

Organ system	Parameters	0	1	2	3	4
Liver	Bilirubin (mg/dL)	<1.2	≥1.2 to ≤2.0	≥2.0 to <6.0	≥6.0 to <12.0	≥12.0
Kidney	Creatinine (mg/dL)	<1.2	≥1.2 to <2.0	≥2.0 to <3.5	≥3.5 to <5 or RRT	≥5.0 or RRT
Brain	Hepatic encephalopathy (HE) grade	No HE	1	2	3	4
Coagulation	International normalized ratio (INR)	<1.1	≥1.1 to <1.25	≥1.25 to <1.5	≥1.5 to <2.5	≥2.5 or platelet <20,000/dL
Circulation	Mean arterial pressure (MAP) (mm Hg)	≥70	<70	Dopamine <5 or dobutamine or terlipressin	Dopamine >5 or epinephrine <0.1 or norepinephrine <0.1	Dopamine >15 or epinephrine >0.1 or norepinephrine >0.1
Lungs	PaO_2/FiO_2 SpO_2/FiO_2	400 >512	301–400 357–512	201–300 214–357	101–200 89–214	≤100 ≤89

(CLIF-SOFA: chronic liver failure-sepsis organ failure assessment; RRT: renal replacement therapy)

TABLE 2: Diagnostic criteria of ACLF as per the European Association for the Study of the Liver (EASL) guideline and its mortality outcome as per severity.

		28-day mortality (%)	90-day mortality (%)
No ACLF	• Patients with no organ failure • Patients with a single "nonkidney" organ failure and no hepatic encephalopathy • Patients with single cerebral failure who had a serum creatinine level <1.5 mg/dL	1.9	9.7
ACLF grade 1	• Patients with single kidney failure • Patients with single nonrenal organ failure (liver, coagulation, circulation or respiration) plus either serum creatinine level ranging >1.5–1.9 mg/dL or grade 1/2 hepatic encephalopathy or both • Patients with single cerebral failure who had a serum creatinine level ranging from 1.5 to 1.9 mg/dL	22.1	40.7
ACLF grade 2	Patients with two organ failures	32	52.3
ACLF grade 3	Patients with three organ failures or more	76.7	79.1

(ACLF: acute-on-chronic liver failure)

https://efclif.com/research-infrastructure/score-calculators/clif-c-of-aclf-ad/.

PROGNOSTIC ASSESSMENT MODELS IN ACUTE-ON-CHRONIC LIVER FAILURE

Acute on chronic liver failure is a dynamic disease. Temporal evolution of ACLF 1 to ACLF 2 or 3 is associated with increased mortality. Whereas, regression in ACLF grade means improvement in organ function, hence has a better outcome. The prognosis of patients admitted to the ICU with ACLF is generally done with specific scoring systems such as CLIF-C ACLFs, COSSH-ACLFs II, and APASL ACLF Research Consortium (AARC) score. Traditional scoring systems such as CTP, MELD, and MELD-Na are nonspecific and do not predict the outcome and need for transplant in a sick ACLF patient. Following are the scoring systems available for cirrhotic patients:

- *CLIF-C ACLFs score:*
  $10 \times (0.33 \times \text{CLIF-C OFs} + 0.04 \times \text{age} + 0.63 \times \ln(\text{WBC}) - 2)$

This widely used prediction model is validated as per the EASL-CLIF consortium CANONIC database and validated for ACLF.[3] The majority of patients in the

Flowchart 1: Management algorithm of ACLF.

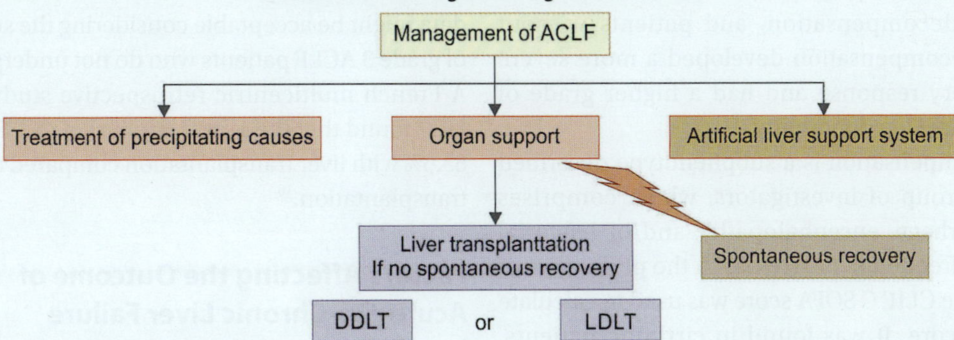

(ACLF: acute-on-chronic liver failure; DDLT: deceased donor liver transplantation; LDLT: living donor liver transplantation)

CANONIC database were alcohol-related CLD, hepatitis C-related CLD; hence, in this subgroup of patients, this score has superior predictive ability compared to MELD, MELD-Na, or the CTP score. The predictive ability of CLIF-C ACLF at 48 hours of admission is better compared to the score at the time of admission, implying the role of sequential measurement of the score in patients with ACLF.[4] A CLIF-C ACLF score ≥70 at 48 hours of ICU admission predicts futility in most studies.[5,6]

APASL ACLF Research Consortium (AARC) score: AARC score identifies patients with ACLF and grades them as per severity, as per the Asian Pacific Association for the Study of the Liver (APASL) definition.[7] AARC-ACLF is a prognostication score for short-term mortality in ACLF patients **(Flowchart 1)**. AARC score <10 has better survival; whereas, a score >11 at admission or after 1 week of hospitalization is associated with poor survival.[8] In patients with alcohol-related hepatitis AARC score helps to identify/classify patients with ACLF.

AARC-ACLF grade three patients have higher 90-day mortality, steroid nonresponsiveness, and extrahepatic organ failure.[9]

- *COSSH-ACLFs II score:*
  1.649 × ln (INR) + 0.457 × HE score + 0.425 × ln (neutrophil) + 0.396 × ln (TBIL) + 0.576 × ln (serum urea) + 0.033 × age).

This score is validated for hepatitis B virus (HBV)-related cirrhosis and found to have higher prognostic accuracy for early short-term mortality[10] in HBV-ACLF patients compared to CLIF-C ACLF, MELD-Na, and outcome of post-liver transplant in this segment of patients in terms of 1-year mortality.[11] It was found that patients with COSSH-ACLF IIs[7-10] had a higher posttransplant 1-year survival benefit compared to patients with scores >10 and <7.

- *HINT score for ACLF:*
  1.48 × HE + 3.92 × ln (INR) + 0.73 × ln (neutrophil) −0.46 × ln (TSH) −5.78.
  [HE = 0 for without HE, 1 for mild HE (grade 1–2), and 2 for severe HE (grade 3–4)].

This is a novel prognostication score[12] in HBV-ACLF patients having comparable prognostic accuracy to COSSH-ACLF score, but higher than CTP, MELD, and CLIF-C ACLF score. TSH value on admission was found to be significantly lower at admission.

- *TACIA score:*
  0.003 × total bilirubin (μmol/L) + 0.036 × age + 0.009 × creatinine (μmol/L) + 0.525 × INR−0.003 × AFP (ng/mL).

A composite score value ≥4.34 indicates poor outcomes in HBV-related ACLF with comparable receiver operating characteristics (ROC) of other ACLF-specific scores.[13]

Analysis of the CANONIC study population had several important characteristics. The differential characteristics of patients with ACLF and non-ACLF were:

- The prevalence of ACLF in patients with acute decompensation (AD) is 30%.
- ACLF patients had higher short-term mortality; 28-day mortality was 15 times higher than patients without ACLF.
- ACLF occurred frequently in relatively younger individuals, and patients with alcoholic cirrhosis, and less frequently with hepatitis C cirrhosis.
- They had a precipitating event such as acute alcoholism or systemic infection
- They were associated with systemic inflammation such as high white blood cell (WBC) and C-reactive protein (CRP), the intensity of inflammation correlates with the severity of ACLF and associated mortality.

- ACLF may develop in patients without a prior history of decompensation, and patients without previous decompensation developed a more severe inflammatory response and had a higher grade of ACLF and associated mortality.

Acute decompensation is a subphenotype described by the same group of investigators, which comprises ascites, hemorrhage, encephalopathy, and/or bacterial infections and frequently progresses to the phenotype of ACLF.[4] The same CLIF C SOFA score was used to calculate the CLIF-AD score. It was found in cirrhotic patients, admitted to the hospital with decompensation but no ACLF, that 3-month mortality is <2% if the CLIF-OF score is ≤45, whereas mortality increases to >30% if the CLIF-C AD score is ≥60.

MANAGEMENT OF ACUTE-ON-CHRONIC LIVER FAILURE

The principles of management of ACLF are threefold given as follows:

1. Treatment of precipitating causes such as infection, gastrointestinal (GI) bleeding, and HBV reactivation
2. Support of failing organs
3. Liver transplantation

The artificial liver support system (ALSS) plays some role in the stabilization of the patients in the process.

A liver transplant is the only definitive option for ACLF when the regenerative capacity of the liver is exhausted. Both cadaveric and living donor liver transplantation may be used with more or less similar posttransplant outcomes. These group of patients mostly have high MELD scores; hence, pretransplant stabilization and support of failing organs and treatment of the precipitating causes (such as infection, GI bleeding, and HBV reactivation) play a vital role in the posttransplant outcome.

OUTCOME OF ACUTE-ON-CHRONIC LIVER FAILURE PATIENTS WITH LIVER TRANSPLANT

The posttransplant outcome in ACLF patients in terms of 1-year graft (78%) and patient survival (82%) is inferior compared to those transplanted without ACLF (92%). Transplant outcome is dependent on the grade of ACLF, with higher grades of ACLF correlating with a higher rate of posttransplant graft loss, patient morbidity, and mortality (1-year mortality for ACLF grade 1, 2, and 3 post-LT are 86%, 81%, and 76%, respectively) along with higher healthcare cost and resource utilisation.[14] However, this data might be acceptable considering the survival of <20% of grade 3 ACLF patients who do not undergo transplant.[15] A French multicentric retrospective study published in 2017 found that the 1-year survival of ACLF 3 patients was 83.6% with liver transplantation compared to 7.9% without transplantation.[16]

Factors Affecting the Outcome of Acute-On-Chronic Liver Failure Post-liver Transplantation

One of the key influences on the outcome of liver transplantation in patients with ACLF is the ability to reduce the severity of ACLF from grade 3 to grade 1 or 2 through pretransplant ICU management, which has been shown to significantly improve posttransplant results.[17] Transplantation for ACLF-3 model (TAM) score helps stratify posttransplant survival in ACLF 3 patients, considering four factors (age >53 years, pre-LT arterial lactate >4 mmol/L, $PaO_2/FiO_2 \leq 200$ mm Hg with mechanical ventilation, and pre-LT leukocyte count ≤10 G/L). A score ≥3 reflects poor posttransplant survival in ACLF 3 patients (8.3% 1-year survival compared to 83.9% 1-year survival in patients with TAM score ≤2).[18] Multiple retrospective studies have evaluated risk factors for poor outcomes post-liver transplant. The need for mechanical ventilation for respiratory issues with a P/F ratio <200 implies unfavorable outcomes. Analysis of data from the CANONIC database showed that pretransplant lactate >4 mmol/L, need for renal replacement therapy (RRT), and multidrug-resistant (MDR) infection pretransplant are independently associated with 1-year posttransplant mortality.[19] As per a consensus statement from 35 experts including intensivists, hepatologists, transplant surgeons, and anesthesiologists, published in 2021, liver transplantation should be deferred or withdrawn in severely frail patients (defined as clinical frailty scale >7), who have ongoing sepsis, or previous infection with pan drug-resistant *Enterobacteriaceae*, and organ failure such as respiratory failure (Pao_2/FiO_2 ratio <150 mm Hg), circulatory failure (norepinephrine dose ≥1 μg/kg/min), and metabolic failure (lactate level ≥9 mmol/L).[20] Apart from that, severe comorbidities [cardiovascular, central nervous system (CNS), and respiratory], active GI bleeding, presence of malignancy, and absence of abstinence also contraindicate liver transplantation in a given setting.[21]

Donor-specific characteristics also play a role in posttransplant outcomes in ACLF. A donor-risk index (DRI) score ≥1.7 was associated with higher long-term mortality post-liver transplant for ACLF patients in the DDLT setting;[22] hence, marginal donors should be used with caution here. Machine perfusion of the liver (MPL) may play a vital role in the coming days to utilize marginal donors more effectively; however, its role has not been validated in clinical trials in high MELD ACLF patients so far.

Living donor liver transplantation (LDLT) is an attractive option for ACLF patients, which expands the donor organ pool and may expedite transplantation in sick ACLF patients without waiting for a cadaver graft. LDLT is the predominant mode of liver transplantation in Asian countries where cadaver organ donation is not as common as in Western countries. Results of studies evaluating posttransplant survival in ACLF following LDLT are comparable to deceased donor liver transplantation (DDLT), and expectedly, patients with ACLF 3 show worse outcomes compared to non-ACLF and low-grade ACLF (1-year survival 70–75% in different studies and higher rate of posttransplant complications.[23-25] Younger donors, less graft steatosis, and a graft-to-recipient weight ratio (GRWR) near 1% contribute to better outcomes in high MELD ACLF patients.[23]

TIMING OF TRANSPLANT AND IDENTIFICATION OF FUTILITY

Prioritization of liver transplantation in the setting of ACLF is an ethical and debatable issue. The current MELD-based organ allocation system may not be accurate in the ACLF setting. The impact of extrahepatic organ failure is not captured in MELD-based scoring system and is inferior for mortality prediction in ACLF compared to specific dynamic scoring systems such as CLIF-C ACLF, AARC-ACLF, or COSSH-ACLF. Investigators of AARC studied the timing of liver transplantation in LDLT setting for the ACLF cohort and found that early stabilization followed by transplantation within day 5 to day 7 of ICU admission provides better outcomes following transplant than waiting >7 days, which led to rebound worsening of the condition and escape beyond the transplant window.[26] Based on the above-mentioned study, APASL guideline recommends early transplantation for ACLF patients with baseline MELD >28, AARC score >10, and advanced HE in the absence of overt sepsis or multiorgan failure.[7]

It is also important to consider the futility of liver transplants in the sickest group of patients, as transplants require exhaustive healthcare resource allocation and invaluable organs. ACLF patients with four or more organ failures, CLIF-C ACLF ≥70 after 48 hours of full organ support has been found to predict mortality with high accuracy.[5] Other contraindications of transplantation are the presence of malignancy, severe comorbidities, absence of abstinence, severe frailty, and age >70 years.

PRETRANSPLANT STABILIZATION OF PATIENTS WITH ACUTE-ON-CHRONIC LIVER FAILURE

Most of the patients with ACLF land up in the ICU before transplant due to their organ failure and related complications. Intensive organ support plays a vital role in downstaging ACLF pretransplant. Early identification of organ dysfunction is important, and interventions to prevent slipping into the "failure" stage improve overall outcomes. The transplant window for this patient group is short; immediate referral of all ACLF patients to a dedicated liver intensive care unit with the facility of a transplant program is suggested.

Treating the Precipitating Factors

The most common precipitating factors for ACLF are acute alcohol intake, infection, GI bleeding, and HBV reactivation. In almost 40% of cases, the precipitating event is not identifiable.[1] Bacterial infection is one of the common triggers, the prevalence of which is approximately 50% in ACLF and >70% in ACLF 3,[27] and leads to worse clinical outcomes. All patients with ACLF should be screened for infection with meticulous clinical examination, and microbiological testing and empirical treatment should be started based on local epidemiology in patients with possible infection. Patients with GI bleeding should get a combination of early endoscopic treatment (variceal ligation or endoscopic sclerotherapy) and vasoconstrictor therapy (terlipressin or octreotide for 2–5 days). All patients with GI bleeding in CLD should receive prophylactic antibiotics. HBV reactivation is treated with nucleoside analogues such as tenofovir, tenofovir alafenamide or entecavir. Early and rapid reduction in HBV DNA levels within 2 weeks is related to the reversal of the progression of ACLF and improvement in survival.[28] A significant proportion of patients with alcoholic hepatitis present with ACLF.[9] Steroids are used in severe alcoholic hepatitis where Maddrey's discriminant function (MDF) is >32 in the absence of contraindications. Given the significant side effect profile of steroids, a dynamic Lille score is used on day 4 and day 7, and values ≥0.45 identify patients with steroid nonresponsiveness[29], where steroids should be discontinued. Steroid responsiveness is also correlated negatively with the number of organ failures in severe alcoholic hepatitis ACLF group (77% for patients without ACLF, 52% for ACLF-1, 42% for ACLF-2, and only 8% for ACLF-3);[30] hence, in ACLF subgroup of alcoholic hepatitis, steroids should be used very cautiously.

Support of Organ System Pretransplant Period

The aim of organ support in patients with ACLF is to prevent further deterioration and improve organ failure score pretransplant.

- *Support of coagulation system:* It is important to avoid unnecessary transfusions in patients with ACLF. We should avoid correction of INR in the absence of bleeding or a planned procedure. Viscoelastic tests [e.g., rotational thromboelastometry (ROTEM) or thromboelastography (TEG)] guided management can help reduce the use of fresh frozen plasma (FFP) and favor the use of other factors such as cryoprecipitate, fibrinogen, prothrombin complex concentrate (PCC), or platelet concentrate in a given clinical setting. Overzealous transfusions lead to transfusion-associated volume overload and transfusion-related acute lung injury (TRALI), which compromise the respiratory parameters. It has also been shown to increase portal pressure and increase the rate of GI bleed. Fibrinogen level should be checked routinely, and it is better to maintain a level of >120 mg/dL in the setting of bleeding.[31]
- *Support of kidney:* Kidney dysfunction is the most predominant extrahepatic organ dysfunction in ACLF patients and an independent predictor of mortality.[1,32] The causes of acute kidney injury are diverse. It may be due to hypovolemia from GI bleed, an overdose of diuretics, diarrhea, large volume paracentesis, use of iodinated contrast media, nephrotoxic medications, bacterial sepsis, parenchymal or glomerular nephropathy, and hepatorenal syndrome (HRS). Early identification of acute kidney injury (AKI) is done as per KDIGO/AKIN criteria.[33] ACLF patients with AKI stages 2 and 3 sometimes may have a protracted course and may progress to stages of AKI, and chronic kidney disease (CKD).[34] Apart from that prevalence of CKD is also rising in patients with end-stage liver disease (ESLD)[35] with the rising number of metabolic-associated fatty liver disease (MAFLD), and this should be kept in mind while evaluating patients' kidney dysfunction for prospective transplantation.

Volume management is the crux in patients with AKI in cirrhosis. The pathophysiology of AKI is complex, but all patients with AKI follow two distinct phenotypes one is "Responsive to volume expansion phenotype" and "Nonresponsive to volume expansion phenotype".[36] Point of care ultrasound (POCUS), Focused cardiac ultrasound (FoCUS), and lung ultrasound with B protocol are three extremely important tools to identify volume status in these patients. HRS is usually treated with albumin, terlipressin, or norepinephrine as per EASL guidelines. It is important to understand that response to vasoconstrictor therapy declines with the number of organ failures at a given time.[37] Two recently published trials (ATTIRE trial,[38] and ALPS trial[39]) showed a higher incidence of pulmonary complications with albumin administration in patients with decompensated cirrhosis. The CONFIRM trial[40] showed a higher incidence of pulmonary complications with terlipressin infusion in patients with HRS. Regular cardiopulmonary assessment may decrease the adverse pulmonary events with albumin and terlipressin in patients with ACLF.[34] All forms of nephrotoxic drugs should be avoided. RRT is used as a traditional indication in patients with ACLF, although the decision is mostly taken as an individualized approach. A preemptive initiation of RRT is strongly recommended in APASL guidelines in patients with ACLF with progressive stage 3 AKI and non-responsive to vasoconstrictive therapy within 12–24 hours.[34] ACLF patients with prospective liver transplantation, RRT may be started as a bridge for stabilization of volume status and metabolic milieu.[33] CRRT is often the preferred mode of RRT in patients with ACLF with stage 3 AKI, considering systemic inflammation a key driver in overall pathophysiology and in the presence of unstable hemodynamics. The dose of CRRT is usually 20–25 mL/kg/h. Regional citrate anticoagulation may be used in ACLF patients requiring CRRT with careful monitoring of acid-base status and "total to ionized calcium ratio" to detect citrate accumulation. Routine measurement of intra-abdominal pressure (IAP) in patients with tense ascites, performing TIPS or extracorporeal liver support for the treatment of AKI is not evidence-based as per current literature.[33] Acute tubular necrosis, as a cause of AKI before transplant, puts patients at risk for post-LT mortality increase and persistent renal dysfunction.[41] AKI in ACLF often has a dismal prognosis, and understanding futility in care is a challenge in patients with grade 3 ACLF requiring RRT. CLIF-C ACLF score >59.5 calculated 48 hours after commencing RRT with the presence of >4 organ failures has been found to have 100% mortality with or without transplant in a recently published study.[42] Patients with grade 1 and 2 AKI should be considered for expedited liver transplantation. RRT is an independent predictor for worse outcomes post-LT (ELITA study[19]); hence, decision for transplant in anuric patients on RRT should be judged extremely carefully and on a case-by-case basis.

- *Support of respiration:* Healthcare-associated pneumonia is a problem in patients with repeated admissions to the hospital due to different causes. TRALI is common in patients with ACLF; it is important to limit transfusion as far as possible. Portopulmonary hypertension, hepatic hydrothorax, and hepatopulmonary syndrome are frequent associations in patients with end-stage liver disease. Restriction of mobility, tense ascites, and frailty add to the inadequate breathing muscle excursion and cause atelectasis. Airway protection is crucial in patients with altered mental status. Lung protective ventilation is the norm for any patient on mechanical ventilation. PPIs are suggested to be used in patients on a ventilator.
- *Support of circulation:* Most patients with decompensated cirrhosis have low SVR, increased cardiac output, and consequent hyperdynamic circulation. They have a low effective circulatory volume due to splanchnic vasodilation. Hyperdynamic circulation is exacerbated in the presence of sepsis or systemic hyperinflammation of ACLF. The presence of cirrhotic cardiomyopathy adds complexity to the whole situation. Diastolic dysfunction is a common association in patients with advanced cirrhosis. Hypovolemia leads to acute kidney injury and a decrease in organ perfusion, and hypervolemia leads to congestive nephropathy, increased extravascular lung volume, and other organ dysfunction. Lactate loses its importance as a marker of organ perfusion in patients with advanced liver failure. $Scvo_2$ is not a reliable marker due to hyperdynamic cardiovascular pathophysiology. Bedside echocardiography (LV/RV function, TR jet, dynamic markers, fluid responsiveness, and clinical parameters is extremely important to individualize volume management protocol. As per recently published APASL guidelines, Balanced crystalloids and 4% or 5% albumin are used as first-line resuscitation fluid in patients with ACLF in the presence of shock.[34] 20–25% albumin is used in the presence of SBP and large-volume paracentesis and volume expansion in HRS in the absence of shock. It is better to be careful with albumin as the use of albumin as a resuscitation fluid for sepsis-induced hypotension in the absence of SBP has been found to cause more pulmonary complications without any survival benefit.[39] Starch-based formulae are generally avoided. Norepinephrine is the first-line vasopressor agent in patients who remain hypotensive despite fluid resuscitation. A target MAP >65 mm Hg has been suggested by SCCM. As a goal of resuscitation.
- *Support of brain:* Hepatic encephalopathy is a common form of decompensation in cirrhosis. Other causes of altered mental status (structural, metabolic, and delirium) should also not be forgotten. Neuroimaging is warranted in patients with focal neurological signs or who fail to improve after standard medical treatment. Routine measurement of ammonia level is not required in critically ill cirrhotic patients in ICU. Unlike ALF, ammonia level does not correlate with the degree of encephalopathy in CLD. Intracranial hypertension from hyperammonemia is not a feature of ACLF. Clinical evaluation of GCS at regular intervals and airway status evaluation is important in patients with altered mentation. Endotracheal intubation is needed when GCS is <9. Benzodiazepine is generally avoided in decompensated cirrhosis. Propofol and opioid-based sedation are predominantly used for sedation purposes. Selective alpha 2 adrenergic agonist (dexmedetomidine) based sedation is sometimes helpful. Specific treatment includes treatment of precipitating factors such as GI bleeding and infection. Lactulose-based therapy and rifaximin help prevent hepatic encephalopathy. Lactulose may be administered per rectal as a retention enema when the oral route cannot be used. Polyethylene glycol (PEG-3350) bowel irrigation solution may be used as an alternative to or in combination with lactulose, and in a recent study, the combination of PEG and lactulose is superior to lactulose alone in ACLF patients in terms of rapid resolution of HE and improved 28-day mortality.[43] While CVVHDF may be used as antiammonia therapy

in patients with ALF, it has not been demonstrated to be useful as antiammonia treatment in patients with ACLF.[44]

- *Prevention of infection:* Multidrug-resistant bacterial and fungal infections are the major cause of posttransplant mortality and morbidity. Careful screening of pretransplant colonization status is helpful in certain cases. Risk factors for MDRO in the posttransplant settings are multiple hospitalization pretransplant, longer ICU stay, high MELD, HCC, Roux-en-Y choledochojejunostomy, perioperative RRT, and bile leak. Invasive fungal infection (IFI) is a concern in transplantation in patients with MELD scores of >30, retransplantation, and need for RRT. Invasive aspergillosis occurs in patients with ACLF who have received corticosteroids or severe alcoholic hepatitis. Prophylactic antifungal is recommended by the International Liver Transplant Society (ILTS) for all high-risk ACLF patients with MELD >30.[45]
- *Nutritional therapy and prehabilitation*: Early ambulation and physical rehabilitation with good nutritional support are the keys to preventing respiratory muscle deconditioning. Enteral nutrition with standard polymeric feed should be continued. Protein restriction or use of branched-chain amino acids is not recommended in critically ill cirrhotic patients in ICU.[44] Patients requiring CRRT should have 1.5–2 g/kg of protein daily prescribed as they are in a high catabolic state.
- *Therapies for promoting hepatic regeneration:* Hepatic regeneration is the only way for recovery of the liver following an acute insult in ACLF patients. Therapy with G-CSF was found in a few initial studies to overcome cirrhosis-associated immune dysfunction (CAID) and offer survival benefits. But the latest large multicentric phase II, randomized open-label trial (GRAFT study[46]) to analyze the effect of G-CSF in patients with ACLF, did not find any survival benefit compared to standard medical therapy, and the study was prematurely terminated for futility.

Hepatocyte transplantation with human allogeneic liver-derived progenitor cells (HALPC, or HepaStem®, Promethera Biosciences, Belgium) is another emerging therapeutic option. A phase 2 clinical trial has shown the safety of HALPC in patients with ACLF at a given intravenous dose.[47] Further proof of concept study in a larger population is warranted.

Modulation of gut dysbiosis by fecal microbiota transplantation is another interesting option in patients with ACLF.[48] Selective gut-specific nonabsorbable antibiotics such as rifaximin and nonantibiotic gut decontaminating products such as Carbalive™ and Dialive™ target to manipulate gut-derived PAMPs and reduce inflammation have shown promise in preliminary studies.[49]

PREOPERATIVE EVALUATION OF CARDIAC FUNCTION IN ACUTE-ON-CHRONIC LIVER FAILURE PATIENTS

Coronary evaluation before transplant in patients with ACLF is challenging and extremely important. A recently published review article from a French center suggested a pragmatic approach for pretransplant coronary evaluation in patients admitted to ICU with ACLF.[50] Noninvasive stress testing is not possible for most of the patients admitted with ACLF. As per the author, all patients should undergo TTE for evaluation of PASP. If PASP is >45 mm Hg, right heart catheterization was suggested to understand the nature of pulmonary hypertension. Along with that, patients with MAFLD-related CLD and patients with ≥3 AHA cardiovascular risk factors (diabetes mellitus, prior cardiovascular disease, left ventricular hypertrophy, age greater than 60 years, smoking, hypertension, and dyslipidemia) were suggested to perform CAD screening with coronary angiography as per the article.

Artificial Liver Support System Therapy

Artificial liver support systems may be of two types: Biological [Extracorporeal Liver Assist Device (ELAD®)] and nonbiological artificial liver (NBAL), which are extracorporeal dialysis-based systems such as Prometheus® system and molecular adsorbent recirculating system (MARS). So far, these devices have not shown improvement in mortality compared to standard medical care in published clinical trials **(Table 3)**. An exception to this is therapeutic plasma exchange (PE). The rationale for the use of ALSS is to reduce cellular damage in ACLF from excessive "cytokine burst" and removal of proinflammatory cytokines and vasoactive substances. In a way, they improve circulatory dysfunction and metabolic profile by decreasing ammonia and bilirubin, correcting coagulation parameters, and creating

TABLE 3: ACLF grading as per APASL guideline.

APASL ACLF Research Consortium (AARC) score					
Point	***Bilirubin***	***HE grades***	***INR***	***Creatinine***	***Lactate***
1	<15	0	<1.8	<0.7	<1.5
2	15–22	I–II	1.8–2.5	0.7–1.5	1.5–2.5
3	>22	III–IV	>2.5	>1.5	>2.5
Score 5–7: ACLF 1; score 8–10: ACLF 2; score 11–15: ACLF 3					

(ACLF: acute-on-chronic liver failure; APASL: Asian Pacific Association for the Study of the Liver; HE: hepatic encephalopathy; INR: international normalized ratio)

an environment for potential hepatic regeneration and recovery. An interesting article from the Chinese liver transplant registry by Ling et al. found that the use of ALSS to decrease pretransplant MELD <30 improves outcome post-liver transplant.[51]

In 2021, Du et al. derived a PALS score taking five parameters (presence or absence of cirrhosis, total bilirubin, PT/INR, presence or absence of infection, and hepatic encephalopathy grade), and developed a predictive PALS grade (score range 0–9 and grade 1–3) to identify who will benefit most with ALSS in hepatitis-B ACLF patients.[52]

TABLE 4: ALSS and role in ACLF.

ALSS devices	***Working principle***	***Clinical studies***	***Outcome and current verdict***
Extracorporeal Liver Assist Device (ELAD® Vital Therapies Inc., San Diego, CA, USA)	Utilizes hepatocytes derived from a hepatoblastoma cell line in the dialysis circuit	• Thompson et al. Phase III RCT. ITT analysis • 203 participants with severe alcoholic hepatitis (AH) • 3–5 days of continuous ELAD therapy plus standard care (SOC) vs. SOC alone	No difference in patient survival[54]
Prometheus® system (Fresenius Medical Care AG, Hamburg, Germany)	Fractionated plasma separation and adsorption (FPSA) approach, facilitates the removal of both albumin-bound and water-soluble toxins	• HELIOS study, ITT analysis • 145 patients with ACLF • FPSA vs. standard medical therapy	• Reduced serum bilirubin • No survival benefit[55]
Molecular adsorbent recirculating system (MARS; Baxter International Inc., Deerfield, IL, USA)	Dialysis circuit containing 600 mL of 20% human albumin with a charcoal column and an anion exchange resin column with a conventional hemodialysis filter.	• RELIEF trial • 189 patients with ACLF • MARS vs. standard medical therapy • Meta-analysis, data from 285 participants from three RCTs • MARS vs. SMC • LIT (MARS <4 session), HIT (MARS >4 session)	• No difference in transplant-free survival at 28 and 90 days[56] • Decrease bilirubin levels and improve HE • No difference in 30-day survival • Improved outcome with HIT compared to LIT in ACLF[57]
Liver dialysis device (DIALIVE, Baxter, USA)	Extracorporeal dual filtration system connected in series, one for ultrafiltration of dysfunctional albumin and cytokines (SepteX kit), another for adsorption of PAMPs, DAMPs and endotoxins (oXiris kit)	• Multicenter RCT in Europe • 32 alcohol related ACLF patients • DIALIVE therapy for 5 days vs. SOC	• Safety was primary end point[58] • No difference in 28-day mortality • Faster resolution in ACLF grade
Double plasma molecular adsorption system (DPMAS)	Uses two columns of neutral macroporous adsorption resin and ion exchange resin to remove macromolecules from plasma	• Systematic review and meta-analysis of 11 articles • DPMAS combined with PE in ACLF patients	• May be an effective treatment in ACLF[59] • No analysis of survival benefit

(ACLF: acute-on-chronic liver failure; ALSS: artificial liver support system; HE: hepatic encephalopathy; PE: plasma exchange; RCT: randomized controlled trial)

PLASMA EXCHANGE AS SALVAGE THERAPY IN PATIENTS WITH ACUTE-ON-CHRONIC LIVER FAILURE

Therapeutic PE is the most promising extracorporeal bridging modality in patients with ACLF to either early transplantation or spontaneous recovery, although this is still not a recommendation as per the American Society of Apheresis. In a recently published meta-analysis on the effect of PE in patients with ACLF, the conclusion remained grey with a remark on the need for further studies to prove survival benefit.[53] However, this is the most commonly used extracorporeal therapy used. In India, currently in patients with ACLF with high MELD for stabilization of organ function before liver transplantation **(Table 4)**.

CONCLUSION

Acute-on-chronic liver failure is a difficult-to-treat condition with a high risk of mortality. Despite having higher posttransplant complications, this is a logical and ethical choice where survival without transplant is minimal. Pretransplant ICU management plays a vital role in organ stabilization and downgrading ACLF grade, which improves posttransplant outcomes. Determining an optimal transplant window is critical in ensuring the best possible outcome for the patient. A careful call needs to be taken with a multidisciplinary approach with intensivists, transplant surgeons, and hepatologists for this purpose. An immediate referral of all ACLF patients to a dedicated liver intensive care unit with the facility of a transplant program is suggested.

REFERENCES

1. Moreau R, Jalan R, Gines P, Pavesi M, Angeli P, Cordoba J, et al. Acute-on-chronic liver failure is a distinct syndrome that develops in patients with acute decompensation of cirrhosis. Gastroenterology. 2013;144:1426-37.e9.
2. Vincent JL, Moreno R, Takala J, Willatts S, De Mendonça A, Bruining H, et al. The SOFA (Sepsis-related Organ Failure Assessment) score to describe organ dysfunction/failure. Intensive Care Med. 1996;22:707-10.
3. Jalan R, Saliba F, Pavesi M, Amoros A, Moreau R, Ginès P, et al. Development and validation of a prognostic score to predict mortality in patients with acute-on-chronic liver failure. J Hepatol. 2014;61:1038-47.
4. Arroyo V, Moreau R, Jalan R, Ginès P. Acute-on-chronic liver failure: A new syndrome that will re-classify cirrhosis. J Hepatol. 2015;62:S131-43.
5. Engelmann C, Thomsen KL, Zakeri N, Sheikh M, Agarwal B, Jalan R, et al. Validation of CLIF-C ACLF score to define a threshold for futility of intensive care support for patients with acute-on-chronic liver failure. Crit Care. 2018;22(1):254.
6. Nagel M, Westphal R, Hilscher M, Galle PR, Schattenberg JM, Schreiner O, et al. Validation of the CLIF-C OF Score and CLIF-C ACLF Score to predict transplant-free survival in patients with liver cirrhosis and concomitant need for intensive care unit treatment. Med. 2023;59(5):866.
7. Sarin SK, Choudhury A, Sharma MK, Maiwall R, Al Mahtab M, Rahman S, et al. Acute-on-chronic liver failure: consensus recommendations of the Asian Pacific association for the study of the liver (APASL): an update. Hepatol Int. 2019;13:353-90.
8. Choudhury A, Jindal A, Maiwall R, Sharma MK, Sharma BC, Pamecha V, et al. Liver failure determines the outcome in patients of acute-on-chronic liver failure (ACLF): comparison of APASL ACLF research consortium (AARC) and CLIF-SOFA models. Hepatol Int. 2017;11:461-71.
9. Maiwall R, Pasupuleti SSR, Choudhury A, Kim DJ, Sood A, Goyal O, et al. AARC score determines outcomes in patients with alcohol-associated hepatitis: a multinational study. Hepatol Int. 2023;17:662-75.
10. Li J, Liang X, You S, Feng T, Zhou X, Zhu B, et al. Development and validation of a new prognostic score for hepatitis B virus-related acute-on-chronic liver failure. J Hepatol. 2021;75:1104-15.
11. Li P, Liang X, Luo J, Li J, Xin J, Jiang J, et al. Predicting the survival benefit of liver transplantation in HBV-related acute-on-chronic liver failure: an observational cohort study. Lancet Reg Heal-West Pacific. 2023;32:100638.
12. Wu D, Sun Z, Liu X, Rao Q, Chen W, Wang J, et al. HINT: a novel prognostic model for patients with hepatitis B virus-related acute-on-chronic liver failure. Aliment Pharmacol Ther. 2018;48:750-60.
13. Wang X, Sun M, Yang X, Gao L, Weng M, Yang D, et al. Value of liver regeneration in predicting short-term prognosis for patients with hepatitis B-related acute-on-chronic liver failure. Biomed Res Int. 2020;2020:5062873.
14. Agbim U, Sharma A, Maliakkal B, Karri S, Yazawa M, Goldkamp W, et al. Outcomes of liver transplant recipients with acute-on-chronic liver failure based on EASL-CLIF Consortium definition: a single-center study. Transplant Direct. 2020;6:E544.
15. Arroyo V, Moreau R, Jalan R. Acute-on-Chronic Liver Failure. N Engl J Med. 2020;382:2137-45.
16. Artru F, Louvet A, Ruiz I, Levesque E, Labreuche J, Ursic-Bedoya J, et al. Liver transplantation in the most severely ill cirrhotic patients: A multicenter study in acute-on-chronic liver failure grade 3. J Hepatol. 2017;67:708-15.
17. Sundaram V, Kogachi S, Wong RJ, Karvellas CJ, Fortune BE, Mahmud N, et al. Effect of the clinical course of acute-on-chronic liver failure prior to liver transplantation on post-transplant survival. J Hepatol. 2020;72:481-8.

18. Artzner T, Michard B, Weiss E, Barbier L, Noorah Z, Merle JC, et al. Liver transplantation for critically ill cirrhotic patients: Stratifying utility based on pretransplant factors. Am J Transplant. 2020;20:2437-48.
19. Belli LS, Duvoux C, Artzner T, Bernal W, Conti S, Cortesi PA, et al. Liver transplantation for patients with acute-on-chronic liver failure (ACLF) in Europe: results of the ELITA/EF-CLIF collaborative study (ECLIS). J Hepatol. 2021;75:610-22.
20. Weiss E, Saner F, Asrani SK, Biancofiore G, Blasi A, Lerut J, et al. When is a critically ill cirrhotic patient too sick to transplant? Development of consensus criteria by a multidisciplinary panel of 35 international experts. Transplantation. 2021;561-8.
21. Sacleux SC, Saliba F. How to optimize the results of liver transplantation for acute-on-chronic liver failure. Life. 2023;13:1152.
22. Sundaram V, Mahmud N, Perricone G, Katarey D, Wong RJ, Karvellas CJ, et al. Longterm outcomes of patients undergoing liver transplantation for acute-on-chronic liver failure. Liver Transpl. 2020;26:1594-602.
23. Moon DB, Lee SG, Kang WH, Song GW, Jung DH, Park GC, et al. Adult living donor liver transplantation for acute-on-chronic liver failure in high-model for end-stage liver disease score patients. Am J Transplant. 2017;17:1833-42.
24. Yadav SK, Saraf N, Choudhary NS, Sah JK, Sah SK, Rastogi A, et al. Living donor liver transplantation for acute-on-chronic liver failure. Liver Transplant. 2019;25:459-68.
25. Singh SA, Pampaniya H, Mehtani R, Jadaun SS, Kumar M, Khurana S, et al. Living donor liver transplant in acute on chronic liver failure grade 3: Who not to transplant. Dig Liver Dis. 2024;56(1):152-8.
26. Choudhury A, Vijayaraghavan R, Maiwall R, Kumar M, Duan Z, Yu C, et al. 'First week' is the crucial period for deciding living donor liver transplantation in patients with acute-on-chronic liver failure. Hepatol Int. 2021;15:1376-88.
27. Fernández J, Acevedo J, Wiest R, Gustot T, Amoros A, Deulofeu C, et al. Bacterial and fungal infections in acute-on-chronic liver failure: prevalence, characteristics and impact on prognosis. Gut. 2018;67:1870-80.
28. Wang J, Ma K, Han M, Guo W, Huang J, Yang D, et al. Nucleoside analogs prevent disease progression in HBV-related acute-on-chronic liver failure: validation of the TPPM model. Hepatol Int. 2014;8:64-71..
29. Louvet A, Naveau S, Abdelnour M, Ramond MJ, Diaz E, Fartoux L, et al. The Lille model: a new tool for therapeutic strategy in patients with severe alcoholic hepatitis treated with steroids. Hepatology. 2007;45:1348-54.
30. Sersté T, Cornillie A, Njimi H, Pavesi M, Arroyo V, Putignano A, et al. The prognostic value of acute-on-chronic liver failure during the course of severe alcoholic hepatitis. J Hepatol. 2018;69:318-24.
31. Liu P, Hum J, Jou J, Scanlan RM, Shatzel J. Transfusion strategies in patients with cirrhosis. Eur J Haematol. 2020;104:15-25.
32. Napoleone L, Solé C, Juanola A, Ma AT, Carol M, Pérez-Guasch M, et al. Patterns of kidney dysfunction in acute-on-chronic liver failure: relationship with kidney and patients' outcome. Hepatol Commun. 2022;6:2121-31.
33. Nadim MK, Kellum JA, Forni L, Francoz C, Asrani SK, Ostermann M, et al. Acute kidney injury in patients with cirrhosis: acute disease quality initiative (ADQI) and International Club of Ascites (ICA) joint multidisciplinary consensus meeting. J Hepatol 2024;81:163-83.
34. Maiwall R, Singh SP, Angeli P, Moreau R, Krag A, Singh V, et al. APASL clinical practice guidelines on the management of acute kidney injury in acute-on-chronic liver failure. Hepatol Int.2024;18:833-69.
35. Kumar R, Priyadarshi RN, Anand U. Chronic renal dysfunction in cirrhosis: a new frontier in hepatology. World J Gastroenterol. 2021;27:990.
36. Banegas-Deras EJ, Mazón-Ruiz J, Romero-González G, Ruiz-Cobo JC, Sanz-García C, Serrano-Soto M, et al. Acute kidney injury and point-of-care ultrasound in liver cirrhosis: redefining hepatorenal syndrome. Clin Kidney J. 2024;17:112.
37. Piano S, Schmidt HH, Ariza X, Amoros A, Romano A, Hüsing-Kabar A, et al. Association between grade of acute on chronic liver failure and response to terlipressin and albumin in patients with hepatorenal syndrome. Clin Gastroenterol Hepatol. 2018;16:1792-800.e3.
38. China L, Freemantle N, Forrest E, Kallis Y, Ryder SD, Wright G, et al. A randomized trial of albumin infusions in hospitalized patients with cirrhosis. N Engl J Med. 2021;384:808-17.
39. Maiwall R, Kumar A, Pasupuleti SSR, Hidam AK, Tevethia H, Kumar G, et al. A randomized-controlled trial comparing 20% albumin to plasmalyte in patients with cirrhosis and sepsis-induced hypotension [ALPS trial]. J Hepatol. 2022;77:670-82.
40. Wong F, Pappas SC, Curry MP, Reddy KR, Rubin RA, Porayko MK, et al. Terlipressin plus albumin for the treatment of type 1 hepatorenal syndrome. N Engl J Med. 2021;384:818-28.
41. Asrani SK, Saracino G, O'Leary JG, Gonzalez S, Kim PT, McKenna GJ, et al. Recipient characteristics and morbidity and mortality after liver transplantation. J Hepatol. 2018;69:43-50.
42. Staufer K, Roedl K, Kivaranovic D, Drolz A, Horvatits T, Rasoul-Rockenschaub S, et al. Renal replacement therapy in critically ill liver cirrhotic patients—outcome and clinical implications. Liver Int. 2017;37:843-50.
43. Ahmed S, Premkumar M, Dhiman RK, Kulkarni AV, Imran R, Duseja A, et al. Combined PEG3350 plus lactulose results in early resolution of hepatic encephalopathy and improved 28-day survival in acute-on-chronic liver failure. J Clin Gastroenterol. 2021;56:E11–9.
44. Nanchal R, Subramanian R, Alhazzani W, Dionne JC, Peppard WJ, Singbartl K, et al. Guidelines for the management of adult acute and acute-on-chronic liver

failure in the icu: neurology, peri-transplant medicine, infectious disease, and gastroenterology considerations. Crit Care Med. 2023;51:657-76.

45. Campos-Varela I, Blumberg EA, Giorgio P, Kotton CN, Saliba F, Wey EQ, et al. What is the optimal antimicrobial prophylaxis to prevent postoperative infectious complications after liver transplantation? A systematic review of the literature and expert panel recommendations. Clin Transplant. 2022;36:e14631.
46. Engelmann C, Herber A, Franke A, Bruns T, Reuken P, Schiefke I, et al. Granulocyte-colony stimulating factor (G-CSF) to treat acute-on-chronic liver failure: A multicenter randomized trial (GRAFT study). J Hepatol. 2021;75:1346-54.
47. Nevens F, Gustot T, Laterre PF, Lasser LL, Haralampiev LE, Vargas V, et al. A phase II study of human allogeneic liver-derived progenitor cell therapy for acute-on-chronic liver failure and acute decompensation. JHEP reports. 2021;3(4):100291. .
48. Sharma A, Roy A, Premkumar M, Verma N, Duseja A, Taneja S, et al. Fecal microbiota transplantation in alcohol-associated acute-on-chronic liver failure: an open-label clinical trial. Hepatol Int 2022; 16: 433-46.
49. Trebicka J, Hernaez R, Shawcross DL, Gerbes AL. Recent advances in the prevention and treatment of decompensated cirrhosis and acute-on-chronic liver failure (ACLF) and the role of biomarkers. Gut. 2024;73:1015-24.
50. Gaudefroy J, Brunet P, Lordier B, Lebas B, Pottecher J. Assessment of liver transplantation eligibility for ACLF patients. J Liver Transplant. 2023;11:100167.
51. Ling Q, Dai H, Zhuang R, Shen T, Wang W, Xu X, et al. Predicting short-term survival after liver transplantation on eight score systems: a national report from China Liver Transplant Registry. Sci Rep. 2017;7(1):42253.
52. Du L, Ma Y, Zhou S, Chen F, Xu Y, Wang M, et al. A prognostic score for patients with acute-on-chronic liver failure treated with plasma exchange-centered artificial liver support system. Sci Reports. 2021;11:1-12.
53. Beran A, Mohamed MFH, Shaear M, Nayfeh T, Mhanna M, Srour O, et al. Plasma exchange for acute and acute-on-chronic liver failure: a systematic review and meta-analysis. Liver Transplant. 2024;30:127-41.
54. Thompson J, Jones N, Al-Khafaji A, Malik S, Reich D, Munoz S, et al. Extracorporeal cellular therapy (ELAD) in severe alcoholic hepatitis: a multinational, prospective, controlled, randomized trial. Liver Transplant. 2018;24:380-93.
55. Kribben A, Gerken G, Haag S, Herget-Rosenthal S, Treichel U, Betz C, et al. Effects of fractionated plasma separation and adsorption on survival in patients with acute-on-chronic liver failure. Gastroenterology. 2012;142:782-9.e3.
56. Bañares R, Nevens F, Larsen FS, Jalan R, Albillos A, Dollinger M, et al. Extracorporeal albumin dialysis with the molecular adsorbent recirculating system in acute-on-chronic liver failure: the RELIEF trial. Hepatology. 2013;57:1153-62.
57. Bañares R, Ibáñez-Samaniego L, Torner JM, Pavesi M, Olmedo C, Catalina MV, et al. Meta-analysis of individual patient data of albumin dialysis in acute-on-chronic liver failure: focus on treatment intensity. Therap Adv Gastroenterol. 2019;12:1756284819879565.
58. Agarwal B, Cañizares RB, Saliba F, Ballester MP, Tomescu DR, Martin D, et al. Randomized, controlled clinical trial of the DIALIVE liver dialysis device versus standard of care in patients with acute-on-chronic liver failure. J Hepatol. 2023;79:79-92.
59. Bai W, Yao C, Mao D, Wu J, Wang K, Wei H, et al. The clinical efficacy of double plasma molecular absorption system combined with plasma exchange in the treatment of acute-on-chronic liver failure: a systematic review and meta-analysis. J Health Eng. 2022;2022:3139929.

CHAPTER 7

Challenges of Perioperative Hemodynamic Management in Liver Transplant Setting

Akila Rajakumar, Amal Francis Sam

INTRODUCTION

Liver transplantation (LT) has become the standard of care for patients with decompensated end-stage liver disease, irreversible fulminant liver failure of any cause, and a few other metabolic disorders.[1] LT can be performed with the graft from a living donor or a deceased donor where it could be a whole graft or a partial split graft. Postoperative hemodynamic management of these patients after LT should be meticulously planned with careful attention to the following: The surgical factors and graft quality and altered pathophysiology in various organ systems, mainly the cardiovascular system. A good functioning graft is essential for smooth patient recovery both in cadaveric and living donor liver transplantation (LDLT),[2] and the graft function essentially determines the postoperative course. The contribution of each of these can be variable postoperatively and poses challenges in the management of such patients.

FACTORS INFLUENCING POSTOPERATIVE MANAGEMENT

Surgery and Graft-related Factors

Liver transplantation is a complex major abdominal surgery, which involves clamping and unclamping of major vessels causing abrupt, sudden variations of preload with the potential for ischemia–reperfusion injury (IRI). As the surgical times are often prolonged, it has inherent risks of large fluid shifts, large volume blood loss, and massive transfusion.

To overcome the shortage of cadaveric organs and waitlist mortality, the transplant community has increased the margins for acceptance of a donor in deceased donor liver transplantation (DDLT) and a smaller volume graft in living donor LT[2] to prioritize donor safety.[3,4] This has led to increasing use of marginal grafts, which increase the likelihood of primary graft dysfunction (PGD). PGD can be in the form of primary nonfunction (PNF) or early allograft dysfunction (EAD). Patients with PNF have unstable hemodynamics, worsening coagulopathy, massive bleeding needing massive transfusion, renal dysfunction, worsening lactatemia, and acidosis. The super urgent listing criteria for retransplantation as accepted by the Organ Procurement and Transplantation Network (OPTN) are PNF of a transplanted liver within 7 days of implantation with aspartate aminotransferase (AST) levels ≥3,000 IU/L and one or both of the following: (1) International normalized ratio (INR)[5] ≥2.5 and (2) acidosis, defined as having an arterial pH ≤7.30 or venous pH of 7.25 and/or lactate ≥4 mmol/L.

Various definitions of EAD have been developed by several authors, but the one proposed by Olthoff et al.[6] is well validated. Presence of one or more of the following variables bilirubin >10 mg/dL, INR >1.6 on postoperative day 7, and AST or alanine aminotransferase (ALT) >2,000 U/L within the first 7 postoperative days was termed as EAD. Small-for-size syndrome (SFSS) is one of the forms of EAD when a partial liver graft is unable to meet the demands of the recipient.[2]

Early graft failure in the form of PNF is an uncommon but very challenging situation. Early recognition of the problem with incorporation of multidisciplinary inputs and anticipation of impending complications are all keys to successful management. Multiorgan dysfunction sets in at the late stages of graft failure. It is, therefore, imperative to identify signs of early graft failure to decide if urgent retransplantation is required and also to identify grafts with potential to recover with meticulous postoperative care.

In the LDLT setting, if the early period after transplantation is well supported with a conducive milieu, the majority of PGD would recover without much consequences.[7] All efforts should be made to extract maximal function of the failing graft and enhance liver regeneration. Optimizing and preventing extrahepatic organ dysfunction is the most important goal.

Other common surgical complications in the postoperative period include vascular issues such as portal vein thrombosis, hepatic vein occlusion or thrombosis, and hepatic arterial thrombosis; biliary issues such as bile leak which is evident in the drain or with the presence of intrahepatic biliary dilatation, bleeding inside the abdomen; and immunological issues such as rejection and graft-versus-host disease and infections all of which can cause hemodynamic instability.

Cardiovascular events have been shown to be the leading nongraft-related cause of 30-day mortality following LT.[8,9] In a study from Australia looking at predictive risk factors for major adverse cardiovascular events (MACE) after LT, hepatorenal syndrome (HRS), beta-blocker use, portopulmonary hypertension (PoPH), and poor functional status were found to be associated with over a twofold higher risk of MACE.[10] In a study from seven academic centers in the United States, a 3.7% incidence of intraoperative cardiac arrest (ICA) with a 1.2% incidence of intraoperative mortality was observed. Risk factors for ICA include body mass index, Model for End-Stage Liver Disease (MELD) score, reperfusion syndrome, reoperation, living donor, and length of surgery.[11] In a study from Pittsburgh, ICA occurred in 68 of 1,238 LT recipients (5.5%), and 90% occurred during the neohepatic phase, causes being reperfusion syndrome and pulmonary thromboembolism. A higher MELD score was found to be the most significant risk factor for ICA. The intraoperative mortality rate was 29.4%, 30-day patient survival rate after ICA was 55.9%, and the 1-year survival rate was 45.6%.[12]

Altered Pathophysiology

Cardiac and Vascular System (Fig. 1)

It has been clearly demonstrated by scintigraphy that distribution of blood volume is altered in cirrhotic patients. They have a relatively low blood volume in the thorax region and substantially increased relative and absolute blood volumes in the splanchnic region.[13] It has also been clearly demonstrated that during volume expansion, the central and arterial blood volume increased significantly only in patients with Child-Turcotte-Pugh (CTP) class A cirrhosis, whereas no significant change occurs in patients with either class B or class C. On the contrary, an increase in noncentral blood volume was observed in patients with class B and C cirrhosis. However, the cardiac output

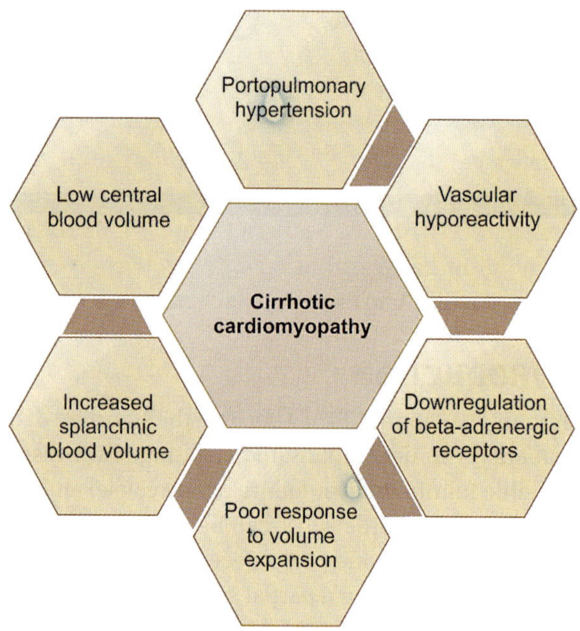

Fig. 1: Altered cardiovascular dynamics in cirrhotic patients.

increased and the systemic vascular resistance decreased, whereas no significant change in mean arterial blood pressure (BP) was seen.[14]

It is now clearly understood that in advanced liver disease, most of the administered intravenous fluids distribute disproportionately to splanchnic vascular beds, increasing splanchnic blood volume without any significant increase in central blood volume and cardiac output.[14] This phenomenon of splanchnic steal results in aggravation of portal hypertension and bleeding with fluid loading, especially during hepatectomy.

Downregulation of beta-adrenergic receptors both in terms of numbers and sensitivity along with high levels of circulating catecholamines has been demonstrated in patients with advanced cirrhosis which is presumed to be the reason for impaired myocardial performance.[15,16] It has also been observed that patients with cirrhosis have vascular hyporeactivity to vasoconstrictors such as norepinephrine and angiotensin II, and antioxidants have been tested and proven to reverse this hyporeactivity.[17]

Cirrhotic cardiomyopathy (CCM) is now been well understood and is defined as a syndrome of depressed cardiac function in the absence of primary heart disease in patients with cirrhosis. The CCM consortium of 2019 has given modified diagnostic criteria for diagnosing CCM based on transthoracic echocardiogram (ECHO) parameters.[18] Prevalence rates reported are 26–81% in decompensated cirrhotics.[19] The systemic vasodilatation seen in cirrhotic patients often masks early systolic dysfunction and the early decrease in contractility by decreasing afterload and increasing preload.[20] The ejection fraction derived from transthoracic ECHO usually overestimates systolic function. It is highly likely that these patients may not manifest signs and symptoms of overt heart failure in the preoperative period because of systemic vasodilation but have the risk of heart failure due to surgical stress, overzealous fluid administration, and the restoration of vascular reactivity and afterload with a functioning new liver.[21,22] It has been presumed that LT is the definitive treatment for CCM, although these effects are not seen until the first year after transplantation.[19,21]

In a single-center retrospective matched cohort study of 141 LT patients, it was observed that patients without CCM had a higher 5-year cardiovascular disease-free survival rate (85.2% vs. 60.7%), with the most pronounced effect on survival observed within the first 90 days post-LT. This highlights the importance of heightened monitoring in the immediate postoperative period and intensive cardiac surveillance post-hospital discharge.[21] A gradual deterioration of diastolic dysfunction associated has been reported in the first 3 months which can be due to natural progression of the disease or cardiotoxicity of calcineurin inhibitors (CNIs).[23] Improvement of all indices of both systolic and diastolic function, cardiac workload, and exercise capacity has been demonstrated from 6 to 12 months after transplantation.[24]

Significant and progressive QTc prolongation has been reported in all patients undergoing LT, and this effect seems more pronounced in patients with baseline prolongation of QTc,[25] which highlights the increased risk of perioperative arrhythmias in these patients with stimuli. Restoration of QTc to normal levels is observed only in 50% of CCM patients within 1 year,[26] suggesting other additional causes.

Caution and careful titration will be required during administration of vasoconstrictors, such as angiotensin II and terlipressin, which increase the left ventricular (LV) afterload by increasing systemic vascular resistance and, thus, unmask a latent LV dysfunction.[27,28] Similarly, vasodilators and other afterload-reducing agents should be used with caution due to the risk of further aggravation of the vasodilatory state.

Portopulmonary hypertension is a serious pulmonary vascular disease secondary to portal hypertension with a reported incidence of 2–10%.[29] PoPH is associated with significant morbidity during the entire perioperative period, major risks being right heart failure and death. Therefore, targeted therapies should be instituted to improve pulmonary hemodynamics and functional capacity, and LT should be offered only to those who respond to therapy.[30] Therapy needs to be continued in the postoperative period to control pulmonary artery pressures and to avoid graft congestion and heart failure. The exact relationship between resolution of PoPH following LT and the use of targeted therapy is not clearly reported.[31] Of all the studies that reported LT in PoPH, a total of 32 out of 46 (70%) of PoPH patients were able to wean off all targeted therapy over a period of 7–25 months following LT.[32]

In various studies, the prevalence of coronary artery disease in patients with end-stage liver disease has ranged from 16.2 to 32.5%,[33,34] which is found to be higher than in the general population and similar to that in patients with diabetes.[35] The prevalence has increased over the years, which reflects the changing profile of an increasingly older patient population undergoing LT.[34]

Other Organ Systems

Respiratory manifestations in patients with liver disease include pleural effusion/hydrothorax, atelectasis due to restrictive effects of pleural effusion and ascites, hepatopulmonary syndrome, and POPH.[36]

Kidneys are very susceptible to dysfunction even with minor insults in these patients. HRS occurs in 20% of patients with ascites.[37] Hyperdynamic circulatory state and the low renal perfusion pressure along with abnormal neurohumoral regulation contribute to renal dysfunction in these patients. Cirrhotic patients have an impairment in solute-free water excretion which can result in hyponatremia.[38]

Relative adrenal insufficiency (RAI) has been reported in nearly half of patients with cirrhosis. They have more profound hemodynamic stability and also a poor response to vasopressors.[39]

HEMODYNAMIC MANAGEMENT IN THE CRITICAL CARE UNIT

Cardiovascular Support

With a good functioning graft, restoration of central blood volume can reverse the vasodilatation seen in these patients and can unmask underlying cirrhotic cardiomyopathy, resulting in cardiac failure. Systemic inflammatory response syndrome (SIRS) could be seen in these patients from the IRI and PGD, and the mediators can cause marked vasodilation and vasoplegia. The clinical picture is indistinguishable from septic shock. Relative endogenous vasopressin deficiency has been demonstrated in patients with liver disease[40] presenting for LT, and this could be the reason for vasodilatory shock seen in these patients, similar to septic shock.

Incidence of post-LT heart failure has been reported to range from 1 to 47%.[41] Cardiac failure occurring within the first 12 hours postsurgery has been associated with a higher risk of multiorgan failure and death.[42] Causes for post-LT heart failure are enumerated in **Box 1**.

Stress (Takotsubo) cardiomyopathy (SCM) is manifested by acute transient LV apical ballooning with severe vasopressor-refractory hypotension. The prevalence of SCM *after* LT is about 0.3%.[43]

A systematic review of the literature and expert panel recommendations conducted in preparation for the ILTS–ERAS4OLT.org Consensus Conference on Enhanced Recovery for Liver Transplantation recommend a moderately restrictive or "replacement only" fluid management protocol fluid regimen, especially during the dissection phase of surgery. Intravascular volume status should be assessed frequently with ECHO parameters and assessment of fluid responsiveness. Sustained hypervolemia should be avoided. The recommendation was also against the use of 130/0.4 hydroxyethyl starch, given the high incidence of acute kidney injury (AKI) in this population.[44] This approach should be extrapolated to the postoperative period as well, consistent with all other major abdominal surgeries.

It has been observed that a more positive cumulative fluid balance at 48 hours after LT increased the development of pulmonary complications,[45] and cumulative positive fluid balance over 4 days after LT was independently associated with the development of AKI and the requirement of renal replacement therapy (RRT).[46] Goal-directed fluid therapy has been shown to reduce the duration of mechanical ventilation in postoperative ileus.[47] A thorough insight into all fluid therapy trials recommends that clinicians should focus on the precision for using invasive or noninvasive approaches at the initial presentation of high-risk patients.[48] Intravenous fluids should be meticulously titrated, keeping in mind the risks of graft congestion versus inadequate tissue perfusion. Attention should be paid to all the losses which occur through the ascitic drains and pleural drains, if any, and this needs to be replaced at a rate depending on the volume status of the patient. In the cohort of patients with PGD and those with underlying cardiopulmonary issues or renal dysfunction, fluids and vasopressor use should be guided by cardiac output monitoring.

Crystalloids can contribute to dilutional coagulopathy and can increase the risk of bleeding. Colloids are recommended in protein-rich drain losses, including ascites. A common ratio for replacement is 8 g of 20% albumin per liter of ascites drained when no other fluids are administered.[49] In patients with bleeding concerns or those with PGD, factor concentrates such as prothrombin complex concentrates, fibrinogen concentrates and recombinant activated factor VII are preferred, whenever possible, for having the advantage of avoiding fluid overload, immunological issues, and lung injury caused by blood products. When used with guidance from point-of-care coagulation tests, these concentrates are found to be safe.[50]

Shock in liver failure is vasodilatory in nature and, therefore, extrapolating evidence from management of septic shock, norepinephrine (NE) is recommended as a first-choice vasopressor in patients with liver disease who remain hypotensive despite fluid resuscitation or those with profound hypotension and tissue hypoperfusion even if fluid resuscitation is ongoing.[51] A target mean arterial pressure of 65 mm Hg has been recommended.[51] Complications such as atrial fibrillation were more common with higher vasopressor-induced BP.[52] Exogenous vasopressin administration has demonstrated a rapid correction of hemodynamics in LT patients who typically have low endogenous levels.[40] Vasopressin restores vascular smooth muscle sensitivity to catecholamines.[53] A synergistic effect between vasopressin and NE has also been demonstrated in vasodilatory shock.[54] Therefore,

BOX 1: Causes of perioperative hemodynamic instability.

- *Acute cardiac failure:*
  - Intracardiac thrombus and pulmonary embolism
  - Worsening cirrhotic cardiomyopathy with surgical stress
  - New-onset ischemia
  - Portopulmonary hypertension—right heart failure
  - Stress cardiomyopathy
  - Transfusion-associated circulatory overload (TACO)
- *Graft issues:* Primary nonfunction/hepatic artery thrombosis/ portal vein thrombosis
- Bleeding
- Infections—predominantly bacterial
- Acute cellular rejection—occasionally presents with fever and tachycardia

a stepwise approach is recommended by adding vasopressin once a specific dose of NE has been reached (approximately 0.2 µg/kg/min).

No specific therapy has been recommended for LV dysfunction in patients undergoing LT.[55] When inotropes are required, dobutamine should be preferred as a first choice.[51] Some limited reports of successful use of mechanical circulatory support such as intra-aortic balloon pump[56] and venoarterial extracorporeal membrane oxygenation (VA-ECMO)[57] encourage their use in LT recipients with acute circulatory collapse if resources and logistics are favorable.

All therapies for PoPH initiated in the preoperative period should be continued into the intraoperative and postoperative period, including inhaled nitric oxide and intravenous agents (prostacyclins and milrinone).[58] There are case reports of successful use of intraoperative VA-ECMO and venovenous ECMO to treat acute increase in pulmonary arterial pressure and right ventricular (RV) dysfunction in the perioperative period and can be considered for use when logistics are feasible.[59]

In LDLT recipients who receive small-for-size grafts, restrictive fluid strategy should be considered along with routine use of cardiac output monitoring, as well as use of pharmacologic portal flow modulation when appropriate beginning from the intraoperative phase to the postoperative period. Postoperatively, these patients should receive proactive monitoring for SFSS and consider for early RRT for avoidance of graft congestion.[60]

The nature of LT surgery and patient cohort with preexisting altered systemic hemodynamics mandates effective hemodynamic monitoring and management for optimal perioperative outcomes. Effective hemodynamic monitoring should translate to appropriate therapeutic interventions for patient-centered outcomes.[61]

In the event of intraoperative catastrophes, there is no doubt that early detection and appropriate intervention are very crucial. This would support the continuing use of the pulmonary artery catheter (PAC)[62] and transesophageal echocardiography (TEE) during LT. TEE can become a standard monitoring modality during LT in the near future as per a recent global survey.[63] TEE provides valuable information for immediate clinical decision making during intraoperative catastrophes. Its role in the postoperative period has not been studied because of logistics. PAC is routinely used in about 90% of all United States centers regardless of the size of the LT program.[64] PAC can be continuously used in the postoperative period.

In a study from Seoul of 1,565 liver transplant cases,[65] monitored with PAC or FloTrac/Vigileo, post-transplant clinical outcomes were not significantly different between the groups with and without PAC, justifying the fact that perioperative hemodynamic management can be performed safely without PAC in most circumstances. On comparing PAC with uncalibrated pulse contour analysis, no improvement in accuracy was achieved even with the fourth-generation FloTrac/Vigileo adult LT.[66] In a study, intermittent cardiac output monitoring with EV1000 system[67] showed a percentage error compared with PAC in the acceptable threshold of 45%. Considering these facts, PAC can be reserved for special circumstances such as PoPH and those patients with advanced cardiopulmonary disorders. **Box 2** gives a choice of hemodynamic monitoring.

Mechanical Ventilation

Preemptive lung protective ventilation strategies are the most effective way of reducing the incidence and severity of acute lung injury (ALI) from any underlying cause. The recent international expert panel-based consensus recommendations for perioperative ventilation[68] recommend protective strategies and to initiate ventilation with a tidal volume of 6–8 mL/kg predicted body weight and positive end-expiratory pressure (PEEP) of 5 cmH_2O. PEEP could then be individualized as per the status of oxygenation. Whenever recruitment maneuvers are required, the lowest effective pressure and shortest effective time or fewest number of breaths are to be used. PEEP up to 15 cmH_2O is associated with preserved hepatic venous outflow and can be used safely in patients following LT.[69]

BOX 2: Choosing hemodynamic monitoring tool in the perioperative period.

Assess the cardiovascular disease activity

- *Low risk:*
  - Arterial cannula and CVC
  - SVV and PPV in ventilated patients
- *Moderate risk:* Above with pulse contour analysis (calibrated/uncalibrated)
- *High risk:* Above with PAC, especially in patients with PoPH

TEE is more surgery specific and should be considered intraoperative in all patients when logistics permit.

(CVC: central venous catheter; PAC: pulmonary artery catheter; PoPH: portopulmonary hypertension; PPV: pulse pressure variation; SVV: stroke volume variation; TEE: transesophageal echocardiography)

Renal Support

It has been observed that even under normal circumstances, there is a significant decline in renal function accompanied by impaired renal oxygenation directly after LT.[70] It is obvious that these changes will be exaggerated during PGD. In patients who develop renal dysfunction, careful attention to be made to volume status, acid-base balance, and other electrolyte disturbances. Those patients with EAD also tend to have higher rates of progression to renal dysfunction and nonrecovery compared to others without EAD.[71]

Early RRT in patients with associated renal dysfunction increases graft and patient survival in patients with acute liver failure (ALF).[72] It has also been well established that continuous RRT (CRRT) is better than intermittent RRT in ALF because of the slower changes in serum osmolality and a smaller effect on arterial pressure, which are thought to preserve cerebral perfusion and avoid fluctuations in hemodynamics and intracranial pressure. This factor needs to be kept in mind during the management of patients with PNF.

Infection Prevention and Control

In addition to immunosuppressive therapy, factors such as mechanical ventilation, invasive lines, and drains increase the risk of infection. Broad-spectrum antibacterial and antifungal, as per the local hospital antibiogram and very stringent infection control measures, should be instituted.

Nutritional Support

Nutritional therapy principles should be similar to other critically ill patients, and we should aim to initiate and establish enteral feeding within 5–7 days after surgery.[73] As in all critically ill patients, this improves gut mucosal integrity and bacterial flora. While parenteral nutrition is an option if enteral feeding is not possible, the risk of infection and cholestasis is increased.

Neurological Support

Primary graft dysfunction can manifest by failure to wake up at the end of surgery in fast-track centers and inappropriate sensorium in other recipients. Patient evaluation should be directed toward excluding and eliminating neurological diseases, which can have a similar presentation as EAD. Posterior reversible encephalopathy syndrome[74] is a relatively frequent entity, which occurs due to uncontrolled hypertension or CNIs in the postoperative period. Therefore, it is imperative that BP should be appropriately managed.

Thromboprophylaxis

As mentioned earlier, these patients are prone to thromboembolic phenomenon as other patients. Titrated anticoagulation prophylaxis has to be started for deep vein thrombosis and also for the venous anastomosis and reconstruction performed. Hepatic arterial thrombosis is a dreaded complication after LT, which also necessitates prophylaxis with anticoagulants and antiplatelets in some centers.

Immunosuppression

Experience over the years has enabled clinicians to choose drugs with less long-term consequences and adverse effect profiles while minimizing rejection episodes.[75] Choice of the immunosuppressive regimen is protocolized for each program, but basic principles are similar. CNIs in combination with steroids have remained the mainstay of immunosuppressive regimens in LT.[76] Interleukin-2 (IL-2) receptor monoclonal antibodies such as basiliximab are used as part of renoprotective strategy in combination with mycophenolate mofetil (MMF) with delayed introduction of low-dose tacrolimus.[77] CNIs can cause dose-independent renal and neurotoxicity.

DEDICATED LIVER INTENSIVE CARE TEAMS

It has been well accepted that designated liver transplant anesthesia teams improve outcomes in LT in terms of reduced blood transfusion, need for mechanical ventilation, and duration of intensive care unit (ICU) stay.[78] The same concept has been extended to liver intensive care in many centers in the world. Designated medical and nursing teams can provide consistent high standards of care.

It is important to identify and assemble a dedicated team of clinical pharmacists, physiotherapists, and nutritional therapists to prioritize and attend to the unique needs of these patients. Continuous quality improvement can be achieved by regular on-the-job training, conducting good quality research and audits, and having academic training programs for all specialists involved in the care of patients after LT.

MULTIDISCIPLINARY INPUT

Care of these patients should emphasize collaborative teamwork for achieving good outcomes. Along with the intensivist, inputs from the transplant surgeons, hepatologists, and infectious disease specialists must be integrated into the daily care plan for these patients.

CONCLUSION

To conclude, proper understanding of the altered pathophysiology in these patients and knowledge of common surgical complications are essential for the intensivists managing these patients. Anticipation and preemptive management of complications as much as possible are essential because of the diminished reserve in these patients. Involving multidisciplinary teams and efficient communication are important factors in the critical care management of LT recipients.

REFERENCES

1. O'Leary JG, Lepe R, Davis GL. Indications for liver transplantation. Gastroenterology. 2008;134(6):1764-76.
2. Kow AWC, Liu J, Patel MS, de Martin E, Reddy MS, Soejima Y, et al. Post living donor liver transplantation small-for-size syndrome: definitions, timelines, biochemical, and clinical factors for diagnosis: guidelines from the ILTS-iLDLT-LTSI consensus conference. Transplantation. 2023; 107(10):2226-37.
3. Lai JC, Feng S, Roberts JP. An examination of liver offers to candidates on the liver transplant wait-list. Gastroenterology. 2012;143(5):1261-5.
4. Barshes NR, Horwitz IB, Franzini L, Vierling JM, Goss JA. Waitlist mortality decreases with increased use of extended criteria donor liver grafts at adult liver transplant centers. Am J Transplant. 2007;7(5):1265-70.
5. Hoeter K, Heinrich S, Wollschläger D, Melchior F, Noack A, Tripke V, et al. The optimal fluid strategy matters in liver surgery: a retrospective single centre analysis of 666 consecutive liver resections. J Clin Med. 2023;12(12):3962.
6. Olthoff KM, Kulik L, Samstein B, Kaminski M, Abecassis M, Emond J, et al. Validation of a current definition of early allograft dysfunction in liver transplant recipients and analysis of risk factors. Liver Transpl. 2010;16(8):943-9.
7. Chae MS, Kim Y, Lee N, Chung HS, Park CS, Lee J, et al. Graft regeneration and functional recovery in patients with early allograft dysfunction after living-donor liver transplantation. Ann Transplant. 2018;23:481-90.
8. VanWagner LB, Lapin B, Levitsky J, Wilkins JT, Abecassis MM, Skaro AI, et al. High early cardiovascular mortality after liver transplantation. Liver Transpl. 2014;20(11):1306-16.
9. VanWagner LB, Serper M, Kang R, Levitsky J, Hohmann S, Abecassis M, et al. Factors associated with major adverse cardiovascular events after liver transplantation among a national sample. Am J Transplant. 2016;16(9):2684-94.
10. Koshy AN, Farouque O, Cailes B, Ko J, Han HC, Weinberg L, et al. Prediction of perioperative cardiovascular events in liver transplantation. Transplantation. 2021;105(3):593-601.
11. Smith NK, Zerillo J, Kim SJ, Efune GE, Wang C, Pai SL, et al. Intraoperative cardiac arrest during adult liver transplantation: incidence and risk factor analysis from 7 academic centers in the United States. Anesth Analg. 2021; 132(1):130-9.
12. Matsusaki T, Hilmi IA, Planinsic RM, Humar A, Sakai T. Cardiac arrest during adult liver transplantation: a single institution's experience with 1238 deceased donor transplants. Liver Transpl. 2013;19(11):1262-71.
13. Kiszka-Kanowitz M, Henriksen JH, Møller S, Bendtsen F. Blood volume distribution in patients with cirrhosis: aspects of the dual-head gamma-camera technique. J Hepatol. 2001;35(5):605-12.
14. Møller S, Bendtsen F, Henriksen JH. Effect of volume expansion on systemic hemodynamics and central and arterial blood volume in cirrhosis. Gastroenterology. 1995; 109(6):1917-25.
15. Gerbes A, Jüngst D, Remien J, Sauerbruch T, Paumgartner G. Evidence for down-regulation of beta-2-adrenoceptors in cirrhotic patients with severe ascites. Lancet. 1986; 327(8495):1409-11.
16. Ma Z, Miyamoto A, Lee SS. Role of altered beta-adrenoceptor signal transduction in the pathogenesis of cirrhotic cardiomyopathy in rats. Gastroenterology. 1996; 110(4): 1191-8.
17. Ferlitsch A, Pleiner J, Mittermayer F, Schaller G, Homoncik M, Peck-Radosavljevic M, et al. Vasoconstrictor hyporeactivity can be reversed by antioxidants in patients with advanced alcoholic cirrhosis of the liver and ascites. Crit Care Med. 2005;33(9):2028-33.
18. Izzy M, VanWagner LB, Lin G, Altieri M, Findlay JY, Oh JK, et al. Redefining cirrhotic cardiomyopathy for the modern era. Hepatology. 2020;71(1):334-45.
19. Chahal D, Liu H, Shamatutu C, Sidhu H, Lee SS, Marquez V. Review article: comprehensive analysis of cirrhotic cardiomyopathy. Aliment Pharmacol Ther. 2021;53(9): 985-98.
20. Liu H, Naser JA, Lin G, Lee SS. Cardiomyopathy in cirrhosis: from pathophysiology to clinical care. JHEP Rep. 2024; 6(1):100911.
21. Izzy M, Oh J, Watt KD. Cirrhotic cardiomyopathy after transplantation: neither the transient nor innocent bystander. Hepatology. 2018;68(5):2008-15.
22. Therapondos G, Flapan AD, Plevris JN, Hayes PC. Cardiac morbidity and mortality related to orthotopic liver transplantation. Liver Transpl. 2004;10(12):1441-53.
23. Therapondos G, Flapan AD, Dollinger MM, Garden OJ, Plevris JN, Hayes PC. Cardiac function after orthotopic liver transplantation and the effects of immunosuppression: a prospective randomized trial comparing cyclosporin (Neoral) and tacrolimus. Liver Transpl. 2002;8(8):690-700.

24. Torregrosa M, Aguadé S, Dos L, Segura R, Gónzalez A, Evangelista A, et al. Cardiac alterations in cirrhosis: reversibility after liver transplantation. J Hepatol. 2005; 42(1):68-74.
25. Shin WJ, Kim YK, Song JG, Kim SH, Choi SS, Song JH, et al. Alterations in QT interval in patients undergoing living donor liver transplantation. Transplant Proc. 2011; 43(1):170-3.
26. Adigun AQ, Pinto AG, Flockhart DA, Gorski JC, Li L, Hall SD, et al. Effect of cirrhosis and liver transplantation on the gender difference in QT interval. Am J Cardiol. 2005; 95(5): 691-4.
27. Krag A, Bendtsen F, Mortensen C, Henriksen JH, Møller S. Effects of a single terlipressin administration on cardiac function and perfusion in cirrhosis. Eur J Gastroenterol Hepatol. 2010;22(9):1085-92.
28. Møller S, Bendtsen F. The pathophysiology of arterial vasodilatation and hyperdynamic circulation in cirrhosis. Liver Int. 2018;38(4):570-80.
29. Navarro-Vergara DI, Roldan-Valadez E, Cueto-Robledo G, Jurado-Hernandez MY. Portopulmonary hypertension: prevalence, clinical and hemodynamic features. Curr Probl Cardiol. 2021;46(3):100747.
30. Savale L, Guimas M, Ebstein N, Fertin M, Jevnikar M, Renard S, et al. Portopulmonary hypertension in the current era of pulmonary hypertension management. J Hepatol. 2020;73(1):130-9.
31. Jose A, Kay D, Elwing JM. Treatment of portopulmonary hypertension (PoPH): a review. J Liver Transpl. 2022;6:100071.
32. Krowka MJ. The liver-lung vascular connection. BRN Rev. 2017;23:204-19.
33. Lee BC, Li F, Hanje AJ, Mumtaz K, Boudoulas KD, Lilly SM. Effectively screening for coronary artery disease in patients undergoing orthotopic liver transplant evaluation. J Transpl. 2016;2016(1):7187206.
34. Patel SS, Lin FP, Rodriguez VA, Bhati C, John BV, Pence T, et al. The relationship between coronary artery disease and cardiovascular events early after liver transplantation. Liver Int. 2019;39(7):1363-71.
35. Prevalence of coronary heart disease—United States, 2006-2010. MMWR Morb Mortal Wkly Rep. 2011;60(40):1377-81.
36. Machicao VI, Balakrishnan M, Fallon MB. Pulmonary complications in chronic liver disease. Hepatology. 2014; 59(4):1627-37.
37. Ginès P, Schrier RW. Renal failure in cirrhosis. N Engl J Med. 2009;361(13):1279-90.
38. Ginés P, Berl T, Bernardi M, Bichet DG, Hamon G, Jiménez W, et al. Hyponatremia in cirrhosis: from pathogenesis to treatment. Hepatology. 1998;28(3):851-64.
39. Piano S, Favaretto E, Tonon M, Antonelli G, Brocca A, Sticca A, et al. Including relative adrenal insufficiency in definition and classification of acute-on-chronic liver failure. Clin Gastroenterol Hepatol. 2020;18(5):1188-96.e3.
40. Wagener G, Kovalevskaya G, Minhaz M, Mattis F, Emond JC, Landry DW. Vasopressin deficiency and vasodilatory state in end-stage liver disease. J Cardiothorac Vasc Anesth. 2011;25(4):665-70.
41. Møller S, Bernardi M. Interactions of the heart and the liver. Eur Heart J. 2013;34(36):2804-11.
42. Eimer MJ, Wright JM, Wang EC, Kulik L, Blei A, Flamm S, et al. Frequency and significance of acute heart failure following liver transplantation. Am J Cardiol. 2008;101(2):242-4.
43. Zmaili M, Alzubi J, Alkhayyat M, Cohen J, Alkharabsheh S, Rana M, et al. Takotsubo cardiomyopathy in orthotopic liver transplant recipients: a cohort study using multi-center pooled electronic health record data. World J Hepatol. 2022;14(2):400-10.
44. Morkane CM, Sapisochin G, Mukhtar AM, Reyntjens KMEM, Wagener G, Spiro M, et al. Perioperative fluid management and outcomes in adult deceased donor liver transplantation—a systematic review of the literature and expert panel recommendations. Clin Transpl. 2022; 36(10):e14651.
45. Kohli M, Garg N, Sindwani G, Tempe D, Pamecha V, Pasupuleti SSR. Effect of positive cumulative fluid balance on postoperative complications after living donor liver transplantation: a retrospective analysis. Indian J Anaesth. 2021;65(5):383-9.
46. Codes L, de Souza YG, D'Oliveira RAC, Bastos JLA, Bittencourt PL. Cumulative positive fluid balance is a risk factor for acute kidney injury and requirement for renal replacement therapy after liver transplantation. World J Transplant. 2018;8(2):44-51.
47. Reydellet L, Blasco V, Mercier MF, Antonini F, Nafati C, Harti-Souab K, et al. Impact of a goal-directed therapy protocol on postoperative fluid balance in patients undergoing liver transplantation: a retrospective study. Ann Fr Anesth Reanim. 2014;33(4):e47-54.
48. Nguyen HB, Jaehne AK, Jayaprakash N, Semler MW, Hegab S, Yataco AC, et al. Early goal-directed therapy in severe sepsis and septic shock: insights and comparisons to ProCESS, ProMISe, and ARISE. Crit Care. 2016;20(1):160.
49. Cardenas A, Gines P, Runyon BA. Is albumin infusion necessary after large volume paracentesis? Liver Int. 2009; 29(5):636-40.
50. Kirchner C, Dirkmann D, Treckmann JW, Paul A, Hartmann M, Saner FH, et al. Coagulation management with factor concentrates in liver transplantation: a single-center experience. Transfusion. 2014;54(10 Pt 2):2760-8.
51. Han X, Davis AM, Parker WF. Managing adult acute and acute-on-chronic liver failure in the ICU. JAMA. 2021; 326(19):1964-5.
52. D'Aragon F, Belley-Cote EP, Meade MO, Lauzier F, Adhikari NK, Briel M, et al. Blood pressure targets for vasopressor therapy: a systematic review. Shock. 2015;43(6):530-9.
53. Landry DW, Oliver JA. The pathogenesis of vasodilatory shock. N Engl J Med. 2001;345(8):588-95.

54. Russell JA, Walley KR, Singer J, Gordon AC, Hébert PC, Cooper DJ, et al. Vasopressin versus norepinephrine infusion in patients with septic shock. N Engl J Med. 2008; 358(9):877-87.
55. Bezinover D, Mukhtar A, Wagener G, Wray C, Blasi A, Kronish K, et al. Hemodynamic instability during liver transplantation in patients with end-stage liver disease: a consensus document from ILTS, LICAGE, and SATA. Transplantation. 2021;105(10):2184-200.
56. Palanisamy AP, Nadig SN, Chedister GR, Dowden JE, Koch DG, Stoll WD, et al. Use of intra-aortic counterpulsation in cardiogenic shock post-liver transplantation. Clin Transpl. 2017;31(7):e13002.
57. Hogen R, Sedra AH, Motamed A, Emamaullee J. The evolving role of ECMO in liver transplantation. Curr Opin Organ Transplant. 2021;26(3):333-8.
58. Krowka MJ, Fallon MB, Kawut SM, Fuhrmann V, Heimbach JK, Ramsay MA, et al. International liver transplant society practice guidelines: diagnosis and management of hepatopulmonary syndrome and portopulmonary hypertension. Transplantation. 2016;100(7):1440-52.
59. Bohman JK, Findlay JY, Krowka MJ. ECMO and POPH: more help for the right heart. Liver Transpl. 2021;27(5):627-8.
60. Chadha R, Sakai T, Rajakumar A, Shingina A, Yoon U, Patel D, et al. Anesthesia and critical care for the prediction and prevention for small-for-size syndrome: guidelines from the ILTS-iLDLT-LTSI consensus conference. Transplantation. 2023;107(10):2216-25.
61. Pinsky MR, Cecconi M, Chew MS, De Backer D, Douglas I, Edwards M, et al. Effective hemodynamic monitoring. Crit Care. 2022;26(1):294.
62. Aurilio C, Sansone P, Barbarisi M, Pota V, Giaccari LG, Coppolino F, et al. Mechanisms of action of carbapenem resistance. Antibiotics. 2022;11(3):421.
63. Bezinover D, Zerillo J, Chadha RM, Wagener G, Blasi A, Johnson T, et al. Use of transesophageal echocardiography for liver transplantation: a global comparison of practice from the ILTS, SATA, and LICAGE. Transplantation. 2024;108(7):1570-83.
64. Schumann R, Mandell MS, Mercaldo N, Michaels D, Robertson A, Banerjee A, et al. Anesthesia for liver transplantation in United States academic centers: intraoperative practice. J Clin Anesth. 2013;25(7):542-50.
65. Jung JY, Sohn JY, Lim L, Cho H, Ju JW, Yoon HK, et al. Pulmonary artery catheter monitoring versus arterial waveform-based monitoring during liver transplantation: a retrospective cohort study. Scientific Rep. 2023;13(1): 19947.
66. Murata Y, Imai T, Takeda C, Mizota T, Kawamoto S. Agreement between continuous cardiac output measured by the fourth-generation FloTrac/Vigileo system and a pulmonary artery catheter in adult liver transplantation. Scientific Rep. 2022;12(1):11198.
67. Vetrugno L, Bignami E, Barbariol F, Langiano N, De Lorenzo F, Matellon C, et al. Cardiac output measurement in liver transplantation patients using pulmonary and transpulmonary thermodilution: a comparative study. J Clin Monit Comput. 2019;33(2):223-31.
68. Young CC, Harris EM, Vacchiano C, Bodnar S, Bukowy B, Elliott RRD, et al. Lung-protective ventilation for the surgical patient: international expert panel-based consensus recommendations. Br J Anaesth. 2019;123(6):898-913.
69. Saner FH, Olde Damink SW, Pavlakovic G, Sotiropoulos GC, Radtke A, Treckmann J, et al. How far can we go with positive end-expiratory pressure (PEEP) in liver transplant patients? J Clin Anesth. 2010;22(2):104-9.
70. Larsson JS, Bragadottir G, Redfors B, Ricksten SE. Renal function and oxygenation are impaired early after liver transplantation despite hyperdynamic systemic circulation. Crit Care. 2017;21(1):87.
71. Wadei HM, Lee DD, Croome KP, Mai L, Leonard D, Mai ML, et al. Early allograft dysfunction is associated with higher risk of renal nonrecovery after liver transplantation. Transplant Direct. 2018;4(4):e352.
72. Knight SR, Oniscu GC, Devey L, Simpson KJ, Wigmore SJ, Harrison EM. Use of renal replacement therapy may influence graft outcomes following liver transplantation for acute liver failure: a propensity-score matched population-based retrospective cohort study. PLoS One. 2016;11(3): e0148782.
73. Plauth M, Bernal W, Dasarathy S, Merli M, Plank LD, Schutz T, et al. ESPEN guideline on clinical nutrition in liver disease. Clin Nutr. 2019;38(2):485-521.
74. Evans L, Rhodes A, Alhazzani W, Antonelli M, Coopersmith CM, French C, et al. Surviving sepsis campaign: international guidelines for management of sepsis and septic shock 2021. Intensive Care Med. 2021;47(11):1181-247.
75. European Association for the Study of the Liver. EASL clinical practice guidelines: liver transplantation. J Hepatol. 2016;64(2):433-85.
76. Wiesner RH, Fung JJ. Present state of immunosuppressive therapy in liver transplant recipients. Liver Transpl. 2011;17 Suppl 3:S1-9.
77. Neuberger JM, Mamelok RD, Neuhaus P, Pirenne J, Samuel D, Isoniemi H, et al. Delayed introduction of reduced-dose tacrolimus, and renal function in liver transplantation: the 'ReSpECT' study. Am J Transplant. 2009;9(2):327-36.
78. Hevesi ZG, Lopukhin SY, Mezrich JD, Andrei AC, Lee M. Designated liver transplant anesthesia team reduces blood transfusion, need for mechanical ventilation, and duration of intensive care. Liver Transpl. 2009;15(5):460-5.

CHAPTER 8

Anesthetic Considerations in Liver Transplant Surgery and How does it Impact Postoperative Outcome?

Ambreen Sawant, Aaditya A Prabhudesai

INTRODUCTION

Decompensated liver cirrhosis is a multisystem disorder with extrahepatic organ involvement during the disease. Anesthetizing a patient for liver transplantation (LT) requires a thorough understanding of the altered physiology associated with liver dysfunction; the extent of systemic involvement; and stewardship in hemodynamic monitoring, fluid, and acid-base management. A command on coagulation and bleeding management, along with skills for invasive procedures such as vascular cannulations, transesophageal echocardiography (TEE), enhances the quality of care. Moreover, older and sicker candidates with multiple comorbidities are being transplanted, making it an uphill and challenging task for the anesthesiologists. The quality of perioperative care remains vital for optimal graft function, overall outcome, and patient survival. Preoperative optimisation, prehabilitation and intraoperative managemnt plays vital role in overall post operative outcome.

PATHOPHYSIOLOGY OF END-STAGE LIVER DISEASE

End-stage liver disease (ESLD) is a systemic disorder **(Flowchart 1)** with extrahepatic organ damage of varying degrees.[1]

Splanchnic arteriolar vasodilation is a key feature of decompensated liver disease, leading to blood pooling, hypovolemia, and compensatory mechanisms such as activation of the renin-angiotensin-aldosterone system (RAAS), vasopressin system, and sympathetic nervous system (SNS), which result in vasoconstriction, sodium retention, ascites, kidney dysfunction, and hepatorenal syndrome (HRS). HRS is considered a subset of acute kidney injury (AKI) in cirrhotic patients with ascites and is diagnosed when there is no response to diuretic withdrawal and plasma expansion with albumin in the absence of shock or nephrotoxic drugs. HRS negatively impacts waitlist mortality, and LT is the curative treatment.

Flowchart 1: Pathophysiology of end-stage liver disease.

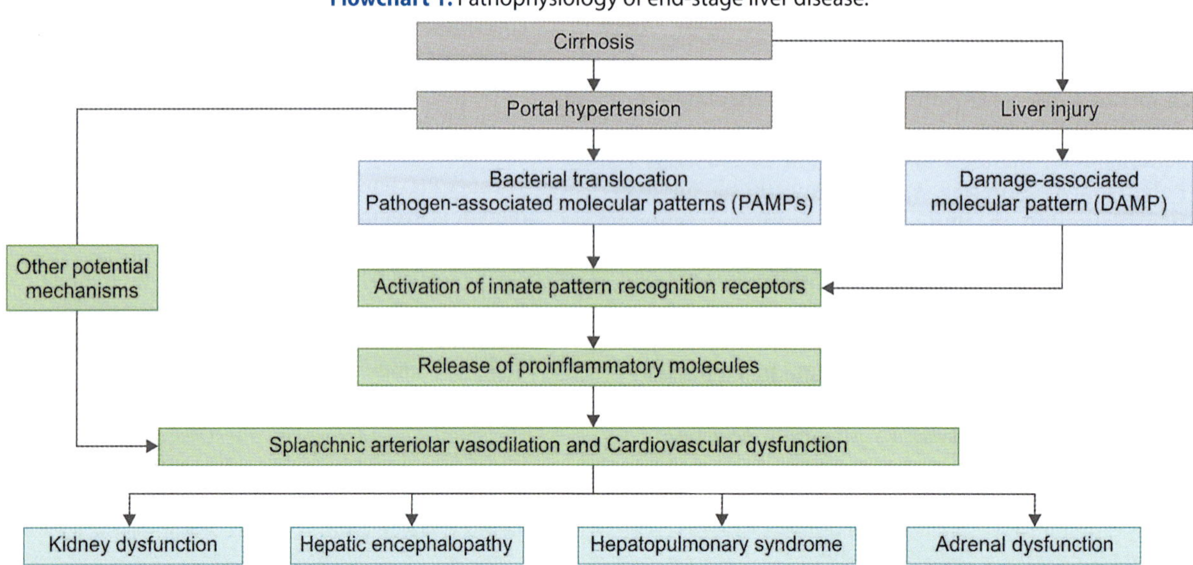

Source: Reproduced from European Association for the Study of the Liver 2018.[1]

Preoperative optimization and bridging to transplantation are challenging, with renal replacement therapy serving as a potential perioperative rescue, though its side effects must be considered. In selected cases where AKI persists for >6 weeks, with a documented glomerular filtration rate (GFR) of ≤25 mL/min every 7 days or ongoing dialysis dependence, simultaneous or subsequent liver-kidney transplantation may be considered as a treatment option.

Cirrhotic cardiomyopathy (CCM) results from the combination of hypervolemia, maladaptation of RAAS and SNS, and uncleared vasodilatory molecules such as nitric oxide (NO), leading to peripheral vasodilation and reduced systemic vascular resistance (SVR).[2]

The current definition for CCM involves systolic dysfunction, defined as ejection fraction <50% or global longitudinal strain (GLS) <18% and/or a diastolic dysfunction that includes three of four variables, left atrial volume index (LAVI) <34 mL/m^2, E/e′ >15, tricuspid regurgitation velocity >2.8 m/s, and septal e′ velocity <7 cm/s.

The emerging pandemic of obesity has put metabolic-associated steatotic liver diseases (MASLD) related chronic liver disease (CLD), a rising cause of ESLD. MASLD and diabetes have a high association with coronary artery diseases (CADs) and may need advanced cardiac evaluation before transplant. While the hemodynamic and metabolic profile accompanied with patient inactivity does not allow manifestations of overt CAD, this may present in the postoperative period and combination with immunosuppression.[3]

The respiratory system is uniquely affected in decompensated cirrhosis, and the two unique complications with significant perioperative implications are hepatopulmonary syndrome (HPS) and portopulmonary hypertension (PoPH). HPS has its own challenges in perioperative management. This discussion is beyond the scope of this chapter. Identification of HPS in preoperative evaluation, documenting alveolar arterial oxygen gradient, intra pulmonary shunts are essential. Intraoperative strategies include nitric oxide therapy. In selected cases, extra corporeal oxygenation may be required. The use of NO in immediate post operative ICU proves to be essential for optimal oxygenation and prevention of hypoxic injury to the graft.

Mild PoPH (mPAP 25–35 mm Hg) and moderate PoPH (mPAP 35–45 mm Hg) can be considered for transplant after 2–4 weeks of treatment with pulmonary vasodilators. Severe PoPH (mPAP >45 mm Hg) remains a contraindication to LT.

Hepatic hydrothorax is asymptomatic in most cases. Massive effusion can sometimes cause respiratory distress with lung collapse, requiring drainage and optimization of the lung function before LT. Persistent preoperative hydrothorax can lead to trapped lung syndrome and higher postoperative morbidity and mortality.[4]

Immune dysfunction leads to increased susceptibility to infection, further accentuated with the use of immunosuppression medications, especially with multiple indwelling catheters and lines in these patients.

End-stage liver disease rebalances the *coagulation system* to a new threshold, leaving the static tests of coagulation practically of no use to guide transfusion. Liver dysfunction has been traditionally associated with coagulopathy; however, with an improved understanding of coagulation physiology, ESLD is now considered a state of altered coagulation with a risk of both thrombosis and bleeding.[5] Dynamic tests of coagulation such as thromboelastogram (TEG) and rotational thromboelastometry (ROTEM) have become essential monitoring tools to guide transfusion in this population, closely reflecting in vivo coagulation and shorter turnaround time (TAT).

Encephalopathy is a very common decompensation of liver disease, often occult, recovering posttransplant. The presence of hepatic encephalopathy (HE) significantly reduces the anesthetic requirement in proportion to the grades of encephalopathy.[6] On-table extubation is usually not considered in the presence of preoperative significant encephalopathy.

Common metabolic and electrolyte abnormalities are hyponatremia, hypo/hyperkalemia, hypomagnesemia, mixed metabolic acidosis, hypocalcemia, and hyperglycemia, all needing continuous monitoring and management in the perioperative period.

Preoperative Evaluation of the Recipient

Liver transplantation is a complex abdominal surgery that carries significant risks, including fluid shifts and bleeding. A comprehensive preoperative evaluation is conducted for all recipients, often involving a multidisciplinary team to assist in decision-making. Each organ system is assessed, and risk stratification is performed accordingly. The primary goal of these tests is not only to determine surgical fitness but also to identify any absolute contraindications to the procedure, such as severe PoPH, infections, or the spread of extrahepatic carcinoma in cases of hepatocellular carcinoma (HCC). Timing is extremely crucial, as too much delay leads to worsening decompensation, and too early transplant without proper optimization of physiological reserve leads to worse post-LT outcome.

The preanesthesia consultation starts with a detailed history that covers the etiology, progression, decompensations, and any other comorbidities. The severity of liver disease is commonly categorized using scores such as Child–Pugh, model for end-stage liver disease (MELD) for adults, and pediatric end-stage liver disease (PELD) models for pediatric patients.

The biochemistry panel typically includes a complete blood count, liver and renal function tests, as well as an in-depth evaluation of coagulopathy status, including prothrombin time (PT)/international normalized ratio (INR), fibrinogen, D-dimers, and clotting tests such as TEG and ROTEM. Lung evaluation includes clinical examination, pulse oximetry, chest radiographs, and, when necessary, high-resolution computed tomography (CT) scans and pulmonary function tests (PFTs). Diffusing capacity of the lungs for carbon monoxide (DLCO) can help rule out interstitial lung diseases, while a technetium-99m-labeled macroaggregated albumin (MAA) scan is done to assess severity in case of HPS.

Cardiac assessment involves evaluating functional capacity, a resting electrocardiogram (ECG), and an echocardiogram. Current guidelines recommend that patients older than 60 years (or 50 years in India), diabetics, and those with metabolic-associated fatty liver disease (MASLD) undergo further evaluation with a CT coronary angiogram or standard coronary angiography due to their increased risk of CAD. Dobutamine stress echocardiography (DSE) and myocardial perfusion imaging can be used, although their reliability is limited since patients often have a reduced heart rate (HR) response, making these tests potentially inconclusive.[3] Coronary artery calcium scoring (CaCS) can be helpful in high-risk patients when deciding whether to proceed with invasive coronary angiography (preoperative cardiac evaluation has been discussed in detail in the chapter 3).

ANESTHESIA MANAGEMENT OF LIVER RECIPIENT

Recipient surgery is divided into three phases, and each comes with its unique challenges **(Flowchart 2)**.

1. *Dissection/preanhepatic phase:* It starts from skin incision to clamping of the main portal vein. The liver is dissected from all its attachments and removed after clamping the major inflow and outflow vessels. This phase can be associated with significant fluid shifts due to drainage of ascites, bleeding (surgical/coagulopathic), liver manipulation, and traction on inferior vena cava (IVC), causing reduced preload, with subsequent hemodynamic changes. In case of any previous abdominal surgery, the duration of this phase may be extended, and the blood loss may increase. The main concern in this phase is to keep up with fluid shifts and electrolytes. Here, goal-directed fluid management plays a pivotal role.
2. *Anhepatic phase:* This is a phase of complete absence of liver function, characterized by hemodynamic, coagulation, and metabolic disturbances. It starts with clamping of the portal vein and ends with reperfusion of the new graft. This phase can be quite dynamic with challenges of coagulopathy, acidosis, electrolyte imbalance, hypoglycemia, and hypothermia when prolonged. The IVC is either partially or completely clamped, causing further hemodynamic compromise due to poor venous return and, hence, reduced cardiac output (CO). Patients without significant portal hypertension or portosystemic collaterals poorly tolerate portal vein clamping, often needing portocaval/mesocaval shunt. Maintaining the

Flowchart 2: Intraoperative phases in liver transplantation surgery.

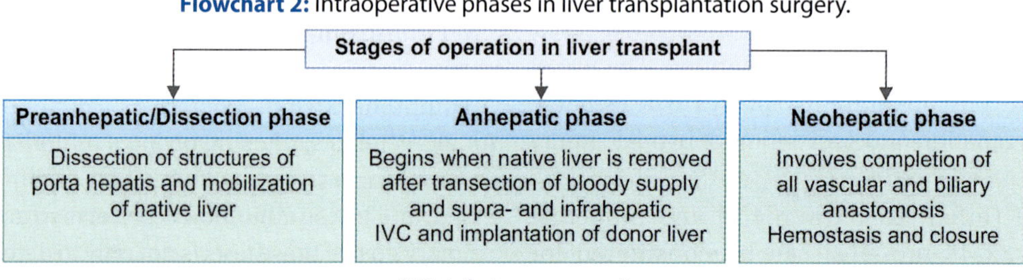

(IVC: inferior vena cava)

end organ perfusion, e.g., cerebral perfusion, remains an indispensable goal usually guided by mean arterial pressure (MAP).

The absence of liver from the circulation aggravates acidosis and poses a risk of hypoglycemia and dyselectrolytemia, especially hypocalcemia and hyperkalemia. Serially performed arterial blood gases (ABGs) can provide the pH, partial pressure of oxygen (pO_2), partial pressure of carbon dioxide (PCO_2), bicarbonate, sodium, potassium, chloride, ionized calcium, hemoglobin or hematocrit, and, most importantly, lactates.

An adequate fluid balance is necessary to maintain the circulating volume but not to cause overload that can increase bleeding due to the exaggeration of portal hypertension. Adequate fluid rescussitation with appropriate choice of the fluid (including 5% or 20% Albumin and/or Blood or blood product reamin necessary prerequisite of optimal homeostasis in anhepatic phase. The extent and duration of IVC clamp, duration of anhepatic reflects in kidney functions in post operative period.)

3. *Neohepatic phase:* This phase begins with the initiation of portal flow to the new graft and is the main event of the recipient surgery. The hallmark of this phase is the postreperfusion syndrome (PRS), defined by significant hypotension occurring as the reduction in MAP >30% from the baseline, within the first 5 minutes of opening the portal vein and sustained for >1 minute.[7] A sudden rush of cold, acidotic blood into the new graft causes transient depression of myocardial contractility and chronotropy, along with systemic vasodilation, resulting in significant to sometimes profound hemodynamic changes. Arrhythmias, including asystole, have been reported during reperfusion. Bleeding can occur from vascular anastomosis during this phase. The phase is characterized by heparin-like molecules from the cold graft worsening the coagulopathic field. Graft dysfunction can present as coagulopathy, new onset, or persistence of the deranged coagulation. PRS is more commonly seen in extended-criteria cadaveric grafts. Appropriate combination of inotropes (noradrenaline or vasopressin) and intravenous fluid remain key to maintain the circulatory volume and end organ perfusion. The postoperative recovery from damage caused by reactive oxygen species may be reduced by use of scavenging molecules like methyl prednisolone (dose remains dependent on variables like etiology of liver disease, decompensations, severity of the disease and weight), 20% mannitol and at times infusion of *N*-acetyl cysteine.

After the completion of the vascular anastomosis, the last phase of recipient surgery is completed with biliary anastomosis. Early indicators of a functioning graft are improving metabolic and hemodynamic parameters, urine output, presence of bile, and maintenance of blood sugar level and temperature. The importance of ABG analysis is again highlighted here, as the single investigation panel provides important information. The metabolic acidosis is corrected after the new liver starts functioning. This is reflected in the normalizing (decreasing) trend of the lactates and bicarbonates. These are also some of the first signs of the early graft function. This remains one of the criterion for on table or early extubation.

INDUCTION AND MAINTENANCE OF ANESTHESIA

Cirrhosis alters the pharmacodynamics (p/d) and pharmacokinetics (p/k) of anesthetic drugs, as the liver remains the major site for xenobiotic metabolism.[8] A transplant anesthesiologist should be well acquainted with drug metabolism in his armamentarium in the operating room (OR). Hypoalbuminemia, HE, fluid and water retention with reduced central plasma volume, and hyperdynamic circulation all influence anesthetic drug levels. Bioavailability of anesthetic agents is greatly increased due to the above factors, reducing the dosage requirement.

The most preferred induction regimen includes intravenous (IV) propofol along with short-acting opioids and muscle relaxants. The liver is very efficient at propofol metabolism, with a blood extraction ratio of 90% as long as the hepatic perfusion is maintained. Extrahepatic sites account for 40% of clearance. Hepatic metabolism is mainly through glucuronidation, followed by renal excretion, making it an excellent choice even in cirrhotic patients. Etomidate can be used in patients with left ventricular dysfunction.

Short-acting opioids such as fentanyl or remifentanil are commonly used. Fentanyl is the most preferred and has an excellent safety profile when used in prescribed doses, including infusions. Remifentanil is an excellent choice for infusion due to its ester hydrolysis, allowing rapid titration of doses and facilitating fast-tracking, including OR extubation. The major disadvantage of remifentanil is the lack of residual analgesia.

Atracurium and cisatracurium are commonly used nondepolarizing muscle relaxants. Sharing the metabolic pathway through Hoffman elimination and ester hydrolysis, cisatracurium has a longer onset of action but with much less histamine release, better cardiovascular stability and superior potency.[9] Vecuronium is not used due to its hepatic metabolism. Rocuronium can be used for induction, chiefly in rapid sequence induction (RSI). With advent of suggamadex, use of rocuronium has become safer and more common.

Indications for RSI remain standard. The presence of tense ascites does not necessitate RSI.

Maintenance of anesthesia with a balanced technique using a combination of inhalational agents, short-acting muscle relaxant, and opioid is routinely preferred. The use of total intravenous anesthesia (TIVA) using propofol, opioid, and muscle relaxant can achieve better hemodynamic control over inhalational agents. Most inhalational agents used in modern anesthesia practice are hepatosafe. The modern anesthesia machines have revolutionised the intraoperative management of long surgeries like LT using low flows that overall reduces amount of inhalational agent required. Infusions of short-acting muscle relaxants such as atracurium and opioids such as fentanyl and remifentanil help with fast tracking.

Preoxygenation during induction is a good practice to follow and can be particularly useful in patients with tense ascites, moderate to large hydrothorax, and HPS with hypoxemia. One should be extremely gentle during laryngoscopy and intubation, more so in a coagulopathic recipient. Mucosal trauma can cause significant oozing and crust formation, swelling, and edema. Upper airway edema is a common occurrence in sicker recipients and can exacerbate postextubation, causing hoarseness and stridor, adding to postoperative morbidity, and tissue handling should be more respectful. Insertion of Ryle's tube can rarely cause a rupture of esophageal varices and needs careful handling.

Patient Positioning and Temperature Management

The importance of proper positioning and padding cannot be emphasized enough, with long surgical hours, hypotension, poor skin quality with preexisting edema, and the presence of ecchymoses all adding up to the risk of skin peeling and its consequence in the postoperative period. Temperature control using a multipronged approach with the use of fluid warmers, warming blankets and hemotherm, and forced air warmers (Bair Hugger) is recommended. Hypothermia can worsen coagulopathy. The use of a pneumatic compression device is a standard of care against deep vein thrombosis (DVT) prophylaxis. Routine eye care is advised.

Concept of Volume Restriction

The concept of volume restriction is based on maintaining low central venous pressure (CVP) to prevent liver congestion by minimizing blood loss and reducing the need for transfusions. Elevated CVP can increase splanchnic venous pressure, which can be harmful, particularly for patients with splanchnic vein thrombosis. However, this strategy has its limitations, especially in patients with advanced liver cirrhosis, where a decrease in arterial blood volume and a hypovolemic, hyperactive circulation are common. CVP is not a reliable indicator of actual volume status in cirrhotic patients due to the increased extracellular fluid volume and elevated right atrial pressures. In cases of HRS, traditional CVP targets often fail to accurately assess hypovolemia. Fayed et al. investigated the effects of low CVP and transesophageal Doppler-guided fluid management on blood loss and transfusion requirements during LT.[10] Their comparison showed that while fluid management guided by transesophageal Doppler resulted in slightly less blood loss, packed red blood cell and platelet use was not significantly different, but it did lead to lower colloid use and higher norepinephrine administration. Urine output was significantly lower in the low CVP group during the preanhepatic phase, and lactate levels were notably higher at the end of the anhepatic phase.

Even if the side effects are disregarded, the prophylactic transfusion of blood products can lead to volume overload, raising CVP, and contributing to increased bleeding. Preemptive phlebotomy in the preoperative period can reduce total circulatory volume, thereby decreasing the need for transfusions, as shown in one study.[11] However, it is important to avoid hypoperfusion during fluid restriction to protect kidney function and ensure adequate blood flow to vital organs. Abnormal blood flow, a factor in Virchow's triad, can trigger thrombosis. Kidney injury in the T surgeries is multifactorial and unavoidable. But all efforts must be directed to minimize the same. Thus appropriate fluid theapy is pivotal in limiting the kidney injuty. Immunosuppression with tacrolimus may worsen the course. In some selected cases use of nephroprotective drugs like basiliximab may warranted.

HEMODYNAMIC MONITORING

Recipient surgery is a state of rapidly changing hemodynamics associated with large fluid shifts due to drainage of ascites, traction and handling of the liver, clamping of major vessels such as IVC and portal vein (PV), bleeding and coagulopathy, and, rarely, severe vasoplegia.[9]

The already stressed cardiovascular system of cirrhosis is burdened further during surgery, making it a daunting task to manage hemodynamics. A monitor with continuous inputs on the volume status, myocardial function, organ perfusion, and peripheral oxygen delivery would help maintain homeostasis and guide fluid therapy. This is in addition to the routine monitoring recommended by the American Society of Anesthesiologists (ASA) during surgeries. There is no universal protocol for hemodynamic monitoring in recipients, and it varies from center to center. Also, each center is tailored to patient care to achieve cost-effectiveness. There are varieties of CO monitors available.

Standard Monitoring

As per the ASA guideline, five-lead ECG, pulse oximetry, noninvasive blood pressure (NIBP), and temperature monitoring are routine for all surgeries.

Invasive Monitoring

- A CVP monitor was commonly used by recipients. The use of CVP to guide fluid management is obsolete as CVP is confounded by so many factors (IVC clamp, portal vein clamp, liver handling, diastolic dysfunction, and bleeding) and may not be a true reflection of the volume status. The major use of the CVP trend is to avoid graft congestion and dysfunction.[9]
- Invasive blood pressure measurement, either using radial (peripheral) or femoral/brachial (central) approach, is mandatory in all recipients. In LT, peripheral and central arterial pressures do not correlate well, especially postreperfusion, severe vasodilation, and vasoplegia. Femoral cannulation is safe in experienced hands; complications such as uncontrolled bleeding with hematoma and femoral aneurysm have been reported and can add to the morbidity.[12,13] The preferred route varies according to the institutional and personal preferences of the lead anesthetist. As a general rule, in sicker patients, it is advisable to use the femoral/brachial pressure measurements for central pressures for better monitoring.

CARDIAC OUTPUT MONITORING

Recipient surgery is a state of rapidly changing hemodynamics that needs a closer look at the CO and tissue perfusion. CO is dependent on preload, afterload, and myocardial contractility. Various techniques of CO monitoring that have evolved over the last few decades are based on pulse contour analysis and the thermodilution technique. They vary from noninvasive to invasive. Most of these monitors measure the CO, cardiac index (CI), SVR, and tissue oxygen delivery.

PULMONARY ARTERY CATHETER

Pulmonary artery catheter (PAC) allows the measurement of central venous and pulmonary artery occlusion pressure (PAOP) and is used as a surrogate marker of left ventricular end-diastolic volume (LVEDV) to estimate preload status. Pulmonary artery (PA) catheters can also be used for CO monitoring using the intermittent thermodilution technique, which requires the injection of cold saline solution into the right atrium, and CO is calculated based on the change in temperature of the blood reaching the thermistor at the tip of the catheter using a complex algorithm. It is considered the gold standard for CO but is operator-dependent. The major drawback in liver transplant is during reperfusion when a large amount of cold blood enters the right heart and can underestimate the actual CO.[12] The new generation of PAC allows for continuous CO monitoring, which uses heat instead of cold solution using a thermal filament at PAC tip and calculates temperature drop at distal arterial thermistor in a placed in a central arterial cannula. The limitations of reperfusion remain the same. It can also measure mixed venous oxygen saturation (SvO_2). However, SvO_2 is not reliable as a marker of perfusion during liver transplant due to the surge of desaturated blood during reperfusion.

Though PAC is the gold standard for CO monitoring and is quite safe in experienced hands, it is invasive with its procedural risks, and its use is recommended in a selected group of patients for better outcomes. Perhaps the most genuine indication for PAC use in liver transplant is in patients with PoPH. Mild and moderate POPH patients are not contraindicated for LT but still have high mortality during the perioperative period and need PA pressure monitoring. It can also help in triaging patients cleared pre-LT by unmasking worse PA pressures in the OR before surgery.

CARDIAC OUTPUT USING PULSE CONTOUR ANALYSIS

The left ventricular stroke volume (SV) creates an arterial wave in the vascular tree and is proportional to the CO, which equals to SV × HR. This waveform is used to calculate CO using a complex algorithm. The various CO monitors used are FlowTrac/Vigileo/Volume View (Edward Lifesciences, Irvine, CA, United States), PiCCO (Pulsion Medical System, Munich, Germany), LiDCO (LiDCO Plus, Cambridge, United Kingdom), and, the very latest in the series, HemoSphere (Edward Lifesciences).

PiCCO derives CO by combining the principle of pulse contour analysis and transpulmonary thermodilution technique. PiCCO catheter is an arterial line with a thermistor at the end. It requires jugular venous access along with femoral/brachial access. A cold saline solution is injected in the central venous access, and temperature difference is detected by the thermistor, which is used to calculate the CO. PiCCO has a very comprehensive list of cardiopulmonary parameters along with SV, CO, CI, and SVR; preload indices such as global end-diastolic volume (GEDV) and intrathoracic blood volume (ITBV); and measure of lung water, extravascular lung water (EVLW), indicator of pulmonary edema after initial calibration. Continuous CO is calculated using arterial waveform analysis. In patients undergoing liver transplants, PiCCO-derived CO measurements have been found to correlate well with the gold standard of CO monitoring with PAC thermodilution technique.

Volume View and FlowTrac do not require initial calibration and provide CO using pulse wave analysis. It can be used even with peripheral arterial access. The volume view provides information parameters such as CO, CI, SV, and SVR along with a marker for fluid responsiveness, i.e., stroke volume variation (SVV). Tissue oxygen delivery is a derived parameter and can be calculated using hemoglobin values. The major disadvantage of the volume view is its ineffectiveness during caval clamping and severe vasoplegia with a peripheral arterial line during LT; the values may not correlate with the CO.

However, it should be noted that CO monitoring based on arterial waveform analysis is less accurate in liver transplant settings. For accurate monitoring, continuous transpulmonary thermodilution technique with PAC or TEE is more reliable.[12]

TRANSESOPHAGEAL ECHOCARDIOGRAM

The use of TEE is becoming a common practice for intra-operative CO monitoring. It not only gives information on CO and the volume status but also is a useful guide about myocardial contractility, ventricular dysfunction, intracardiac and pulmonary thrombus formation, systolic anterior mitral leaflet motion leading to left ventricular outflow tract obstruction, and other valvular pathologies. The disadvantages are the need for special training, trauma during insertion, and, very rarely, the rupture of a large esophageal varix, which can result in catastrophic bleeding. Despite challenges and the need for the learning curve, there has been a growing interest in its use in the last few years. Trauma while intubation can be reduced or avoided by the use of video laryngoscope, and insertion of the probe under direct vision. In LT, four midesophageal views are commonly used, thus avoiding the need for distal insertion of the TEE probe, safeguarding to some extent against rupture of esophageal varices. These views are (1) midesophageal four-chamber view, (2) midesophageal right ventricle inflow–outflow tract, (3) aortic valve long-axis view, and (4) midesophageal left ventricle long-axis view.[14] The use of TEE may provide unique, dynamic, robust, and detailed information, pivotal in optimal patient care in the perioperative phase. TEE can be used widely after establishing the safety, quality, and efficacy. Appropriate patient selection remains another area of further study.

BISPECTRAL INDEX

The anesthetic requirement of cirrhotic patients is lower than that of other normal patients receiving anesthesia. Depth of anesthesia monitoring helps with the targeted delivery of anesthetic agents, TIVA, and eventually in fast tracking of these patients for immediate/early extubation. However, with the prevalent use of gas monitors to measure the minimum alveolar concentration (MAC) of anesthetic agents, the need for bispectral index (BIS) monitoring is gradually declining, but it can be useful in acute liver failure with raised intracranial pressures. Some clinicians use BIS to titrate lower dial settings and lower MAC value for appropriate depth of anesthesia.

Bispectral index characteristically increases in the neohepatic period, suggesting adequacy of early graft function.[15]

Fluid Management

Fluid management is central to intraoperative recipient care. Liberal fluid use can result in cumulative weight gain postsurgery, tissue and pulmonary edema resulting in increased ventilation days, ICU days, and hospital stay.[16] Alternatively, restrictive fluid therapy may increase the risk for AKI in the background of other confounding factors such as long ischemia times, cross-clamping of vena cava, immunosuppression medications, and preexisting AKI. Goal-directed fluid therapy (GDFT) helps in achieving better fluid and hemodynamic management in these patients. Balanced salt solutions (BSSs) are preferred. The advantage of BSS is the presence of acetate and its liver-independent metabolism compared to Ringer's lactate (RL), which contains lactate as the base and is dependent on the liver for its metabolism. The use of normal saline (NS) in large quantities can cause hyperchloremic acidosis. Albumin is the preferred colloid. The use of albumin reduces total crystalloid infusion. It is also known to have an anti-inflammatory effect. Albumin replacement is needed to the tune of 7–8 g/L of ascites drained.

Cost remains a concern with its usage. Synthetic colloids do not offer any advantage; in fact, they have major concerns of AKI (starches), interference with coagulation, fibrinolysis, and, rarely, anaphylaxis.

There are no established guidelines for IV fluid management in LT. This should be tailored to the patient's fluid and electrolyte status, ongoing blood loss, and coagulopathy based on the stage of surgery. CO monitors can be a useful tool for GDFT in skilled hands. As per the literature, SVV and pulse pressure variations (PPVs) are more sensitive indicators for monitoring end-diastolic volumes in the left and right ventricles in the dissection phase. PPVs are unreliable once IVC is clamped during anhepatic phase. These tools are also unreliable if tidal volume is <8 mL/kg, driving pressures are <20 cmH_2O, and in the presence of cardiac arrhythmias.[12]

Bleeding and Coagulation Management

Management of bleeding and coagulopathy is one of the challenging aspects of recipient care in the OR. The discussion of the rebalanced state of coagulation[5] in CLD is beyond the scope of this chapter. The advanced liver disease rebalances the coagulation, and it is not always a state of hypocoagulation. In vivo model of coagulation that is initiation, amplification, and propagation helps understand the pathophysiology and balanced coagulation in CLD.

The traditional tests used to assess the coagulopathy may not necessarily predict coagulation disorder. In many patients, focal venous thrombosis (portal venous thrombosis) and bleeding states, e.g., variceal bleed, melena, coexist in decompensated patients with deranged fibrinogen, platelets, etc. Static tests such as PT/INR, platelet count, and serum fibrinogen have long TAT and do not reflect the dynamic state of coagulation during a bleed, with no information on fibrinolysis. Hence, the transfusion of blood and components should be guided by the patient's preoperative coagulation status and hemodynamics in combination with the bleeding. TEG and ROTEM are better guides for in vivo coagulation and, hence, transfusion, perioperative **(Fig. 1)**. Both have shorter TAT, provide point-of-care testing, closely mimic in vivo coagulation, guide product usage, and help in preventing unwanted transfusion with its associated hazards. The use of dynamic tests of coagulation has significantly reduced overall transfusion in liver recipients.

Thromboelastogram is one of the most widely used point-of-care tests. TEG (Haemonetics Corporation, USA) measures the elastic property of fibrin from its formation to complete dissolution. Both TEG and ROTEM graphically express the viscoelastic changes of blood during the clotting process.

The point-of-care coagulation tests (POCTs), a real-time visual display, have advantage over the traditional tests in aspect of faster TAT, evaluation of blood as a wholesome unit for clot formation and strength (evaluation

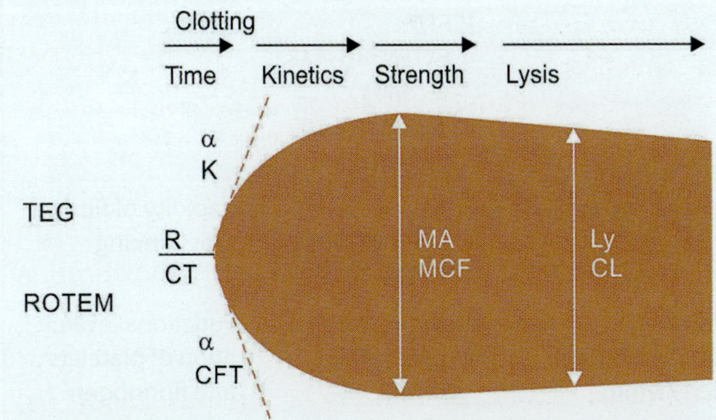

Fig. 1: Point-of-care coagulation tests. Comparison of TEG versus ROTEM. (CFT: clot formation time; CT: clotting time; MA: maximum amplitude; MCF: maximal clot firmness; ROTEM: rotational thromboelastometry; TEG: thromboelastogram)
Source: Reproduced from Clevenger V and Mallett SV.[17]

of the function of clotting factors, platelets, and red cells), leading to overall reduction of excessive transfusion. The POCT underscores that as the measurement of coagulation is done under artificial conditions (kaolin cuvette), the training and competency curve is much longer, being expensive and requiring stringent quality checks.

It is beyond doubt that the number of transfusions has reduced with increasing usage of POCT for coagulation. The data are slowly accumulating. By and large, prolonged R time (Time taken for formation of fibrin strands) of 10 minutes may be due to coagulation factor deficiencies and/or dysfunction or anticoagulants, requiring fresh frozen plasma (FFP) correction, usually in a dose of 10 mL/kg of dry weight **(Table 1)**. Reduced α-angle and increased K time signify platelet deficiency, platelet aggregation dysfunction, and deficiency of dysfunction of fibrinogen. Decreased MA may be caused by platelet deficiency, antiplatelet therapies, or disturbed coagulation factor and/or fibrin formation. In ROTEM, INTEM tracing gives ideas to intrinsic pathway, EXTIM gives ideas to extrinsic pathway, FIBTEM trace provides information about the contribution of fibrinogen in clot formation, HEPTEM trace uncovers coexistent coagulopathy in the presence of systemic heparinization, ECATEM trace diagnoses activity of direct thrombin inhibitors, and APTEM trace diagnoses fibrinolysis. In comparison to TEG, ROTEM has the added advantage of differentiating the need for platelets versus cryoprecipitate (by looking at EXTEM and FIBTEM tracing). Increased Ly30 in TEG may be due to hyperfibrinolysis, which can be treated with the use of Σ-amino caproic acid and its derivatives like tranexamic acid.

TABLE 1: Comparison of interpretation of TEG and ROTEM data.

Thromboelastography (TEG)	***Rotational thromboelastometry (ROTEM)***	***Importance***
R (reaction time): 4–8 minutes	*Clotting time (CT):* • EXTEM: 42–74 seconds • INTEM: 137–246 seconds	Concentration of soluble clotting factors in the blood
K time: 1–4 minutes	*Clot formation time (CFT):* • *EXTEM:* 46–148 seconds • INTEM: 40–100 seconds	Measure of clot kinetic
Alpha angle 47–74°	*Angle:* • EXTEM: 63–81 • INTEM: 71–82	Rapidity of fibrin cross-linking
Maximum amplitude (MA): 55–73 mm	*Maximal clot firmness (MCF):* • EXTEM: 49–71 mm • INTEM: 52–72 mm	Functional evaluation of platelets and fibrinogen concentrate
CL30, CL60	LY30, LY60	Clot stability and fibrinolysis

The Sonoclot measurements detect viscoelastic changes in whole blood, allowing the Sonoclot® Analyzer (Sienco, Inc.) to measure the kinetic forces involved in fibrin formation and clot development. It provides comprehensive information on hemostasis, along with a qualitative graph called the Sonoclot Signature and quantitative values such as clot rate (CR) (the maximum slope during initial fibrin polymerization and clot formation), activated clotting time (ACT), and platelet function results.

Blood and blood product transfusion comes with significant cardiopulmonary consequences such as TRALI, TACO; impacting early endotracheal extubation and post operative pulmonary complications. It also increases the risk of post-transplant infections and sepsis adding to the length of ICU and hospital stay.

Point-of-Care Laboratory Tests

Routine monitoring of oxygen levels, hemoglobin, and other metabolic parameters is essential during LT. Serial ABG testing can be easily done with a bedside monitor at regular intervals during surgery. ABGs provide critical information about the extracellular milieu, including acid–base changes, electrolytes, lactate trend, and ventilation. The major concern during the dissection and anhepatic phase is hypoglycemia, and, hence, a glycemic check is vital.

END OF SURGERY AND FAST-TRACKING

Liver transplantation surgeries, irrespective of live or deceased donation, are now considered for on-table or early endotracheal extubation, early mobilization, and enteral feeding, and fast-tracking has become a standard practice. This has proven to improve the perioperative outcome in terms of reduced rates of respiratory infections, early return of bowel movemnts and resumption of enteral feeding, reduced ICU stay.

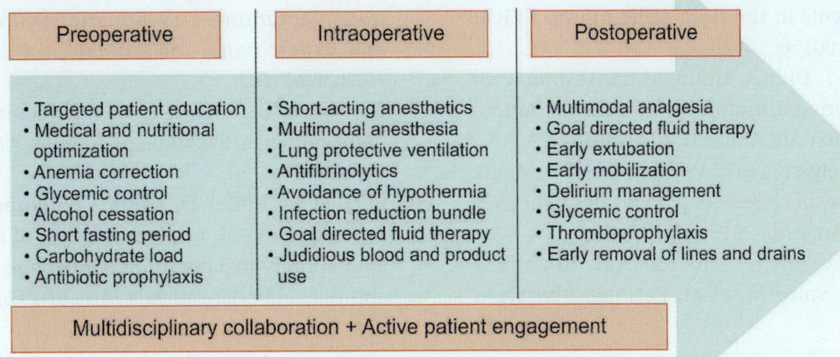

Fig. 2: Components of early recovery after liver transplantation (ERAL). *Source:* Persico M et al.[18]

Many centers have started implementing perioperative principles-based early recovery after liver (ERAL) transplantation protocol **(Fig. 2)**.[18] The advancement in surgical and anesthesia techniques and the gradual advancement in overall knowledge of the field are reflected in fewer blood and blood product transfusions, shorter overall length of stay, earlier discharges, lesser post operative complications and better outcome.

CONCLUSION

Liver transplantation surgeries are becoming common, and the recipient inclusion criterion is widening. This makes the anesthesia more challenging. The concerns for anesthesia in LT include age, etiology, medical status of advanced liver disease, multisystem involvement and decompensations, comorbidities, duration of surgery, and graft function. The considerations revolve around hepato and nephron protective anesthesia, multimodal analgesia, early extubation, and rehabilitation after improving graft function. Advancements of techniques, intricate and detailed preparedness, and management have made early recovery after LT possible.

REFERENCES

1. Angeli P, Bernardi M, Villanueva C, Francoz C, Mookerjee RP, Trebicka J, et al. EASL Clinical Practice Guidelines for the management of patients with decompensated cirrhosis. J Hepatol. 2018;69:406-60.
2. Izzy MJ, VanWagner LB. Current concepts of cirrhotic cardiomyopathy. Clin Liver Dis. 2021;25:471-81.
3. Cheng XS, VanWagner LB, Costa SP, Axelrod DA, Bangalore S, Norman SP, et al. Emerging evidence on coronary heart disease screening in kidney and liver transplantation candidates: a scientific statement from the American Heart Association: endorsed by the American Society of Transplantation. Circulation. 2022;146:E299-324.
4. Melamed KH, Dai D, Cuk N, Markovic D, Follett R, Wang T, et al. Preoperative trapped lung is associated with increased mortality after orthotopic liver transplantation. Prog Transplant. 2021;31:47-54.
5. Driever EG, Stravitz RT, Zhang J, Adelmeijer J, Durkalski V, Lee WM, et al. VWF/ADAMTS13 imbalance, but not global coagulation or fibrinolysis, is associated with outcome and bleeding in acute liver failure. Hepatology. 2021;73:1882-91.
6. Weissenborn K. Hepatic encephalopathy: definition, clinical grading and diagnostic principles. Drugs. 2019;79:5-9.
7. Gao Q, Cai JZ, Dong H. A review of the risk factors and approaches to prevention of post-reperfusion syndrome during liver transplantation. Organogenesis. 2024;20:2386730.
8. Sahinovic MM, Struys MMRF, Absalom AR. Clinical pharmacokinetics and pharmacodynamics of propofol. Clin Pharmacokinet. 2018;57:1539-58.
9. Brezeanu LN, Brezeanu RC, Diculescu M, Droc G. Anaesthesia for liver transplantation: an update. J Crit Care Med. 2020;6:91.
10. Fayed NA, Yassen KA, Abdulla AR. Comparison between 2 strategies of fluid management on blood loss and transfusion requirements during liver transplantation. J Cardiothorac Vasc Anesth. 2017;31:1741-50.
11. Massicotte L, Thibeault L, Roy A. Classical notions of coagulation revisited in relation with blood losses, transfusion rate for 700 consecutive liver transplantations. Semin Thromb Hemost. 2015;41:538-46.
12. Rudnick MR, de Marchi L, Plotkin JS. Hemodynamic monitoring during liver transplantation: a state of the art review. World J Hepatol. 2015;7:1302-11.

13. Rocca GD, Rocca AD. Hemodynamic monitoring in liver transplantation patients in the third millennium. J Liver Transplant. 2023;11:100156.
14. Hansebout C, Desai T, Dhir A. Utility of transesophageal echocardiography during orthotopic liver transplantation: a narrative review. Ann Card Anaesth. 2023;26:367-79.
15. Restoux A, Grassin-Delyle S, Liu N, Paugam-Burtz C, Mantz J, Guen ML. Pilot study of closed-loop anaesthesia for liver transplantation. Br J Anaesth. 2016;117:332-40.
16. Morkane CM, Sapisochin G, Mukhtar AM, Reyntjens KMEM, Wagener G, Spiro M, et al. Perioperative fluid management and outcomes in adult deceased donor liver transplantation—a systematic review of the literature and expert panel recommendations. Clin Transplant. 2022;36:e14651.
17. Clevenger B, Mallett SV. Transfusion and coagulation management in liver transplantation. World J Gastroenterol. 2014;20:6146-58.
18. Persico M, Miller D, Way C, Williamson M, O'Keefe K, Strnatko D, et al. Implementation of enhanced recovery after surgery in a community hospital: an evidence-based approach. J Perianesthesia Nurs. 2019;34:188-97.

CHAPTER 9

Immediate Surgical Complications Post-liver Transplant

Prashant Kadam, Gaurav Gupta

INTRODUCTION

Liver transplantation is the treatment of choice for end-stage liver disease, with a 1-year survival reaching 96% and a 10-year survival of 71% in the posttransplant period.[1] However, the surgical steps and techniques are complex, and nearly two thirds of patients develop surgical complications in the postoperative period, many of which can be life-threatening if not promptly identified and managed.

Following liver transplantation, most patients are closely monitored in intensive care units (ICU) to assess their metabolic and electrolyte status as well as graft synthetic function. Advances in perioperative care and a deeper understanding of postoperative complications, combined with advancements in imaging techniques, have resulted in early detection and treatment of complications, leading to improved prognoses for patients.

Surgical complications can broadly be categorized into two basic types: (1) Vascular complications and (2) biliary complications.

VASCULAR COMPLICATIONS

Hemorrhage

Postoperative hemorrhage is a common complication after liver transplant (LT), affecting up to 5% of the LT recipients, occurring within 48 hours of the transplant procedure.[2] Reoperation to arrest the ongoing bleed or for evacuation for hematoma is necessary in 8–27% of LT recipients,[3] leading to substantial use of resources and higher postoperative mortality. Bleeding posttransplant can be attributed to various factors. Common surgical sources of postoperative hemorrhage include the resected liver bed, gall bladder bed, cystic artery, and small veins that drain into the vena cava. During recipient hepatectomy, special care should be taken around the adrenal gland, as injury to it can lead to recurrent bleeding after surgery. Additionally, hemorrhage can also arise from the vascular anastomoses formed during the procedure. Important medical factors include portal hypertension and preexisting varices in the recipient, the presence of coagulopathy including thrombocytopenia, hypocalcemia, hemodilution, and delayed graft function.

The diagnosis is primarily clinical, with signs including hypotension, tachycardia, drainage, decreased mixed central venous oxygen saturation, and worsening kidney function. Percutaneous drains may fail if hemorrhage occurs >2 days after transplantation, even if placed correctly. In such cases, abdominal distension becomes the prominent clinical sign. An abdominal ultrasound (US) may reveal sub- or perihepatic hematomas and intraperitoneal fluid. CT angiogram scans can help distinguish between intrahepatic hematomas, which are more concerning, and less dangerous extrahepatic hematomas, as well as conditions like liver abscesses or malperfused areas. Hemodynamically stable patients may be conservatively managed if imaging, like US or CT angiogram rules out ongoing bleeding or a significant and expanding hematoma. Reoperation is typically indicated if more than four to six units of packed red blood cells are required within 24 hours or if the patient experiences hemodynamic instability.

Hepatic Artery Thrombosis

Hepatic artery thrombosis (HAT) is one of the most feared and serious complications that has the potential to cause graft loss, morbidity, and mortality after liver transplantation. Its incidence ranges from 2% to 15% with a higher incidence in pediatric and living donor liver transplantation (LDLT). The overall mortality rate of HAT is 33.3%, varying from 0% to 80%, and was notably higher in adults compared to children.[4] Hence, salvaging the graft is a priority considering the limited supply of organs available for transplantation.

TABLE 1: Causes of hepatic artery thrombosis.

Surgical causes	*Nonsurgical causes*
Technical errors	Duration of cold ischemia time
The use of conduits	Hypercoagulable state
Pediatric recipient	ABO Incompatibility
Type of graft (whole size vs. reduced size)	Acute rejection in the first week posttransplantation
Retransplantation	Low recipient weight
Prolonged operation time	Prior TACE procedure
Multiple arterial anastomoses Arterial variants: difficult anastomosis	CMV (+) donor to CMV (–) recipient

(CMV: cytomegalovirus; TACE: transcatheter arterial chemoembolization)

Based on the timing of its presentation, it is differentiated into early HAT (eHAT: within 1 month of transplantation) and delayed or late HAT (dHAT; anytime thereafter).

The risk factors can be attributed to technical, donor, and recipient factors. Though surgical techniques have been associated with the occurrence of eHAT, several nonsurgical causes have also been implicated **(Table 1)**.

Early HAT results in hepatic parenchymal ischemia leading to severe allograft dysfunction which is characterized by a sudden elevation of liver enzymes, lactic acidosis, sepsis, multiorgan failure, and even death. The transplanted liver solely depends on arterial blood flow from the hepatic artery, unlike the native liver, which receives its blood supply from a network of collaterals (mainly phrenic arteries) in addition to the hepatic artery. As a result, the transplanted liver is unable to sustain a major loss of arterialized blood flow secondary to HAT. The formation of arterial collateral vessels may happen as a result of a gradual decrease in hepatic arterial blood flow, leading to a less severe clinical progression in delayed HAT. dHAT may be asymptomatic and found following investigations for deranged liver function tests (LFTs) or have an indolent course depicted by relapsing fevers and cholangitis. As the hepatic artery is the main supply of oxygenated blood flow to the extrahepatic biliary tree, dHAT can also result in diffuse biliary strictures, leaks, and liver abscesses secondary to ischemic cholangiopathy.

Diagnosis

Doppler ultrasound (DUS) of the liver is routinely used for monitoring the hepatic arterial blood flow in the postoperative setting and is the modality of choice for early diagnosis of HAT. The sensitivity and specificity of Doppler sonography for HAT have been reported to range from 54% to 92% and from 64% to 88%, respectively.[5] The absence of an arterial signal or a significantly increased resistive index (RI) is suggestive of a HAT. However, a false positive finding can be present in a setting of hypotension, arterial spasm, small caliber artery, severe parenchymal edema, or technical factors such as patient positioning, abdominal dressings, bowel gas, or ascites which can limit the Doppler examination. In case of inconclusive findings on a Doppler examination, a CT or a conventional angiography may be done. Early diagnosis is of paramount importance in managing HAT after surgery, as it enables prompt intervention and reduces the risk of graft loss.

Management

Depending on the manner and timing of the presentation post-transplantation, the management options include revascularization (surgical or endovascular), retransplantation, or conservative management. Revascularization is more successful when the diagnosis is made early, thus eliminating the need for retransplantation in an already limited donor pool. Surgical revascularization is the treatment of choice for eHAT when the diagnosis is made within 7 days of a transplant. After dismantling the arterial anastomosis, a thrombectomy is performed, followed by reanastomosis of the hepatic artery. In cases where reanastomosis is technically challenging or the arterial flow is inadequate, an aortic conduit can be considered via a supraceliac or infrarenal approach.

Advances in endovascular interventions now make it possible to manage HATs when the diagnosis is made >7 days posttransplant, as long as there is no organ necrosis, sepsis, or other signs indicating an urgent need for retransplantation. It is, however, more likely to be successful if the thrombosis is partial or incomplete. These interventions include intra-arterial thrombolysis and transluminal angioplasty with or without stent placement. Failure or rethrombosis necessitates repeat endovascular intervention or surgical revascularization.

Failure of surgical revascularization calls for urgent listing of the patient for retransplantation. Patients who received a retransplantation for HAT had significantly better results compared to those who underwent retransplantation for other indications.[6]

Hepatic Artery Stenosis

Hepatic artery stenosis (HAS) is defined as the narrowing of the transverse diameter of the hepatic artery. It occurs in about 2–15% of LTs and can occur either at the anastomotic site (59%), graft HA (38%), or recipient HA (2%).[7] Severe HAS is defined as peak systolic velocity >400 cm/s in the prestenotic segment and low RI <0.5 and presence of parvus tardus waveform in the poststenotic segment on DUS. Confirmation of the diagnosis should be done by a CT angiography, with narrowing exceeding 50% of the transverse diameter being deemed as significant HAS. Patients may be asymptomatic with deranged LFTs, but they can also present with biliary complications, cholangitis, or worsening graft function. Saad et al. highlighted the strong correlation between the progression of untreated significant HAS to HAT with an incidence rate of 65% at 6 months; hence, significant HAS should be promptly treated.[8] As soon as the diagnosis is confirmed, patients are started on antiplatelet medications.

Endovascular interventions or surgical revision of the arterial anastomosis are used to manage HAS. Endovascular interventions include percutaneous transluminal balloon angioplasty (PTBA) with or without stent placement. The incidence of arterial rupture in patients undergoing PTBA is typically in the range of 6–12%, therefore, it is avoided in the first three weeks following transplantation.[9] Surgical management comprises of revision of the anastomosis by primary resection and reanastomosis, interposition of artery or vein grafts.

Portal Vein Thrombosis

The incidence of portal vein thrombosis (PVT) can range from 0.3% to as high as 4% (in pediatric transplants and adult LDLTs).[10] Most commonly, it is attributed to technical issues like discrepancy in size and caliber of the donor and recipient portal vein causing stenosis, redundancy, kinking, tension across the anastomosis, and use of interposition vein grafts. Other risk factors include PVT before transplant, previous splenectomy, presence of large portosystemic shunts, hypercoagulable state, and children with biliary atresia.

As with HAT, PVT too is classified as early PVT (if PVT was detected within 30 days of transplantation) or late PVT (if PVT was detected >30 days after transplantation or if early PVT persisted beyond 30 days) based on its timing of presentation. Early complete PVT in the initial 72 hours after transplantation manifests as severe allograft dysfunction. Late PVT presents with features of portal hypertension such as abdominal pain, ascites, gastrointestinal/variceal bleeding, and elevated liver transaminases.

Diagnosis can be made by the absence of flow in the portal vein on a DUS examination. This can further be confirmed by nonopacification of the portal vein on a contrast-enhanced CT scan.

Management

For patients presenting with early complete PVT within 72 hours posttransplant with signs of graft dysfunction, an urgent surgical revision of the portal vein anastomosis following portal vein thrombectomy is indicated. If redundancy or kinking of the vein is the causative factor, revising the anastomosis after trimming the excess vein and ensuring proper alignment should be sufficient to resolve the condition. If this fails to adequately revascularize the graft, then the patient should be considered for urgent retransplantation.

For early PVT (>3 days and <30 days) endovascular intervention in the form of percutaneous thrombolysis (percutaneous or transhepatic approach) and stent placement may be considered. Success rates for various endovascular approaches vary from 68% to 100%, while the associated mortality and morbidity rates range from 0% to 11%, respectively.[11]

Asymptomatic patients with late PVT and normal LFTs can be kept under close surveillance and managed conservatively with systemic anticoagulation. In patients with late PVT and with complications of portal hypertension, endovascular interventions are successful in 60% of the cases, provided the PVT is limited to Yerdel types 1, 2, and 3. Surgical portosystemic shunts should be created in case of failure of endovascular intervention if the superior mesenteric vein or the splenic vein is patent.

Portal vein thrombosis is associated with poor survival without treatment, but prompt diagnosis and proper management can lead to good outcomes in terms of morbidity and mortality.

Portal Vein Stenosis

The incidence of portal vein stenosis (PVS) is <1% of transplanted patients. Most of the cases are asymptomatic, however, significant PVS can lead to recurrent portal hypertension manifested by ascites and variceal bleeding. Significant PVS is characterized as a stenotic segment with a diameter <5 mm or when the stenosis exceeds

50% and the velocity ratio between the anastomotic and preanastomotic segment is more than three times. DUS and CT angiography can confirm the diagnosis. Given delayed presentation, management is largely done via endovascular intervention. The recommended treatment is percutaneous transhepatic balloon angioplasty, which is successful in 70–80% of patients.[12]

Vascular Outflow Complications

Hepatic venous outflow obstruction (HVOO) is a serious complication that can cause graft loss after liver transplantation, particularly if it manifests in the immediate postoperative period. Stenosis or thrombosis of the inferior vena cava (IVC) can occur in 2–6% of transplanted patients depending on the type of anastomosis,[13] and its incidence is reported to be higher in the LDLT setting.

It can present as abdominal pain and/or distension, increased drain output, ascites, pleural effusion, peripheral edema, biochemistry showing worsening LFTs, and imaging findings of an engorged or congested liver. The presentation can be early or late in the postoperative course. It can also present as acute Budd–Chiari syndrome in the form of graft dysfunction and ascites within 48 hours of transplant surgery. Delayed presentation can be due to intimal hyperplasia or perivascular fibrosis.

Early HVOO is usually attributed to technical issues such as a tight anastomosis, discrepancy in the donor and recipient cava diameter, twisting or kinking of the anastomosis, or an intimal flap. External compression by a hematoma or hypertrophic liver graft can also lead to IVC compression. The resultant graft edema or hypertrophy further contributes to the degree of outflow obstruction, setting up a vicious cycle.

A DUS finding showing a reduced monophasic flow (<10 cm/sec) should raise suspicion of HVOO, and a persistent triphasic pattern virtually excludes the possibility of obstruction. CT or MRI venography can be done to help reach a diagnosis. In case of equivocal findings on imaging, a formal hepatic venography can be done, which can measure the pressure gradient across the anastomosis. A gradient of 3 mm Hg is considered diagnostic, but sometimes it is not possible to measure the gradient when there is an outflow obstruction.

Endovascular therapy like balloon angioplasty can be considered; however, multiple sessions of angioplasty may be required as the patency rate after a single balloon dilatation is around 40–60%.[14] Stenting eliminates the necessity for frequent angioplasties and boasts higher success rates ranging from 73% to 90%.[15] Nevertheless, it has the potential risks of stent thrombosis or migration. The angioplasty procedure can theoretically disrupt the vascular anastomosis, leading to life-threatening bleeding.

Surgical cavoplasty is rarely performed nowadays owing to the high success rates of endovascular therapies. It is not only technically challenging but also dangerous because of the short length of the suprahepatic cava. Ultimately, if rescue strategies for HVOO fail or in the event of acute Budd–Chiari syndrome, retransplantation is the only option.

BILIARY COMPLICATIONS

Rightly called as the "Achilles heel" of liver transplantation, biliary complications are the most common complications following orthotopic liver transplantation (OLT) with an incidence ranging from 2% to 19%.[16] They are a major cause of significant postoperative morbidity and mortality following OLT. The most common biliary complications are bile leak and biliary stricture. These complications depend on the type of graft: Deceased donor liver transplant (DDLT) [donation after brain death/donation after cardiac death (DBD/DCD)] versus LDLT, the technique of anastomosis (choledochocholedochotomy vs. Roux-en-Y hepaticojejunostomy), and the duct used for reconstruction. Some surgeons may place a T-tube in the bile duct when they anticipate a difficult biliary reconstruction. This also allows for easy access to radiological intervention or monitoring of bile output. Understanding the various techniques for biliary reconstruction is crucial for diagnosing and managing biliary complications.

Biliary Leak

In DDLT, the incidence of biliary leak (BL) is 7.8%, while in LDLT, it is 9.5%.[17] The majority of the BLs occur in the immediate postoperative period, but they can be observed up to 6 months after liver transplantation. They can occur at the anastomotic site (most common), at the cut surface of the liver (in LDLT/reduced grafts/pediatric transplants), or after T-tube removal. As the bile duct epithelium is completely dependent on the hepatic artery for its blood supply, a HAT in the immediate postoperative setting causes necrosis of the bile duct with complete dehiscence of the biliary anastomosis. They can be asymptomatic, but patients can present with abdominal pain, fever, or signs suggestive of peritonitis. Abdominal drains may or may not demonstrate bile in the drain. Biochemistry may reveal deranged LFTs, and imaging in the form of US, CT, or MRI can demonstrate fluid collections, ascites, or a frank bile leak. A BL in a Choledocho-choledotomy or duct-to-duct anastomosis is usually investigated with an endoscopic retrograde cholangiopancreatography (ERCP), which can reveal contrast extravasation at the site of BL. A sphincterotomy with a plastic biliary stent successfully treats BL in 94% of cases.[18] For a BL in a transplanted patient with Roux-en-Y hepaticojejunostomy reconstruction, percutaneous transhepatic cholangiogram (PTC) with internal-external biliary drain is usually the treatment modality of choice. If endoscopic or interventional radiology procedures are unsuccessful or not feasible, then relaparotomy with revision of the anastomosis is indicated.

Biliary Strictures

Biliary strictures account for around 40% of all biliary complications, making them the most common complications after liver transplantation.[19] Its incidence is much higher in LDLT (28–32%) compared to DDLT (5–15%).[20] Other contributing factors are related to surgical reconstruction techniques (choledochocholedochotomy vs. Roux-en-Y hepaticojejunostomy), use of a T-tube, development of HAT, and ischemic lesions affecting the biliary ducts. Biliary strictures may be categorized as anastomotic or nonanastomotic. Anastomotic strictures (AS) are the more prevalent type and typically are extrahepatic in location, specifically at the site of the biliary anastomosis, while nonanastomotic strictures (NAS) can occur at various locations within the biliary tree, including both extrahepatic and intrahepatic sites. Around 70% of the biliary strictures are diagnosed within 6 months of the transplant surgery.[21] Patients may present with jaundice, abdominal pain, and fever. Biochemistry reveals deranged LFTs with a cholestatic pattern. US with Doppler is the first investigation modality of choice which, in addition to assessing the caliber of the biliary system, can also assess the liver parenchyma and vasculature. As its sensitivity is low (38–66%) to detect biliary obstruction, a magnetic resonance cholangiopancreatography (MRCP) followed by ERCP or PTC should be performed.[20] ERCP with balloon dilatation and placement of a plastic stent have good long-term success rates which varies between 64% and 100%;[22] however, the majority of patients may require multiple sessions of ERCP at frequent intervals (once every 2–3 months) with stent exchange. Surgery with refashioning of the biliary anastomosis is required in case of failure of endoscopic intervention. Endoscopic treatment outcomes for non-anastomotic biliary strictures following liver transplantation have shown variability, yielding somewhat less favorable success rates (55–75%)[20] compared to endoscopic treatment for anastomotic strictures. Around 50% of patients with NAS require transplantation or succumb to complications.[20]

CONCLUSION

Liver transplant is the only lifesaving procedure for patients with end-stage liver disease and acute liver failure. Postoperative surgical complications are a common and significant cause of morbidity and mortality following liver transplantation. Despite its complexity and potential complications, recent advancements in anesthesia and critical care have led to significant improvements in outcomes. Early diagnosis and treatment of postoperative complications are essential to ensure better graft and patient survival.

REFERENCES

1. Adam R, McMaster P, O'Grady JG, Castaing D, Klempnauer JL, Jamieson N, et al. Evolution of liver transplantation in Europe: report of the European Liver Transplant Registry. Liver Transpl. 2003;9(12):1231-43.
2. Agostini C, Buccianti S, Risaliti M, Fortuna L, Tirloni L, Tucci R, et al. Complications in post-liver transplant patients. J Clin Med. 2023;12(19):6173.
3. Ertel AE, Wima K, Chang AL, Hoehn RS, Hohmann SF, Edwards MJ, et al. Risk of reoperation within 90 days of liver transplantation: a necessary evil? J Am Coll Surg. 2016;222(4):419-28.
4. Bekker J, Ploem S, de Jong KP. Early hepatic artery thrombosis after liver transplantation: a systematic review of the incidence, outcome and risk factors. Am J Transplant. 2009;9(4):746-57.
5. Horrow MM, Blumenthal BM, Reich DJ, Manzarbeitia C. Sonographic diagnosis and outcome of hepatic artery thrombosis after orthotopic liver transplantation in adults. AJR Am J Roentgenol. 2007;189(2):346-51.
6. Lui SK, Garcia CR, Mei X, Gedaly R. Re-transplantation for hepatic artery thrombosis: a national perspective. World J Surg. 2018;42(10):3357-63.
7. Piardi T, Lhuaire M, Bruno O, Memeo R, Pessaux P, Kianmanesh R, et al. Vascular complications following liver transplantation: a literature review of advances in 2015. World J Hepatol. 2016;8(1):36-57.

8. Saad WE, Davies MG, Sahler L, Lee DE, Patel NC, Kitanosono T, et al. Hepatic artery stenosis in liver transplant recipients: primary treatment with percutaneous transluminal angioplasty. J Vasc Interv Radiol. 2005;16(6):795-805.
9. Rajakannu M, Awad S, Ciacio O, Pittau G, Adam R, Cunha AS, et al. Intention-to-treat analysis of percutaneous endovascular treatment of hepatic artery stenosis after orthotopic liver transplantation. Liver Transpl. 2016; 22(7): 923-33.
10. Khalaf H. Vascular complications after deceased and living donor liver transplantation: a single-center experience. Transplant Proc. 2010;42(3):865-70.
11. Cavallari A, Vivarelli M, Bellusci R, Jovine E, Mazziotti A, Rossi C. Treatment of vascular complications following liver transplantation: multidisciplinary approach. Hepatogastroenterology. 2001;48(37):179-83.
12. Saad WE. Portal interventions in liver transplant recipients. Semin Intervent Radiol. 2012;29(2):99-104.
13. Darcy MD. Management of venous outflow complications after liver transplantation. Tech Vasc Interv Radiol. 2007; 10(3):240-5.
14. Shimata K, Sugawara Y, Honda M, Ikeda O, Tamura Y, Hayashida S, et al. Efficacy of repeated balloon venoplasty for treatment of hepatic venous outflow obstruction after pediatric living-donor liver transplantation: a single-institution experience. Pediatr Transplant. 2019;23(6): e13522.
15. Weeks SM, Gerber DA, Jaques PF, Sandhu J, Johnson MW, Fair JH, et al. Primary Gianturco stent placement for inferior vena cava abnormalities following liver transplantation. J Vasc Interv Radiol. 2000;11(2 Pt 1):177-87.
16. Raza A, Omer A, Iqbal S, Gudsoorkar V, Koduru P, Krishnan K. Efficacy of nasobiliary tubes and biliary stents in management of patients with bile leak after liver transplantation: a systematic review. Clin Endosc. 2019;52(2):159-67.
17. Akamatsu N, Sugawara Y, Hashimoto D. Biliary reconstruction, its complications and management of biliary complications after adult liver transplantation: a systematic review of the incidence, risk factors and outcome. Transpl Int. 2011;24(4):379-92.
18. Sendino O, Fernandez-Simon A, Law R, Abu Dayyeh B, Leise M, Chavez-Rivera K, et al. Endoscopic management of bile leaks after liver transplantation: an analysis of two high-volume transplant centers. United European Gastroenterol J. 2018;6(1):89-96.
19. Villa NA, Harrison ME. Management of biliary strictures after liver transplantation. Gastroenterol Hepatol (NY). 2015;11(5):316-28.
20. Sharma S, Gurakar A, Jabbour N. Biliary strictures following liver transplantation: past, present and preventive strategies. Liver Transpl. 2008;14(6):759-69.
21. Jarlot-Gas C, Muscari F, Mokrane FZ, Del Bello A, Culetto A, Buscail E, et al. Management of anastomotic biliary stricture after liver transplantation and impact on survival. HPB (Oxford). 2021;23(8):1259-68.
22. Dai SC, Goldberg D, Agarwal A, Ma GK, Yam C, Ahmad NA, et al. Endoscopic therapy is effective for recurrent anastomotic biliary strictures after orthotopic liver transplantation. Ann Hepatol. 2017;16(6):924-31.

CHAPTER 10

Post-liver Transplant Liver-related Complications (Nonsurgical)

Vaishali Solao

INTRODUCTION

Post-liver transplant care is an essential part of perioperative care and crucial in ensuring good graft functions and patient outcomes. Apart from routine hemodynamic, respiratory, and fluid status optimization, monitoring for medical and/or surgical complications are two major aspects of postoperative care. A sound understanding of the surgical steps, intraoperative events, and preoperative status is very important toward comprehensive postoperative care. Local complications related to the liver in the early postoperative phase are an important cause of mortality and morbidity, and early recognition and best therapeutic steps are essential to avoid graft or patient loss.

ROUTINE POSTOPERATIVE MONITORING FOR DETECTION OF HEPATIC COMPLICATIONS

Hemodynamics

Patients on transfer to the critical care unit will require fluid resuscitation. It is routine practice to have some form of dynamic hemodynamic monitoring [FloTrac/PiCCO (Pulse index Continuous Cardiac Output)] in situ to assist postoperative resuscitation. In extubated patients, echo-guided resuscitation is most advisable. Perioperative hemodynamic management has been covered in detail in a separate chapter of this book.

Drain Output

Drain quality and quantity in the postoperative phase are a good window to pick up complications such as hemorrhage, bile leaks, or chylous ascites. Patients who have massive ascites thereby severe portal hypertension preoperatively are expected to have high drain output postoperative also. The function of the drains in the first 3 days is to monitor for primary postoperative hemorrhage, and later in second week for detecting bile leak. In the presence of severe preoperative portal hypertension, daily drain output can sometimes exceed 2 L creating fluid electrolyte imbalance, and the intake needs to be appropriate to avoid postural hypotension or prerenal azotemia. If possible, drains can be removed if the primary hemorrhage is ruled out, but this approach is seldom successful as repeated ascitic tapping is then required to avoid leaking fluid from the surgical wound. Portal hypertension gradually resolves in 4–6 weeks posttransplant by which time drains dry up. High drains are also suggestive of small-for-size syndrome (SFSS) in appropriate circumstances. At times abrupt increase in drain output is indicative of tertiary peritonitis, serial drain cell count can help detect tertiary peritonitis. Drain bilirubin higher than serum bilirubin is indicative of a bile leak, either from duct-to-duct anastomosis or from hepaticojejunostomy site, whatever the case may be.

Arterial Blood Gas

Postoperative acid–base balance needs to be monitored closely for the first 48 hours. Acidosis, especially lactic acidosis, is expected in an immediate postoperative period which gradually resolves over the next 12–24 hours as the graft function gradually picks up. Hypoxemia should be avoided as it adds to graft injury.

Liver Function Test and International Normalized Ratio

Interpretation of liver function test (LFT) in the first 5–7 days postoperative phase needs a thorough understanding of the preoperative donor status, intraoperative events, and natural history of the postoperative course. Aspartate transaminase/serum glutamic oxaloacetic transaminase (AS/SGOT) and alanine aminotransferase/serum glutamic pyruvic transaminase (ALT/SGPT) can be high in marginal donors or donation after cardiac death (DCD) depending on the donor status preretrieval.

Living donor liver transplantation (LDLT) being a far more controlled surgery, the enzyme elevations in immediate postoperative period in the next 12 and 24 hours are modest unless there is severe ischemia-reperfusion injury (IRI). After the first 24–48 hours, the SGOT and SGPT start a downward trend. Rise and fall in serum bilirubin is multifactorial and it depends on preoperative serum bilirubin. Alkaline phosphatase starts rising once the liver starts regenerating, usually at day 5–7. Prothrombin time and international normalized ratio (PT/INR) and fibrinogen are crucial for measuring the graft function postoperative. In the immediately postoperative period, the PT/INR is a reflection of intraoperative blood loss and intraoperative blood product transfusions. After 12 hours, INR is a good reflection of graft function. INR starts to improve as graft functions improve and time to normalization varies in each individual based on graft-to-recipient weight ratio (GRWR), transplanted graft function, and steatosis of graft. There are several reasons for persistent abnormalities in liver enzymes and bilirubin in post-liver transplants. The common causes are enumerated in **Table 1**.

TABLE 1: Causes of persistent altered liver function test post-liver transplantation.

Vascular causes	• Hepatic artery thrombosis • Portal vein thrombosis • Outflow issues in transplanted graft causing segmental congestion
Immunological	• Rejection • Ischemia–reperfusion injury
Biliary	Bile leak, Biliary obstruction
Sepsis	• Bacterial infection (most common infective cause in the first 2 weeks) • Fungal infection • Donor-derived infection
Viral infection	• CMV, HSV, Varicella reactivation • Flare-up of hepatitis B and C, if inadequately treated
Graft issue	• Primary nonfunction (PNF) of graft • Delayed graft function, early allograft dysfunction (EAD) • Small-for-size syndrome (SFSS) • Marginal donor graft
Other causes	• Drug-induced liver injury • Systemic hypotension causing ischemic hepatitis • Cardiac dysfunction causing congestive hepatopathy

(CMV: cytomegalovirus; HSV: herpes simplex virus)

Flowchart 1 illustrates a simplified schematic algorithm for approaching differentials in case of altered LFT.

Liver Doppler

Daily liver Doppler in the first 3–5 days post-liver transplant is crucial to diagnose vascular complications such as hepatic artery thrombosis (HAT), portal vein thrombosis, or hepatic outflow obstruction.

POSTOPERATIVE MEDICAL HEPATIC COMPLICATIONS

Graft-related Complications Post-liver Transplant

Primary Nonfunction

Definition: Primary nonfunction (PNF) is defined by the Organ Procurement and Transplantation Network (OPTN) based on the presence of aspartate aminotransferase (AST) activity ≥3,000 U/L and at least one additional criterion: INR ≥2.5, arterial blood pH ≤7.3, venous blood pH ≤7.25, and lactate concentration ≥4 mmol/L within 7 days after transplantation.[1] This definition is not absolute and considerable research is being conducted to identify PNF. PNF indicates that the graft never functioned after transplantation and remains universally fatal unless retransplanted.

Incidence: The incidence of PNF varies, depending on the definition, from about 2% to over 9%.[2]

Pathophysiology: The pathophysiology behind PNF is not entirely understood, although several grafts, donor, and host-related factors have been postulated to contribute. Donor factors such as old age, graft quality (steatosis), longer cold ischemia time and warm ischemia time, DCD donors, and a high degree of recipient Model for End-Stage Liver Disease (MELD) score are some of the reasons responsible.[3] DCD donors, along with older donors, donors with high BMI, or those with steatotic grafts are classified as so-called extended criteria donors (ECDs). PNF incidence is higher in the ECD transplants. Identifying PNF early and relisting the patient for a super-urgent deceased donor liver transplantation (DDLT) is the only solution. PNF qualifies for super urgent listing in India and most countries with a robust DDLT program.

Management: As the patient awaits a liver, he or she will have to be supported with continuous renal replacement therapy (CRRT), plasma exchange vasopressors,

Flowchart 1: Algorithmic approach for etiology in case of altered LFT post-liver transplantation.

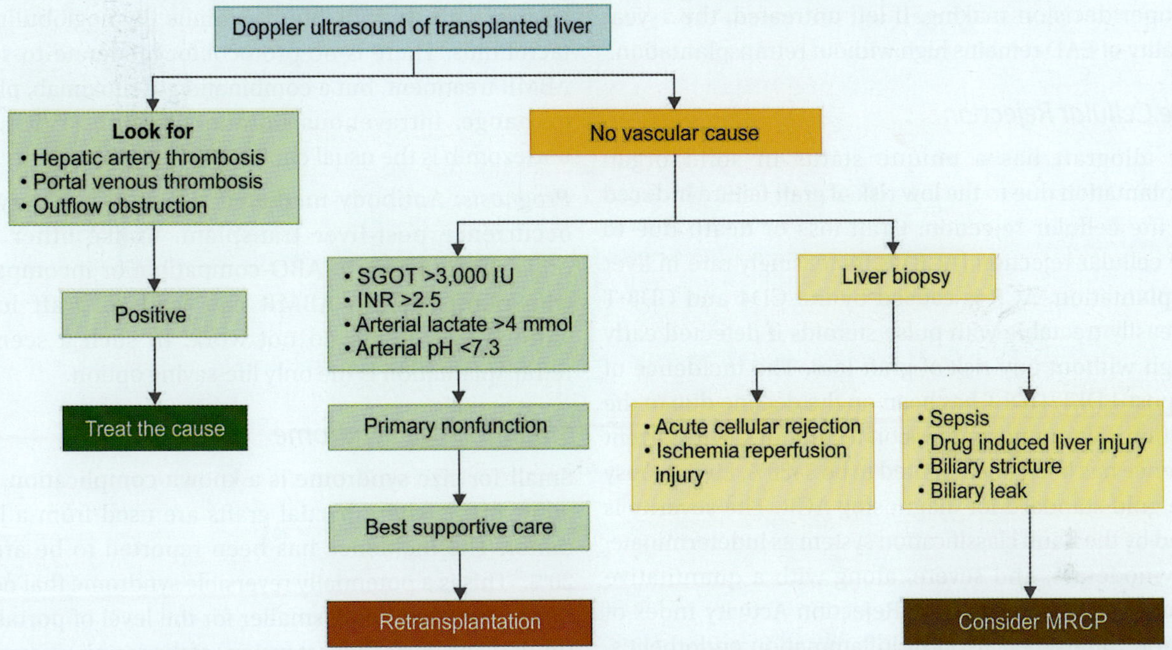

(INR: international normalized ratio; LFT: liver function test; MRCP: magnetic resonance cholangiopancreatography; SGOT: serum glutamic oxaloacetic transaminase)

antibiotics, and antifungals as per local antibiogram and supported by strict infection control measures that prevent the development of new infections in the recipient.

Early Allograft Dysfunction

Definition: Early allograft dysfunction (EAD) is a less severe form of graft dysfunction compared to PNF. Like PNF, EAD has multiple definitions used all over the world. Unlike PNF, most EAD patients can survive without transplantation. The most accepted definition is the one postulated by Olthoff et al. EAD can be diagnosed by meeting at least one of the following criteria: Bilirubin concentration ≥10 mg/dL on day 7, INR value ≥1.6 on day 7, and AST or ALT >2,000 U/L in the first 7 days after transplantation.[4] There has been considerable criticism of static binary definitions and so researchers have been promoting dynamic score, which have a better sensitivity and specificity of predicting need for retransplantation. One such score is the liver graft assessment following transplantation (L-GrAFT) score. Although the L-GrAFT model showed excellent accuracy in determining 3-month graft failure in a single-center study, it still remains to be externally validated in a more diverse condition worldwide.[5]

Incidence: Donation after cardiac death transplants have a higher rate of EAD compared to donation after brain death (DBD). EAD is also known to occur in LDLT. A single large study from the Mayo Clinic reported an incidence of 26.5%.[6]

Pathophysiology of early allograft dysfunction: Ischemia-reperfusion injury to the graft is a major contributory factor to the pathology of EAD. IRI is relatively rare in LDLT, but the incidence increases with the use of extended donor criteria in DBD. The injury to the hepatocytes due to ischemia is then exaggerated by reperfusion. The use of normothermic regional perfusion (NRP) or normothermic machine perfusion (NMP) in DCD organs has been shown to decrease the incidence of IRI. IRI leads to graft dysfunction, biliary strictures, and graft rejection. NRP is an exciting evolving technique to utilize more and more marginal donors without increasing the risk of IRI due to marginal donors. Graft steatosis is also a huge risk factor for EAD. In LDLT, a graft steatosis of >30% is considered unsuitable for donation. In DBD and DCD donors, if the biopsy shows >30% steatosis, the organ is usually rejected. NMP offers a great solution to explore utilizing these organs, which would be rejected due to steatosis.

Management: Early allograft dysfunction may recover spontaneously over a duration if the recipient is sepsis-free in the duration of recovery. Rarely, EAD may require retransplantation, and dynamic daily assessment helps in proper decision-making. If left untreated, the 1-year mortality of EAD remains high without retransplantation.[6]

Acute Cellular Rejection

Liver allograft has a unique status in solid organ transplantation due to the low risk of graft failure induced by acute cellular rejection. Graft loss or death due to acute cellular rejection (ACR) is increasingly rare in liver transplantation. ACR is caused by the CD4 and CD8 T cells easily treatable with pulse steroids if detected early enough without any risk of graft loss. The incidence of ACR post-LDLT/DDLT has been on the decline due to the evolution of immunosuppression techniques. The current incidence has been documented to be 5–20%. Liver biopsy is the gold standard for diagnosing ACR. The severity is graded by the Banff classification system as indeterminate, mild, moderate, and severe, along with a quantitative scoring system known as the Rejection Activity Index of rejection.[7] Biopsy reveals portal inflammation, endothelitis, and bile duct injury. The advisable immunosuppression regime is a combination of calcineurin inhibitors (CNIs), steroids, and mycophenolate mofetil (MMF). Maximum immunosuppression is required in the first 3 months when the risk of ACR is highest. Most centers would target Tacrolimus levels between 5 and 8 ng/L and cyclosporin levels between 80 and 100 μg/mL.

Acute Antibody-mediated Rejection

Acute antibody-mediated rejection (ABMR) post-liver transplant is a very rare and difficult-to-diagnose condition. The exact incidence is still unknown, as this is still in its infancy in the world of liver transplants. Human leukocyte antigen II (HLA II) expression on hepatocytes is less as compared to other solid organs, and the Kupfer cells help mop up the antibodies, making liver a highly unlikely target for ABMR. However, more and more reports of ABMR are being reported post-liver transplant, and our understanding is improving. ABMR is caused by preformed antidonor antibodies, ABO incompatibilities, or de novo antibodies that develop after transplant. A positive donor-specific antibody (DSA) along with classical endothelium and microthrombi and a positive C4d staining on biopsy suggests ABMR.[8]

Management: The most effective method is prevention by reducing exposure preoperatively to blood and blood products. This may, however, be very difficult in cirrhosis with variceal or coagulopathic bleeds. Mild ABMR is treated with steroids plus or minus thymoglobulin and tacrolimus. There is no protocol for moderate-to-severe ABMR treatment, but a combination of rituximab, plasma exchange, intravenous immunoglobulin (IVIG), and bortezomib is the usual choice.

Prognosis: Antibody-mediated rejection is a very rare occurrence post-liver transplant, unlike other solid organ transplants. In ABO-compatible or incompatible transplants, acute ABMR can lead to graft loss if various treatments do not work. In such a scenario, retransplantation is the only life-saving option.

Small-for-size Syndrome

Small-for-size syndrome is a known complication post-adult LDLT where partial grafts are used from a living donor. The incidence has been reported to be around 20%.[9] This is a potentially reversible syndrome that occurs due to the graft being smaller for the level of portal flow (underlying portal hypertension) of the recipient, resulting in shear injury to the endothelium, capillary leakage, and graft hepatocytes injury. The optimal liver size for a recipient is decided by the GRWR of ≥0.8% (or graft volume standard liver volume ratio of ≥40%).

Definition: The most accepted definition is the one proposed by Hernandez et al.[10]

- Size and flow prerequisite: GRWR <0.8 + PVF >250 mL/min/100 g
- Any two of the following:
  - Total bilirubin >5 mg/dL [lasts for 3 consecutive days within the first postoperative week or on postoperative days (POD) 14]
  - INR >2 (lasts for 3 consecutive days within the first postoperative week)
  - Ascites >1 L (lasts for 3 consecutive days within the first postoperative week or on POD 14) or ascites >0.5 L (POD 28)
  - Encephalopathy grade III–IV
- Absence of technical, infectious, or immunological causes

Pathophysiology: Portal hyperperfusion and consequent shear stress of blood flow through the sinusoids are above the optimum needed for hepatic regeneration and responsible for SFSS. Hence, intraoperative measurements of portal pressures and flow after implantation are an essential step to predict SFSS and mitigate it by using flow diversion steps.

Management and prognosis: In anticipated SFSS, inflow modulation of the portal flow is the best-recommended step to avoid the risk of developing SFSS in postoperative period. Inflow modulation, splenic artery ligation, splenectomy, and ligation of large collaterals in case of low portal flow are some of the surgical techniques used to decrease the risk of SFSS. Once SFSS is established, medical management remains the only solution in the hope of slow hepatic regeneration. Adequate infection control, good nutrition, and avoiding sepsis help the graft slowly grow and survival after SFSS is possible. Preventive strategies such as portocaval shunt, splenic artery ligation, or splenectomy, and various intraoperative steps taken to mitigate the risk of SFSS (anticipated/unanticipated). Sepsis is the most common cause of mortality secondary to SFSS. Posttransplant, selective splenic artery embolization is an effective way to regulate portal venous flow and can be utilized as treatment of SFSS.

Drug-induced Hepatotoxicity

Drug interactions and their potential side effects present a significant therapeutic challenge for transplant recipients. Close attention is required to manage possible interactions between immunosuppressive medications and the wide variety of other drugs typically prescribed. These interactions may either enhance the toxicity of a drug or diminish the immunosuppressive effects, leading to liver injury due to rejection. The most common drugs involved in liver injury were antibiotics (48%), followed by immunosuppressive medications (14%), lipid-lowering agents (7%), antivirals (7%), and antifungals (3%). Among these, trimethoprim-sulfamethoxazole (TPM-SMX) was the most frequently implicated drug, accounting for 38% of cases.[11] A key aspect of managing DILI is to prevent re-exposure to the drug that may have caused the liver injury.

CONCLUSION

Optimal perioperative care is as crucial as the surgery itself for good outcomes post-liver transplantation. As critical care specialist taking care of a posttransplant patient, a good understanding of possible complications and interpretation of various tests is of paramount importance. Critical care specialists have a crucial role, therefore, in the mammoth team sport called liver transplantation.

REFERENCES

1. OPTN. (2025). OPTN Policy 9.1 A. [online] Available from https://optn.transplant.hrsa.gov. [Last accessed May, 2025].
2. Masior L, Grąt M. Primary nonfunction and early allograft dysfunction after liver transplantation. Dig Dis. 2022;40(6):766-76.
3. Johnson SR, Alexopoulos S, Curry M, Hanto DW. Primary nonfunction (PNF) in the MELD era: an SRTR database analysis. Am J Transplant. 2007;7(4):1003-9.
4. Olthoff KM, Kulik L, Samstein B, Kaminski M, Abecassis M, Emond J, et al. Validation of a current definition of early allograft dysfunction in liver transplant recipients and analysis of risk factors. Liver Transpl. 2010;16:943-9.
5. Agopian VG, Harlander-Locke MP, Markovic D, Dumronggittigule W, Xia V, Kaldas FM, et al. Evaluation of early allograft function using the liver graft assessment following transplantation risk score model. JAMA Surg. 2018;153(5):436-44.
6. Lee DD, Singh A, Burns JM, Perry DK, Nguyen JH, Taner CB. Early allograft dysfunction in liver transplantation with donation after cardiac death donors results in inferior survival. Liver Transpl. 2014;20(12):1447-53.
7. Demetris A, Batts K, Dhillon A, Wight D, Williams J, Yamabe H. Banff schema for grading liver allograft rejection: an international consensus document. Hepatology. 1997;25:658-63.
8. Lee M. Antibody-mediated rejection after liver transplant. Gastroenterol Clin North Am. 2017;46(2):297-309.
9. Bharathy KG, Shenvi S. Portal hemodynamics after living-donor liver transplantation: management for optimal graft and patient outcomes—a narrative review. Transplantology. 2023;4(2):38-58.
10. Hernandez-Alejandro R, Sharma H. Small-for-size syndrome in liver transplantation: New horizons to cover with a good launchpad. Liver Transpl. 2016;22:33-6.
11. Jiménez-Pérez M, González-Grande R, García-Cortés M, Andrade RJ. Drug-induced liver injury after liver transplantation. Liver Transpl. 2020;26(9):1167-76.

CHAPTER 11

Noninfectious Complications After Liver Transplant

Shabala Paul, Zubair Umer Mohamed

INTRODUCTION

Liver transplantation (LT) has proven to be a boon for patients suffering from irreversible liver disease, including acute and chronic liver failure. In the last few decades, there has been significant progress in the early and long-term management of patients who have undergone the procedure, with a dramatic improvement in their life expectancy. It has been shown to restore their quality of life to one that is comparable with the general population, with only minor limitations. The 5- and 10-year survival rate after LT has been reported as 73 and 71%, respectively, and comparable both in the West and Asia.[1] Results after LT have improved due to advancements in operative technique, immunosuppressive therapy, and better perioperative care. Thus, knowledge of complications that emerge following surgery, early and accurate establishment of diagnosis, and prompt institution of appropriate interventions are essential for optimal patient and graft outcome.

The liver is a major center of activity in the body, with complex interactions that occur with most physiological systems, and thus, the changes after LT are reflected in these as well. It is subjected to a number of insults in the perioperative period, ranging from hypoxia, hypotension, ischemia and reperfusion injury, and the institution of vasoactive drugs, to name a few. In addition, several donor factors such as hepatic steatosis, hemodynamic variations, and size of the allograft and surgical factors such as hemorrhage, vascular and biliary anastomotic issues, as well as immune-mediated responses can affect the outcome after an LT. It is imperative that one anticipate and recognize these complications in a timely manner for appropriate management and good outcomes thereafter.

POSTOPERATIVE COMPLICATIONS AFTER ORTHOTOPIC LIVER TRANSPLANT

Complications after LT can be broadly categorized as immediate complications and intermediate to long-term complications **(Table 1)**.

Post-liver transplant surgical complications, medical hepatic complications, and infection-related complications have been discussed in dedicated

TABLE 1: Postoperative complications.

Immediate	
Allograft dysfunction	• Primary nonfunction • Delayed graft function • Small for size syndrome • Acute cellular rejection • Drug hepatotoxicity
Surgical complications	Postoperative hemorrhage
Vascular complications	• Hepatic artery thrombosis • Portal vein thrombosis • Hepatic venous outflow obstruction
Biliary complications	• Bile leak or fistula • Bile duct stricture
Medical complications	• Hemodynamic instability • Cardiovascular complications • Pulmonary complications • Renal dysfunction • Neurological changes
Intermediate and long-term complications	
Allograft dysfunction	• Rejection • Chronic (ductopenic) rejection • Antibody-mediated rejection • Biliary strictures • Anastomotic and nonanastomotic strictures
Recurrence of initial disease	MASH/alcohol/autoimmune, PBC, and PSC
Systemic	• Infections • Dermatological issues post-liver transplant • Metabolic syndrome/obesity/hypertension/diabetes • Hyperlipidemia • Malignancy/lymphoma/skin cancer

(MASH: metabolic dysfunction-associated steatohepatitis; PBC: primary biliary cirrhosis; PSC: primary sclerosing cholangitis)

chapters in this book. In this chapter, we explore various noninfectious extrahepatic systemic complications that arise following a liver transplant.

Hemodynamic Instability Post-liver Transplant

Multiple overlapping and dynamic reasons can cause patients to present with HDI. These can range from coagulopathy causing diffuse bleeding to surgical bleeds, postreperfusion syndrome, poor graft function, vasoplegic shock, preexisting cirrhotic cardiomyopathy, arrhythmias due to electrolyte abnormalities, and left ventricular (LV) or right ventricular dysfunction. Addressing the primary cause, using fluids and vasopressors to maintain organ perfusion, and transfusion of blood and blood products in the setting of hemorrhage are the mainstays of management.

Cardiovascular Complications

Cardiovascular complications are the leading cause of nongraft-related morbidity and mortality following LT. The spectrum of cardiovascular involvement in end-stage liver disease has been described in previous chapters, highlighting the importance of a detailed preoperative cardiovascular evaluation in a multidisciplinary approach. Cardiovascular complications arise in patients post-orthotopic liver transplantation (OLT) either due to worsening of preexisting cardiac pathology or new onset cardiac issues arising out of significant stress of the major surgery **(Table 2)**. The identification of predisposing factors is important in the preoperative period.

Cirrhotic cardiomyopathy refers to cardiac dysfunction in patients with end-stage liver disease without prior heart conditions. LT is a life-saving treatment for end-stage liver disease. A study by Kim et al. found that 1 year after LT, cardiac function improved, with significant recovery in parameters such as left ventricular ejection fraction (LVEF), left ventricular end-diastolic diameter (LVEDD), global longitudinal strain (GLS), and global circumferential strain (GCS). Additionally, the QTc interval was normalized, demonstrating substantial cardiovascular recovery following LT.[2] On the other hand, LT poses a significant stressor on the cardiovascular system in the perioperative period due to large fluctuations in preload and afterload, potentially triggering ischemic and nonischemic coronary events several days after transplant. In patients with significant flow-limiting coronary obstruction or medically refractory angina, percutaneous coronary intervention (PCI) is required pretransplant. Percutaneous coronary intervention (PCI) is required pretransplant. Some patients may not be suitable for PCI before a liver transplant due to bleeding risks precluding the use of dual antiplatelets, or have unsuitable coronary anatomy, or diffuse coronary disease. These patients face high perioperative risks if treated with either cardiac surgery or liver transplant alone. In such cases, simultaneous liver transplant and cardiac surgery can be considered as long as there are no contraindications such as LV dysfunction.

TABLE 2: Post-liver transplant cardiac complications.

	Diagnosis	*Cause*
Ischemic		
ACS: STEMI, NSTEMI, cardiac arrest	• ECG changes • Regional wall motion abnormality in 2D-echocardiography • Cardiac biomarkers	• Preexisting coronary artery disease • Type 2 myocardial infarction • Coronary vasospasm from tacrolimus, systemic vasopressors
Nonischemic		
Arrhythmias	• Atrial fibrillation • Ventricular or atrial ectopics • Supraventricular tachycardia (SVT) • Ventricular arrhythmia • Severe bradycardia	• Preexisting coronary artery disease • Electrolyte disturbances • QTc prolongation • Invasive line related
Congestive heart failure	• Dyspnea • Hypoxia • Pulmonary infiltrates • ECHO finding • Biochemical markers	• Preexisting coronary artery disease • Preexisting diastolic dysfunction (cirrhotic cardiomyopathy) • Preexisting valvular dysfunction • Volume overload • Stress (takotsubo) cardiomyopathy

(ACS: acute coronary syndrome; ECG: electrocardiogram; ECHO: echocardiogram; NSTEMI: non-ST-elevation myocardial infarction; STEMI: ST-elevation myocardial infarction)

Ischemic Coronary Events

The common risk factors for ischemic coronary events following OLT are the presence of metabolic disease [diabetes mellitus (DM), dyslipidemia, obesity, metabolic syndrome, MASLD as cause of cirrhosis], history of pretransplant coronary artery diseases (CAD), positive stress test, and the presence of pretransplant hepatorenal syndrome (HRS)[3] and chronic renal disease. Apart from this, type 2 myocardial infarction from demand-supply mismatch, acute coronary vasospasm from systemic vasoconstrictors, and a supratherapeutic level of tacrolimus have also been reported in the medical literature.[4] It is important to note that dobutamine stress echocardiography has shown low sensitivity (28%) for screening coronary artery disease despite having high specificity (82%) when compared to the gold standard, coronary angiography.[5] Early postoperative cardiac events are linked to reduced survival in LT recipients, regardless of the presence or severity of CAD. Patients with significant obstructive CAD should undergo preoperative revascularization for optimal outcomes.

Heart Failure

After LT, peripheral vascular resistance and blood pressure rise quickly. In predisposed patients, these changes can trigger acute heart failure, potentially resulting in pulmonary edema. Usually, acute heart failure following OLT develops within hours to days of LT and is majorly nonischemic in nature.[6] Perioperative fluid overload, associated valvular pathology, arrhythmia, and renal dysfunction predispose patients to heart failure.

Takotsubo cardiomyopathy is a dreaded complication in post-liver transplant recipients (LTRs), with a mortality rate as high as 30.4%.[7] A large retrospective review found that takotsubo cardiomyopathy is associated with higher pretransplant Model for End-Stage Liver Disease (MELD) scores, renal insufficiency, sarcopenia, and a history of significant alcohol abuse.[8] Common complications of takotsubo cardiomyopathy include cardiogenic shock with multiorgan involvement, arrhythmia, and LV failure. 2D echocardiography is diagnostic with a drop in LVEF, apical ballooning, and basal hypercontractility with acute mitral regurgitation, LV outflow tract obstruction (LVOTO) and acute dilatation of the left atrium. Coronary angiogram reveals nonobstructive flow. Management is supportive, although some case reports suggest the use of mechanical circulatory support devices such as left ventricular assist device (LVAD) and venoarterial extracorporeal membrane oxygenation (VA-ECMO) for unloading of heart and systemic hemodynamic support. In most cases, the condition is reversible, with complete recovery of LV function over the long term.

Reverse takotsubo cardiomyopathy is a similar condition that results in transient wall-motion abnormalities leading to apical or basal hypokinesia.

Arrhythmia

Postoperative atrial fibrillation (POAF) occurs in a significant number of liver transplant patients and is linked to higher mortality, graft failure, prolonged hospital stays, and stroke.[9] Independent risk factors for the development of POAF are age, MELD score, prior atrial fibrillation, persistent dyselectrolytemia, presence of CAD and valvular heart diseases, higher severity of illness, sepsis, and use of terlipressin. POAF most commonly occurs within the first 24–72 hours after surgery.

In LTRs with arrhythmia, rate and rhythm control agents may be used, but interactions with immunosuppressive medications should be considered, and QT interval should be assessed regularly. If these agents are ineffective, alternatives such as direct current cardioversion or catheter ablation can be considered. The long-term anticoagulation decisions should be guided by stroke risk assessment by CHA2DS2-VASc score versus evaluation of bleeding risk by HAS-BLED score.

Pulmonary Complications

The definitions of postoperative pulmonary complications (POPCs) and postoperative respiratory failure (PRF) are not uniform. Different studies and centers have their own metrics to define those entities. As a standard knowledge, POPCs include respiratory failure of any degree, postsurgical pulmonary infection, pulmonary edema, atelectasis (at least moderate degree) of lungs hampering gas exchange, development of pneumothorax, and pleural effusion (at least moderate degree). A recent retrospective analysis found the incidence of POPC above 50% after living donor liver transplant using these parameters as metrics to define the entity.[10] PRF has been defined as the requirement of mechanical ventilation longer than 48 hours after surgery in one research article,[11] although there are different threshold that exists regarding the duration (24 hours to 7.5 days) to define PRF. The incidence of PRF varies from 11 to 42% as per different literatures, and the study cited in this text quoted an incidence of 36% following liver transplant. There are numerous factors preoperatively, intraoperatively, and postoperatively that can influence the development of POPCs. These are enumerated in **Box 1**. Apart from the recipient native lung status, two important parameters playing a vital role in the development of POPC are the function of the new liver graft as captured with the Model for Early Allograft Function (MEAF) score and surgical complexity during the transplant.

A "trapped lung" is a condition in which a section of the lung cannot reexpand properly due to prolonged preoperative hepatic hydrothorax lasting for months or chronic, nonresolving pleural effusions following OLT. This restriction in lung expansion occurs because of a thick, fibrous layer on the visceral pleura. The presence of a trapped lung, whether due to preoperative or postoperative factors, has been associated with higher morbidity, increased healthcare utilization, and a negative impact on overall post-transplant survival.[12,13]

BOX 1: Common factors for POPCs.[14]

Preoperative risk factors:
- Age, female sex, and high body mass index (BMI)
- Smoking history and diabetes mellitus
- *Preexisting pulmonary pathology:* Chronic obstructive pulmonary disease, congestive heart failure, pneumonia, asthma, hepatic hydrothorax, portopulmonary hypertension, emphysema, and abnormal spirometry
- Hepatopulmonary syndrome
- Severity of liver disease, pretransplant model for end-stage liver disease (MELD) score
- Cirrhotic encephalopathy, left ventricular ejection fraction percentage; systolic pulmonary artery pressure; and diastolic dysfunction
- Cerebral dysfunction
- Acute renal failure, preoperative requirement of hemofiltration
- Albumin level in the recipient
- Preoperative ventilator support, MARS use, deceased donor organ, increased cold ischemia time (CIT), balance of risk (BAR) score, extended criteria donor (ECD)

Intraoperative risk factors:
- Surgery (wide incision)
- Fluid infusion volumes
- Transfusion requirements (packet red blood cells, fresh frozen plasma, and platelets) perioperative fluid balance
- Prolonged intraoperative hypotension
- Fluid retention
- Bleeding volumes
- Tidal volume, PEEP setting in ventilator, and driving pressure during intraoperative phase
- Requirement of venovenous bypass, portocaval anastomosis
- Surgical time

Postoperative risk factors:
- Excessive fluid administration
- Duration of postoperative mechanical ventilation
- Acute rejection
- Acute renal failure, creatinine at the third POD requirement of hemofiltration or hemodialysis
- Hypoproteinemia
- Onset of renal insufficiency
- Poor myocardial function
- Right hemidiaphragm paralysis
- More exposure to nosocomial agents
- Significant decline in recipient's immune function
- Surgical complications
- Reinterventions
- Model for Early Allograft Function, MELD at the third postoperative day

(PEEP: positive end-expiratory pressure; POPCs: postoperative pulmonary complications)

A low tidal volume ventilation strategy with restricted driving pressure is the key for any patient on invasive mechanical ventilation. Early extubation is a crucial element in reducing POPCs, ICU stay, and speeding patient recovery. The evaluation of readiness for extubation relies on various static measures, despite the fact that the dynamic nature of the weaning process makes it challenging to predict its success with certainty. Extubation failure is more common in patients who struggle to manage excessive tracheal secretions due to ineffective coughing or who experience respiratory fatigue resulting from poor cooperation or malnutrition. In some patients who do not completely fulfill the criteria for safe extubation, noninvasive ventilation (NIV) and extubation to high flow nasal cannula with adequate flow setting have been shown to be beneficial in accelerating the weaning process. Noteworthy to mention that, patients having PRF experience less survival to discharge following liver transplant.[11]

Renal Dysfunction

Acute kidney injury (AKI) is a frequent and serious complication following liver transplantation (LTx), with recent reviews indicating that the incidence of postoperative AKI in LTRs ranges from 15 to 40%.[15] About 15% of patients with AKI need renal replacement therapy (RRT). Risk factors are listed in **Table 3**.

A recent meta-analysis has shown that AKI after LT is associated with higher morbidity, prolonged hospital stays, and, in some cases, an increased risk of mortality. The need for dialysis within the first 7 days after LT has been shown to predict post-transplant mortality.[17,18]

A recent retrospective analysis suggests that AKI following LT could be a potential risk factor for the development of de novo chronic kidney disease (CKD) during long-term post-transplant follow-up.[19]

Identification of risk factors and taking preemptive measures to prevent AKI remains crux in the entire management. Preoperatively, volume expansion, discontinuation of nephrotoxic drugs, treating HRS with terlipressin, albumin, midodrine, and RRT have been shown to reduce the incidence of AKI. Similarly, intraoperative avoidance of hypotension can also contribute to reducing the incidence of postoperative AKI. Side-clamping of inferior vena cava (IVC) is preferable to full clamping during vascular anastomosis.

Postoperatively, volume management is crucial. Dynamic assessment of LV preload responsiveness and noninvasive LA pressure assessment provide clues to intravascular volume status. In many centers, invasive hemodynamic tools such as estimation of pulse contour-based cardiac output analysis, estimation of global end-diastolic volume (GEDV), and extravascular lung water calculation are frequently adopted to guide

TABLE 3: Factors associated with the development of AKI post-LT.[16]

Pretransplant comorbidities	*Donor and recipient factors*	*Intraoperative factors*	*Postoperative factors*
• HRS and non-HRS-AKI • CKD • Preoperative dialysis • Advanced age • Overweight and obesity • Hypertension • Diabetes • Anemia, low albumin • Nephrotoxic medications • Alcoholic liver disease • MASLD cirrhosis • Hepatitis B • Hepatitis C • Hepatocellular carcinoma • High MELD • ALF, ACLF	• Donor >60 years • Donor BMI ≥30 kg/m^2 • ABO incompatible grafts • Cold ischemia time • Warm ischemia time • Deceased donor graft • Donation after cardiac death • Extended-criteria graft	• Hypotension, hypovolemia • Postreperfusion syndrome • Hepatic ischemia-reperfusion injury (HIRI) • Inotropic/vasopressor use • Blood loss and transfusion requirements • Oliguria • Complete caval clamping • Duration of anhepatic phase • Duration of surgery	• CNIs • Nephrotoxic medications • ICU stay >3 days after LT • Duration of mechanical ventilation after LT • High volume infusion of chloride liberal fluid • Diuretics • Early allograft dysfunction • CMV infection • New-onset sepsis • Vascular and biliary complications

(ACLF: acute-on-chronic liver failure; AKI: acute kidney injury; ALF: acute liver failure; BMI: body mass index; CKD: chronic kidney disease; CMV: cytomegalovirus; CNI: calcineurin inhibitor; HRS: hepatorenal syndrome; LT: liver transplantation; MELD: model for end-stage liver disease)

fluid administration protocol in challenging settings. Immunosuppressive agents such as the calcineurin inhibitors (CNIs) are known to have nephrotoxicity. The mechanism is related to renal artery vasoconstriction and the development of thrombotic microangiopathy. Minimization of CNI use has been proven to reduce this incidence. One strategy is to administer short-term induction immunosuppression in the form of a polyclonal or monoclonal antibody, followed by delayed initiation of CNI. Another standard strategy is to utilize mycophenolate mofetil (MMF) in combination with CNIs and/or an mTOR inhibitor strategy to allow for CNI dose minimization. At some point, these patients may need RRT to maintain fluid and electrolyte balance, but there is no consensus on the timing of initiation or optimal mode of RRT. Additionally, aggressive control of comorbidities such as hypertension (HTN) and DM and regulation of salt intake is also needed post-LT.

Neurological Complications

As many as 30% of patients develop neurological complications after LT.[20,21] Altered mentation is the most common neurological issue post-OLT.

There are several risk factors for central nervous system (CNS) complications in the post-transplant period. The following neurological conditions are encountered commonly and should be remembered **(Table 4)**:

- *Chronic preoperative hyponatremia:* It may lead to osmotic demyelination syndrome (ODS). Due to massive fluid shifts or rapid correction of hyponatremia, post-LT patients are susceptible to the development of central pontine myelinolysis (CPM), displaying stupor and spastic quadriparesis. Rarely, they may develop intracranial hemorrhage. Traditionally, an immediate preoperative serum sodium of <125 mmol/L and a rise in serum sodium by >12 mmol/L in 24 hours are considered to be two strong risk factors for ODS.[22] A retrospective analysis found perioperative delta sodium (calculated as the difference between the maximum serum sodium within 48 hours after the transplant and the lowest sodium level within seven days prior to the transplant) to be a significant risk factor for post-OLT CNS complications for every 5 mmol/L increase in delta sodium, the odds of experiencing CNS complications post-OLT rise by 47%.[23]

TABLE 4: Common neurological complications post-liver transplant.[21,26]

Neurological complications	***Frequency (%)***
Symptomatic neurological complications: • *Seizures:* Focal or generalized • *Ischemic stroke:* Vascular risk factors • Intracranial and subdural bleed related to coagulopathy • PRES related to hypertension, calcineurin inhibitors, and renal dysfunction • Osmotic demyelination related to rapid shift in sodium • *CNS infections:* Meningoencephalitis	15
Neurocognitive complications: (Encephalopathy, altered mentation, delirium, agitation, delusion, hallucinations, and headache) • Related to chronic liver disease and underlying cardiovascular risk factors and neurodegenerative diseases • *Related to medications:* CNIs, antibiotics	30
ICU-acquired weakness: Critical illness neuropathy and myopathy; preexisting sarcopenia	3–4

(CNIs: calcineurin inhibitors; PRES: posterior reversible encephalopathy syndrome)

- *Drug-induced CNS injury:* Immunosuppressive medications such as CNIs (cyclosporine and tacrolimus) are the common offending agents. In the early post-transplant period, there is a greater risk of CNI neurotoxicity due to higher doses, intravenous use, and impaired blood-brain barrier. Clinical manifestations of CNI toxicity are accompanied by raised tacrolimus or cyclosporine levels, but symptoms may present even with normal serum levels. Hypomagnesemia and hypocholesterolemia may also increase the risk of toxicity. It typically manifests with tremor, headache, and encephalopathy. The presence of altered consciousness and cortical blindness may imply posterior reversible encephalopathy syndrome (PRES) with characteristic findings on magnetic resonance imaging (MRI) of the brain with an increased T2-signal posteriorly in white matter. PRES is associated with reversible vasogenic subcortical edema. There is no specific therapy for CNI neurotoxicity other than symptomatic treatment (e.g., antiepileptics for seizure management), and with dose reduction or switching to alternative immunosuppressants.

Apart from this, corticosteroids and antibiotics such as cefepime and carbapenems may often lead to CNS symptoms. Corticosteroids may increase the risk of critical illness myopathy, or precipitate steroid myopathy, mood disorders, or psychosis. Rarely, corticosteroid use can cause epidural lipomatosis, which may show up as radiculopathies or compressive myelopathy.

- *Sepsis:* Often present with altered sensorium and should always be ruled out in any post-transplant patients with altered sensorium.
- Persistent hepatic dysfunction due to delayed allograft function can cause chronic post-transplant hepatic encephalopathy (HE). Patients with preexisting Wilson's disease may have asterixis and Parkinson-like features.
- Post-transplant renal dysfunction can cause uremic encephalopathy.
- Other metabolic problems such as hypoglycemia and dyselectrolytemia
- Opportunistic CNS infections are rare but well described in medical literature, including human herpesvirus 6 (HHV-6) infection, herpes simplex virus, varicella-zoster virus (VZV), JC virus, fungal, and bacterial infections.
- Coagulopathy is another risk factor predisposing to hemorrhagic stroke.
- Old age, the presence of vascular risk factors may lead to ischemic stroke.

In all forms of neurological issues, it is important to differentiate the structural brain problem causing CNS symptoms from systemic and metabolic causes leading to encephalopathy. The structural brain issues are more abrupt in onset and are often associated with focal signs. Mentation should be objectively monitored with the Glasgow Coma Scale (GCS), and pupillary symmetry and sizes should be assessed periodically. It is imperative to keep control of the airway, as aspiration in post-transplant is often life-threatening. Brain MRI provides clues to structural brain pathologies. Electroencephalogram (EEG) plays a crucial role in differentiating between toxic metabolic encephalopathy and nonconvulsive status epilepticus (NCSE).

Although the outcome of transplantation is usually not affected by neurologic complications, additional morbidity may delay recovery. Additionally, opportunistic infections and immunosuppressant neurotoxicity may complicate the management of immunosuppression and effective prevention of allograft rejection.

Impact of Pretransplant Hepatic Encephalopathy on Post-transplant Outcomes

Hepatic encephalopathy can be categorized into three types based on the underlying liver condition: Type A HE occurs in patients with acute liver failure, type B HE in those with portosystemic shunting but no intrinsic hepatocellular disease, and type C HE, which is the most common, in patients with cirrhosis and cirrhosis-related portosystemic shunting. A retrospective analysis found that mortality after deceased donor LT was significantly higher in the HE group compared to the non-HE group, with the hazard ratio for mortality in the HE group about twice that of the non-HE group. Survival was notably lower in patients having severe HE preoperatively.[24] However, studies have demonstrated that HE is reversible in the long term following LT, and cognitive function improves for the majority of patients within 5 years post-transplant.[25]

Dermatological Issues Following Liver Transplantation

Patients with chronic liver diseases are often associated with multiple skin manifestations. In most cases, the preexisting conditions improve post-liver transplant.[27] For example, Kayser–Fleischer rings in the case of Wilson's disease, livedo reticularis from primary hyperoxaluria, panniculitis from alpha-1 antitrypsin deficiency; cryoglobulinemia, porphyria cutanea tarda, leukocytoclastic vasculitis, and lichen planus from hepatitis C virus (HCV); Raynaud's phenomenon and acanthosis nigricans in the case of primary biliary cholangitis; and photosensitivity from erythropoietic protoporphyria improve after liver transplant.

There are certain dermatological conditions that provide clues to underlying sinister pathology. Like patients with graft-versus-host disease (GVHD) present with typical skin rash along with systemic symptoms.[28] Infection with herpes simplex, herpes zoster, cytomegalovirus, Epstein–Barr virus (EBV), and Parvovirus B19 has its characteristic dermatological manifestations. Apart from this, corticosteroids are associated with steroid dermopathy, CNIs may lead to gingival hyperplasia, folliculitis, and hypertrichosis. Everolimus can lead to slow healing of a surgical incision, and rituximab may lead to urticaria, itch, rash, stomatitis, alopecia, and flushing. MMF may cause acne and erosive stomatitis.

LONG-TERM COMPLICATIONS POST-LIVER TRANSPLANT[29]

Rejection

- *Late acute cellular rejection (ACR)* is generally defined as ACR occurring 1–6 months after LT. This T-cell-mediated inflammatory response typically arises after a reduction in immunosuppressive therapy, often due to insufficient immunosuppression. It is most frequently identified through asymptomatic elevations in transaminases. A definitive diagnosis requires histopathology showing at least two of the following features: (1) portal inflammation, (2) bile duct damage, and (3) subendothelial inflammation in portal and hepatic venules (endotheliitis). Treatment for late ACR depends on the severity of biochemical and histopathological findings and may involve increasing the dose of immunosuppressive agents (e.g., CNIs) with or without pulse steroid therapy. In severe, steroid-refractory cases, lymphocyte-depleting therapy using antithymocyte globulin may be necessary. Early recognition and treatment of late ACR have been shown to reduce the risk of chronic rejection (CR) and improve both graft and patient survival **(Fig. 1)**.

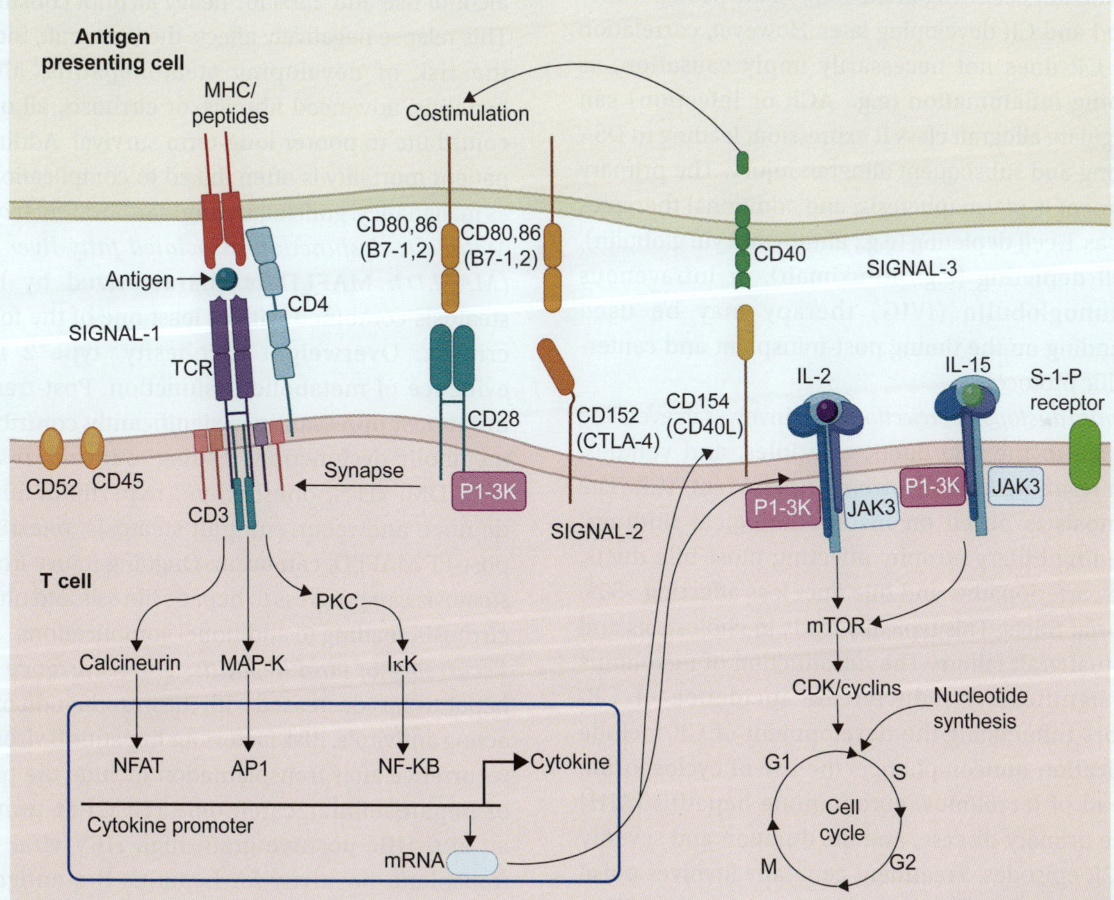

Fig. 1: Multiple signalling pathways of T-cell proliferation: The first signal is activated when major histocompatibility complex (MHC) bound antigen is presented to T cell via T-cell receptor (TCR) by the antigen presenting cell (APC). Engagement of CD80 (B7-1) and CD86 (B7-2) on the APC, with CD28 receptor of T-cell leads to costimulation (Signal-2). Various signal transduction pathways (calcineurin, RAS- [MAP-K] pathway, and the nuclear factor-kappa B [NF-κB] pathway) lead to the expression of many cytokines like interleukin-2 and interleukin-15. These cytokines then activate the "mammalian target of rapamycin" (mTOR) pathway which is the final pathway for T-cell proliferation (signal-3). (TCR: T-cell receptor; PKC: protein kinase C; MAP-K: mitogen-activated protein kinase; IκK: I kappa B kinase; NFAT: nuclear factor of activated T cells; AP-1: activating protein 1; mRNA: messenger ribonucleic acid; JAK3: Janus kinase 3; S-1-P: sphingosine-1-phosphate; PI 3-K: phosphoinositide 3 kinase; CDK: cyclins-dependent protein kinase).

Source: Sánchez–Fueyo, Alberto et al. Immunologic Basis of Graft Rejection and Tolerance Following Transplantation of Liver or Other Solid Organs. Gastroenterology, Volume 140, Issue 1, 51 - 64.e2

- *Antibody-mediated rejection (AMR)* is becoming increasingly recognized as a significant cause of liver allograft dysfunction. The liver was traditionally thought to be protected from AMR due to factors such as (1) the dense sinusoidal network that absorbs antibodies, (2) secretion of soluble human leukocyte antigen (HLA) 1 to neutralize antibodies, and (3) the liver's regenerative ability. AMR diagnosis involves a positive donor-specific antibody (DSA) screen, the exclusion of other causes, and characteristic histology, including complement component 4d (C4d) staining. Presentation of AMR varies, with early graft dysfunction occurring in the immediate postoperative period and CR developing later. However, correlation with CR does not necessarily imply causation, as ongoing inflammation (e.g., ACR or infection) can upregulate allograft class II expression, leading to DSA binding and subsequent allograft injury. The primary treatment is plasmapheresis, and additional therapies such as T-cell depleting (e.g., antithymocyte globulin), B-cell depleting (e.g., Rituximab), or intravenous immunoglobulin (IVIG) therapy may be used depending on the timing post-transplant and center-specific protocols.
- *Chronic (ductopenic) rejection (CR)* involves irreversible damage to the bile ducts, arterioles, and venules, often resulting from recurrent or persistent ACR. The diagnosis is based on histopathological findings, including biliary atrophy affecting most bile ducts, foamy arteriopathy, and bile duct loss affecting >50% of portal tracts. This typically leads to cholestasis and eventual graft failure. The introduction of tacrolimus has significantly reduced the incidence of CR. Factors influencing the development of CR include medication noncompliance, the use of cyclosporine instead of tacrolimus, autoimmune hepatitis (AIH) as the primary disease, and the duration and severity of ACR episodes. Treatment generally involves pulse steroid therapy along with increased doses of CNIs. Unfortunately, advanced CR may result in graft failure, requiring retransplantation or palliative care.[29]

Biliary Complications

Biliary complications can be classified into anastomotic or nonanastomotic strictures (NASs). *Anastomotic strictures* (ASs) occur due to technical issues at the anastomotic site, excessive cautery use, or disturbances in the local blood supply. In contrast, *NASs* are multifocal, irregular, and intrahepatic. NAS can result from macroscopic events such as hepatic artery thrombosis (HAT) as well as microscopic causes such as prolonged ischemia or the use of vasopressors. Both types of strictures generally respond well to endoscopic interventions. However, if left untreated, secondary biliary cirrhosis can eventually lead to graft failure over time.[29]

Recurrence of Primary Liver Disease

- *Alcoholism:* Alcohol relapse after LT for alcoholic cirrhosis occurs at an annual rate of about 4.7% for any alcohol use and 2.9% for heavy alcohol consumption. This relapse negatively affects the liver graft, increasing the risk of developing steatohepatitis, alcoholic hepatitis, advanced fibrosis, or cirrhosis, all of which contribute to poorer long-term survival. Additionally, patient mortality is often linked to complications such as malignancy, graft failure, and cardiovascular causes.[30]
- *Metabolic dysfunction-associated fatty liver disease (MAFLD):* MAFLD is characterized by hepatic steatosis combined with at least one of the following criteria: Overweight or obesity, type 2 DM, or evidence of metabolic dysfunction. Post-transplant immunosuppressant use significantly contributes to metabolic dysfunction, leading to insulin resistance (IR), DM, HTN, obesity, and hyperlipidemia. Both de novo and recurrent graft steatosis, referred to as post-LT MAFLD, can occur. Ongoing injury from graft steatosis can progress to hepatic fibrosis and ultimately cirrhosis, leading to additional complications.
- *Recurrence of viral hepatitis:* The recurrence of viral hepatitis has decreased with the introduction of direct-acting antivirals. Risk factors for hepatitis B virus (HBV) recurrence after transplantation include the presence of hepatocellular carcinoma (HCC) at transplant, an anti-HBc-positive graft, high HBV viral load at transplant, positivity for hepatitis B e-antigen, and mutations in the HBV S gene. Tenofovir and entecavir are the preferred antiviral agents. HCV is now curable, reducing concerns about HCV recurrence.
- *Primary sclerosing cholangitis (PSC):* The recurrence rate of PSC after LT is estimated at 8–27%, typically occurring around a median of 4.7 years. A strict diagnosis of PSC requires evidence of intra- or extrahepatic biliary stricturing, beading, or irregularity lasting >90 days, or histological findings consistent

with PSC. Risk factors for recurrence include increased post-transplant inflammatory bowel disease activity, recurrent cholangitis as an indication for transplant, ACR, cholangiocarcinoma prior to transplant, older donor age, high MELD score, and younger recipient age.

- *Primary biliary cirrhosis (PBC):* The recurrence of PBC after LT ranges from 4% to 46%. PBC is a purely histological diagnosis and can negatively impact graft survival and even lead to death.
- *AIH:* The incidence of AIH recurrence is 8–12% within the first year and 36–68% within 5 years post-transplant. Risk factors for recurrence include younger age at transplant (<42 years), donor–recipient sex mismatch, higher pretransplant immunoglobulin G (IgG) levels, longer time from transplant, discontinuation of steroids, type I AIH, HLA-DRB1 3 or 4 positivity, and pretransplant tacrolimus or post-transplant MMF use. Pretransplant levels of antinuclear antibody (ANA) and antismooth muscle antibody (ASMA) do not predict recurrence. Post-transplant, elevated bilirubin at 6 months and elevated liver enzymes at 12 months are associated with a higher recurrence risk. Recurrence typically presents less severely due to immunosuppression, and diagnostic criteria are the same as for primary AIH. Recurrent AIH is associated with graft loss and mortality, with elevated bilirubin at diagnosis increasing the risk of graft loss. Treatment mirrors that of initial AIH, using steroids, antimetabolites, and continued CNIs.

Metabolic Disorders[31]

- *Obesity:* Weight management following LT is essential. Optimizing immunosuppressive therapy, particularly corticosteroids, plays a key role in controlling weight gain. The addition of glucagon-like peptide-1 (GLP-1) receptor agonists, such as semaglutide, liraglutide, and tirzepatide, has shown significant benefits for managing obesity in transplant recipients.
- *Diabetes and new onset diabetes after transplant (NODAT):* Around 38% of post-transplant patients develop diabetes, with approximately 28% experiencing NODAT. Risk factors include immunosuppressive therapy, HCV infection, and steroid use. CNIs can be toxic to pancreatic beta cells. Since hemoglobin A1c (HbA1c) is unreliable in the first 3 months post-transplant due to frequent transfusions and steroid use, managing immunosuppression and minimizing steroid exposure are critical in managing NODAT.
- *Systemic arterial HTN:* More than 50% of LT recipients develop HTN. CNIs are a leading cause of long-term HTN due to their vasoconstrictive effects on both the systemic circulation and the renal vasculature. The first-line treatment is typically calcium channel blockers, such as amlodipine. Caution is needed with nifedipine, as it can interfere with cytochrome P450 3A4, increasing tacrolimus levels. Other antihypertensive medications, such as angiotensin-converting enzyme (ACE) inhibitors, aldosterone receptor blockers, and thiazides, can cause electrolyte imbalances, especially hyperkalemia, when used with CNIs, requiring careful monitoring.
- *Renal dysfunction:* Post-transplant kidney disease can result from pretransplant kidney injury, postoperative acute tubular necrosis (ATN), exposure to CNIs, and conditions such as post-transplant diabetes, HTN, and obesity. Interestingly, LT recipients have the second-highest incidence of postoperative chronic renal failure among nonrenal organ transplant patients, despite having lower CNI exposure. Elevated creatinine levels at 1 year, cyclosporine use, pretransplant diabetes, and post-transplant AKI are strong predictors of progression to end-stage renal disease (ESRD). CNIs contribute to chronic nephrotoxicity. Notably, survival is better for LT recipients who undergo a subsequent renal transplant compared to those on ongoing dialysis.
- *Bone disease:* Osteoporosis affects 12–50% of cirrhotic patients. Post-transplant, steroids significantly accelerate bone loss in nearly all LT recipients within the first 6 months, increasing the risk of low-energy fractures. Older age and cholestatic diseases exacerbate this risk. Preventive strategies include minimizing steroid use, supplementing with calcium and vitamin D, and regular bone density screening to monitor bone health.

Malignancies

- *Nonmelanoma skin cancer:* The development of nonmelanoma skin cancer in transplant recipients is primarily attributed to reduced immune surveillance of tumor antigens and increased susceptibility to UV-induced DNA damage, which is heightened by drugs such as azathioprine compared to MMF. Prevention strategies include minimizing direct exposure to UV rays and ensuring regular dermatological checkups to monitor for suspicious lesions and perform excisions as needed.

- *Kaposi's sarcoma:* Caused by HHV-8, Kaposi's sarcoma is an angioproliferative neoplasm that is 50 times more common in solid organ transplant recipients than in immunocompetent individuals. Management focuses on reducing immunosuppression while maintaining graft safety to balance tumor control and organ rejection risk.
- *Post-transplant lymphoproliferative disorder (PTLD):* PTLD refers to any lymphoma that occurs in transplant recipients and is commonly associated with EBV infection. The incidence is notably higher in pediatric recipients. The primary approach to treatment involves reducing immunosuppression, while more advanced cases may require rituximab. Surgery may also be employed to manage localized lesions.
- *Recurrence of HCC:* The incidence of recurrent HCC is increasing with the expansion of liver transplant criteria beyond the Milan criteria. Factors such as alpha-fetoprotein (AFP)-producing tumors, tumors outside Milan criteria, microvascular invasion, and poorly differentiated tumors are well-established risk factors for recurrence. High levels of CNIs have been linked to an increased likelihood of tumor recurrence and represent a modifiable risk factor.

CONCLUSION

Liver transplantation has become a widely accepted treatment for end-stage liver disease, offering excellent long-term outcomes. This success is largely due to the early detection and effective management of potential complications. Accurate diagnosis is crucial, as the treatment for different complications can significantly impact both graft function and patient prognosis. The differential diagnosis can be challenging due to the overlap in clinical symptoms and laboratory findings across various complications. However, it is essential for clinicians to remain vigilant, recognize potential issues early, and implement appropriate management strategies to promote optimal long-term recovery and graft function.

REFERENCES

1. Ghelichi-Ghojogh M, Rajabi A, Mohammadizadeh F, Shojaie L, Vali M, Afrashteh S, et al. Survival rate of liver transplantation in Asia: a systematic review and meta-analysis. Iran J Public Health. 2022;51:2207-20.
2. Kim HM, Kim HK, Lee JH, Lee YB, Park EA, Park JB, et al. Myocardial structural and functional changes in patients with liver cirrhosis awaiting liver transplantation: a comprehensive cardiovascular magnetic resonance and echocardiographic study. J Cardiovasc Magn Reson. 2020; 22:25.
3. Koshy AN, Farouque O, Cailes B, Ko J, Han H-C, Weinberg L, et al. Prediction of perioperative cardiovascular events in liver transplantation. Transplantation. 2021;105:593-601.
4. Manuel SL, Sapone J, Lin F. Tacrolimus-induced recurrent acute coronary syndrome due to an unknown mechanism. Cureus. 2024;16:e63266.
5. Soldera J, Camazzola F, Rodríguez S, Brandão A. Cardiac stress testing and coronary artery disease in liver transplantation candidates: meta-analysis. World J Hepatol. 2018;10:877.
6. Nazif K, Kubal C, Guglin M. Acute heart failure post liver transplantation: a systematic literature review. J Hear Lung Transplant. 2021;40:S300.
7. Bachayev M, Brereton B, Mondal A, Alli-Ramsaroop BA, Dhakal R, Leon MCB, et al. Takotsubo syndrome in orthotopic liver transplant: a systematic review and pooled analysis of published studies and case reports. Transplant Proc. 2024;56:2075-83.
8. Yataco ML, Difato T, Bargehr J, Rosser BG, Patel T, Trejo-Gutierrez JF, et al. Reversible non-ischaemic cardiomyopathy and left ventricular dysfunction after liver transplantation: a single-centre experience. Liver Int. 2014;34:e105-10.
9. Rachwan RJ, Kutkut I, Hathaway TJ, Timsina LR, Kubal CA, Lacerda MA, et al. Postoperative atrial fibrillation and flutter in liver transplantation: an important predictor of early and late morbidity and mortality. Liver Transplant. 2020;26:34-44.
10. Oh EJ, Kim J, Kim BG, Han S, Ko JS, Gwak MS, et al. Intraoperative factors modifying the risk of postoperative pulmonary complications after living donor liver transplantation. Transplantation. 2023;107:1748-55.
11. Avolio AW, Gaspari R, Teofili L, Bianco G, Spinazzola G, Soave PM, et al. Postoperative respiratory failure in liver transplantation: risk factors and effect on prognosis. PLoS One. 2019;14:e0211678.
12. Melamed KH, Dai D, Cuk N, Markovic D, Follett R, Wang T, et al. Preoperative trapped lung is associated with increased mortality after orthotopic liver transplantation. Prog Transplant. 2021;31:47-54.
13. Cuk N, Melamed KH, Vangala S, Salah R, Miller WD, Swanson S, et al. Postoperative trapped lung after orthotopic liver transplantation is a predictor of increased mortality. Transpl Int. 2022;35:10387.
14. Feltracco P, Carollo C, Barbieri S, Pettenuzzo T, Ori C. Early respiratory complications after liver transplantation. World J Gastroenterol. 2013;19:9271-81.

15. Raja K, Panackel C. Post liver transplant renal dysfunction—evaluation, management and immunosuppressive practice. J Clin Exp Hepatol. 2024;14:101306.
16. Dong V, Nadim MK, Karvellas CJ. Post-liver transplant acute kidney injury. Liver Transpl. 2021;27:1653-64.
17. Thongprayoon C, Kaewput W, Thamcharoen N, Bathini T, Watthanasuntorn K, Lertjitbanjong P, et al. Incidence and impact of acute kidney injury after liver transplantation: a meta-analysis. J Clin Med. 2019;8:372.
18. Berkowitz RJ, Engoren MC, Mentz G, Sharma P, Kumar SS, Davis R, et al. Intraoperative risk factors of acute kidney injury after liver transplantation. Liver Transplant. 2022;28:1207-23.
19. Fabrizi F, Donato MF, Cerutti R, Invernizzi F, Porata G, Frontini G, et al. Acute kidney injury and chronic kidney disease after liver transplant: a retrospective observational study. Nefrol (English Ed). 2022;42:27-35.
20. Živković SA. Neurologic complications after liver transplantation. World J Hepatol. 2013;5:409.
21. Weiss N, Thabut D. Neurological complications occurring after liver transplantation: role of risk factors, hepatic encephalopathy, and acute (on chronic) brain injury. Liver Transplant. 2019;25:469-87.
22. Crismale JF, Meliambro KA, DeMaria S, Bronster DB, Florman S, Schiano TD. Prevention of the osmotic demyelination syndrome after liver transplantation: a multidisciplinary perspective. Am J Transplant. 2017;17:2537-45.
23. Berry K, Copeland T, Ku E, Lai JC. Perioperative delta sodium and post-liver transplant neurological complications in liver transplant recipients. Transplantation. 2022;106:1609-14.
24. Yoon JU, Yoo YM, Byeon GJ, Kim H-J, Choi E-J, Park S, et al. The impact of pretransplant hepatic encephalopathy, model for end-stage liver disease (MELD) scale on long-term survival following deceased donor liver transplantation: a retrospective study. Ann Palliat Med. 2021;10:5171-80.
25. Hopp AE, Dirks M, Petrusch C, Goldbecker A, Tryc AB, Barg-Hock H, et al. Hepatic encephalopathy is reversible in the long term after liver transplantation. Liver Transplant. 2019;25:1661-72.
26. Khalil M, Elbanhawy I, Elsherbiny A, Amer H, Ahmed S. Neurological complications in recipients after living donor liver transplantation. Neurol India. 2020;68:146-51.
27. Yadav DK, Bai XL, Liang T. Dermatological disorders following liver transplantation: an update. Can J Gastroenterol Hepatol. 2019;2019:9780952.
28. Kaur M, Singh N, Mital R, Schenk A, Fisher K, Korman AM, et al. Dermatologic manifestations of acute graft versus host disease after liver transplantation: a case series of 8 patients. JAAD Case Rep. 2023;39:6-13.
29. Odenwald MA, Roth HF, Reticker A, Segovia M, Pillai A. Evolving challenges with long-term care of liver transplant recipients. Clin Transplant. 2023;37:e15085.
30. Kodali S, Kaif M, Tariq R, Singal AK. Alcohol relapse after liver transplantation for alcoholic cirrhosis-impact on liver graft and patient survival: a meta-analysis. Alcohol Alcohol. 2018;53:166-72.
31. Han MAT, Olivo R, Choi CJ, Pyrsopoulos N. De novo and recurrence of metabolic dysfunction-associated fatty liver disease after liver transplantation. World J Hepatol. 2021;13:1991-2004.

CHAPTER 12

Infectious Complications Post-liver Transplant: How to Minimize Risks, Role of Prophylactic Antibiotics and Antifungals, and Early Detection and Management in the Post-transplant Setting

Deepak Govil, Anant Vikram Pachisia, Sweta J Patel

INTRODUCTION

The first successful liver transplant was performed on 27 July 1967 by Dr Thomas Starzl on a 19-month-old girl with hepatocellular carcinoma who survived for 13 months before succumbing to metastasis.[1] Ever since liver transplant has become a standard of care for end-stage liver disease (ESLD) patients. Today, liver transplantation has expanded to many countries with hundreds of programs running worldwide. Despite various advances, infectious complications remain a leading cause of morbidity and mortality in post-liver transplant recipients.[2]

TIMELINE OF INFECTIONS POST-LIVER TRANSPLANT

Almost 80% of liver transplant recipients will develop infections in the first years after the transplant, of which most are treated, but some will die because of the infections.[3] During the first 3 years post-liver transplant, opportunistic infections are the most common cause of death.[4,5] Post-liver transplant, bacterial infections are the most common (up to 60–70%), followed by viral (20–30%) and fungal (20–30%) infections.[5] Common risk factors for bacterial infections in post-liver transplant recipients are listed in **Box 1**.[6]

Infections during the post-transplant period can be divided into three timelines: <1 month, 1–6 months, and >6 months **(Table 1)**.

BOX 1: Risk factors for bacterial infections post-liver transplant.

Common risk factors for bacterial infections in post-liver transplant recipients

- Elderly
- Preoperative hospital stay
- Duration of surgery
- CMV infection
- Number of blood product units transfused
- Retransplantation
- High preoperative MELD and CTP score
- Roux-en-Y bilio-enteric anastomosis
- Hepatic artery thrombosis
- Biliary leak
- Renal replacement therapy
- Hyperglycemia

(CMV: *Cytomegalovirus*; CTP: Child–Turcotte–Pugh; MELD: model for end-stage liver disease)

HOW TO MINIMIZE RISK?

Infections are the most frequent cause of death from 30 to 180 days in the post-transplant period, according to the United Network of Data Sharing (UNOS) database.[8] The primary difference that exists between post-transplant patients and other patients in a healthcare setting is that of immunosuppression and infections related to it. It is crucial to identify, control, decolonize, and eliminate any bacterial, viral, fungal, or parasitic infections in liver transplant patients, as the procedure is major, complex, and lengthy and is performed on patients who are severely ill. The basics of infection prevention should begin preoperatively in prospective liver transplant recipients and are similar to other hospitalized patients. These include hand hygiene practices, screening programs, outbreak investigation, infectious disease epidemiology, isolation practices, appropriate use of personal protective equipment (PPE), vaccination, and invasive device management, which should be continued in the peri and post-transplant period.[9] Additionally, during the peri and postoperative period, the risk of infection can be minimized by using a high-efficiency particulate air (HEPA) filter, frequent air exchanges, and water treatment/*Legionella* screening.

Both prospective liver transplant recipients and donors should be adequately screened for any infections **(Tables 2 and 3)**.

TABLE 1: Timeline of post-liver transplant infections.

Less than 1 month	***1–6 months***	***More than 6 months***
General risk: • Indwelling vascular catheter and urinary catheters • Secondary seeding from an intra-abdominal source • Prior hospitalization, colonization • Disease transmitted from the donor • Mechanical ventilation	*General risk:* • Immunosuppression • Donor+/recipient mismatch status for viruses • Disease transmitted from the donor • Graft rejection • Repeated biliary tract manipulation • Retransplant	*General risk:* Intense immunosuppression for recurrent allograft dysfunction or rejection
• Bacterial infections including MDR organisms, surgical-site infection (10–37%),[7] and *Clostridium difficile* colitis • Candida species infection • Herpes simplex virus infections (herpes labialis or genitalis or disseminated disease)	• Bacterial infections, *Clostridium difficile* colitis • Common opportunistic infections: – *Cytomegalovirus* – Epstein–Barr virus – HHV 6 and 7 – *Aspergillus* – *Nocardia* – *Mycobacterium tuberculosis* – *Pneumocystis jirovecii* – Endemic mycosis – *Toxoplasma gondii*	• With minimal immunosuppression, usual community-acquired infections • Intense immunosuppression will cause infection with opportunistic infections

(HHV: human herpes virus; MDR: multidrug resistance)

TABLE 2: Screening test for donor.

Screening test	***Interpretation of a positive test***
Anti-CMV IgG	Donor accepted
Anti-HIV	Donor rejected
HBsAg	Usually, organ not accepted
Anti-HBc	• Can be used for patients who are HBsAg, Anti-HBc, and Anti-HBs positive • Can be used in recipient without HBV marker, but lifelong surveillance and anti-viral treatment are required
Anti-HBs	If anti-HBc is negative, donor is accepted; If anti-HBc positive, *see above*
Anti-HCV	Usually not accepted

(CMV: *cytomegalovirus*; HCV, hepatitis C virus; HIV: human immunodeficiency virus; IgG: immunoglobulin G; HBsAg: hepatitis B surface antigen; HBc: Hepatitis B core

TABLE 3: Pretransplant screening of recipient.[10,11]

Serological testing	***HAV, HBV, HCV, HIV, CMV, EBV, VZV, HTLV-1, RPR***
QuantiFERON or T-SPOTTB	*Tuberculosis*
Testing in selected cases (not recommended for all the prospective recipients)	• Parasitic infections (strongyloidiasis, Chagas disease, and schistosomiasis) • Endemic mycoses (coccidioidomycosis and histoplasmosis) • Viral infections (WNV)
Based on clinical history, comorbidities, endemic diseases, and local epidemiology	Vancomycin-resistant *Enterococcus* (VRE) and multidrug-resistant (MDR) Gram negative rectal swab

(CMV: *cytomegalovirus*; EBV: Epstein–Barr virus; HAV: hepatitis A virus; HBV: hepatitis B virus; HCV: hepatitis C virus; HIV: human immunodeficiency virus; HTLV-1: human T-lymphotropic virus type 1; RPR: rapid plasma reagin; VZV: varicella zoster virus; WNV: West Nile virus)

VACCINATION

There is growing but limited evidence that vaccinations are safe in immunosuppressed patients, however, they remain underutilized in this group of population. The timing of vaccination is also crucial. The response of vaccination is limited in patients with end-organ disease and during the first 6 months of transplant. While the prospective recipient is awaiting for a suitable donor, this may be the best window for vaccinations. The response to vaccinations may still be suboptimal but still better than when given after transplant.[12,13] As far as live vaccines are concerned, they should be avoided pending further research. Vaccination for liver transplant recipients is detailed in **Table 4**.[14]

TABLE 4: Vaccination for liver transplant recipients.

Vaccination	*Live attenuated (LA) or inactivated (I)*	*Before transplant*	*After transplant*
Anthrax	I	No	No
Bacillus Calmette–Guérin (BCG)	LA	Yes	No
Hepatitis A	I	Yes	Yes
Hepatitis B	I	Yes	Yes
Hemophilus influenzae type B	I	Yes	Yes
Human papillomavirus (HPV)	I	Yes	Yes
Inactivated Polio vaccine	I	Yes	Yes
Influenza	I	Yes	Yes
Mumps/Measles/ Rubella (MMR)	LA	Yes	No
Pertussis (Tdap)	I	Yes	Yes
Rabies	I	Yes	Yes
Streptococcus pneumoniae (conjugate vaccine)	I	Yes	Yes
Streptococcus pneumoniae (polysaccharide vaccine)	I	Yes	Yes
Tetanus	I	Yes	Yes
Varicella (live-attenuated)	LA	Yes	No
Varicella (subunit; Shingrix)	I	Yes	Yes

ANTIBACTERIAL PROPHYLAXIS

Antibacterial surgical prophylaxis is recommended for all patients undergoing liver transplantation. A liver transplant is a long complex surgical procedure that involves multiple anastomoses such as vascular and biliary, predisposing to leaks, peritoneal contamination during Roux-en-Y anastomosis, a large quantity of blood transfusions, etc. The antibacterial prophylaxis should consider any colonization by methicillin-resistant *Staphylococcus aureus* (MRSA), vancomycin-resistant *Enterococcus* (VRE) or carbapenem-resistant organism (CRO), and thus expand the antibacterial spectrum to cover these organisms. Infection rates and recurrences are higher in recipients colonized with multidrug-resistant organisms (MDRO).[15-17] Once established in organ recipients, carbapenem-resistant Enterobacteriaceae (CRE) can have a mortality rate as high as 40%.[18] Decolonization strategies are of questionable benefit except for skin decolonization by chlorhexidine bathing.[19] Each transplant center should develop its antimicrobial prophylaxis regimen depending on the local flora, resistance pattern, and patient profile.

ANTIFUNGAL PROPHYLAXIS

Liver transplant recipients are among the high-risk populations for fungal infection after small bowel and lung transplants. Candidiasis is the most frequent fungal infection post any solid organ transplant, accounting for 50–60% of fungal infections. The common risk factors for fungal infection are hyperglycemia, use of corticosteroids, parenteral nutrition, abdominal surgery, use of broad-spectrum antibiotics, renal dysfunction, need for renal replacement therapy, presence of central venous catheter, and complicated operative course.[20] The risk of infection can also be influenced by the type of anastomosis performed during a liver transplant. For instance, recipients with choledochojejunostomy have a higher likelihood of developing candidiasis compared to those with a choledocho-choledocho anastomosis.[21] Bloodstream candidiasis is more common than intra-abdominal candidiasis.[22] Like bacterial infections, institutions should develop their antifungal prophylaxis depending on the common local species and resistance pattern. According to the 2019 guidelines from the American Society of Transplantation, solid organ transplant recipients who are at high risk for invasive fungal infections (IFIs) should receive postoperative antifungal prophylaxis with either fluconazole (400 mg daily) or a lipid formulation of amphotericin B (3–5 mg/kg intravenously daily).[23] The use of echinocandins for IFI prophylaxis is also reasonable and is not nephrotoxic like amphotericin B.[24] Routine prophylaxis for *Pneumocystis jirovecii* is questionable with one recent study showing an incidence of 1 infection per 1,000 patients.[25] Many centers do not give routine prophylaxis and this practice can vary from center to center.

DETECTION AND MANAGEMENT OF INFECTIONS POST-TRANSPLANT

Bacterial Infections

In the past 20 years, there has been a rise in the prevalence of Gram-negative bacilli that produce extended-spectrum beta-lactamases (ESBL), with 40% of Escherichia coli, 60% of *Acinetobacter baumannii*, 55% of *Stenotrophomonas maltophilia*, and 51% of *Pseudomonas* isolates exhibiting multidrug resistance.[26]

Diagnosis

Cultures from appropriate sites like blood, tissue, intra-abdominal fluid, or bronchoalveolar lavage remain the gold standard for diagnosing bacterial infections. The FilmArray blood culture identification panel multiplex tests for sepsis have been available for more than a decade now. Recent data suggests that they may be superior to blood cultures in detecting infection with a much shorter turnaround time.[27] Given the increasing incidence of MDRO, the four most prevalent carbapenemases, i.e., OXA-48, New Delhi metallo-beta-lactamase (NDM), Verona integron-encoded metallo-beta-lactamase (VIM), and *Klebsiella pneumoniae* carbapenemase (KPC) should also be evaluated in appropriate Gram-negative bacterial cultures. Also, it is important to identify MRSA and VRE organisms in the culture for appropriate antibiotic selection.

Diagnostic testing for *Clostridium difficile* is illustrated in **Flowchart 1**.

Management

The most important thing apart from administering antimicrobials is source control. The use of antibiotics should be judicious and most antibiotics used in the post-liver transplant period are the same as those used during the pretransplant period. However, in certain conditions, extra caution should be used while selecting antibiotics **(Table 5)**.

Flowchart 1: *Clostridium difficile* infection workup.

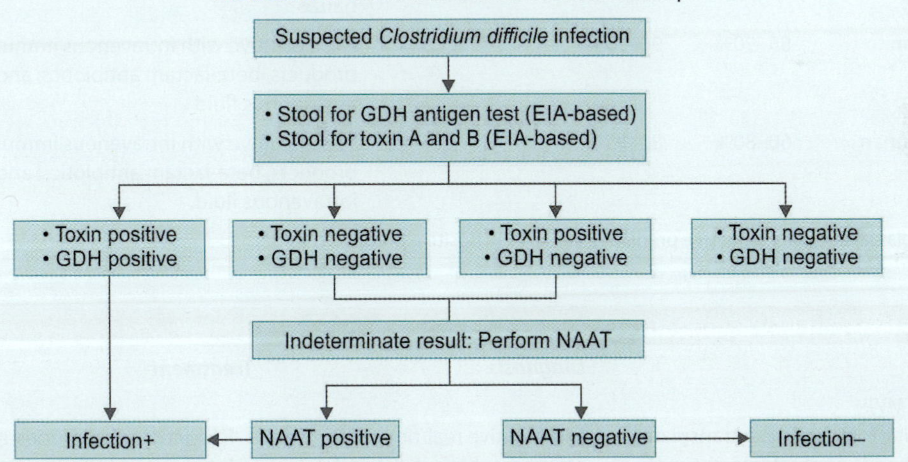

(EIA: enzyme immunoassay; GDH: glutamate dehydrogenase;; NAAT: nucleic acid amplification testing)

TABLE 5: Antibiotics according to resistance profile.

Bacterial resistance profile	*Antibiotics*
MRSA	Vancomycin, linezolid, teicoplanin, daptomycin, tigecycline (high dose for blood stream infection), and ceftaroline
VRE	Linezolid, daptomycin, tigecycline (high dose for blood-stream infection), and dalbavancin
NDM/NDM+ OXA-48	Ceftazidime–avibactam + aztreonam,[28,29] polymyxin/colistin
OXA-48	Ceftazidime–avibactam and polymyxin/colistin

(MRSA: methicillin-resistant *Staphylococcus aureus*; NDM: New Delhi metallo-beta-lactamase; VRE: vancomycin-resistant *Enterococcus)*

Fungal Infections

Diagnosis

As for bacterial infections, the cultures from the appropriate site remain the gold standard for diagnosing a fungal infection. Also, the FilmArray blood culture identification panel multiplex tests can be used for fungal infections with similar advantages. There are certain biomarker-based tests, which can also be performed for suspected fungal infections **(Table 6)**.[30]

Management

Candida infections (81%) are the most common followed by *Aspergillus* (16%) and *Cryptococcus* (3%).[31] Infection with non-Albicans *Candida* species is on the rise, with 68% of infections caused by them.[32] Another problem area is a rapid rise in *Candida auris* infections, which have a high risk of horizontal transmission and are usually multidrug resistant. Any case of *Candida auris* infection/colonization should be promptly isolated and strict infection-control protocol should be followed.[33,34]

Immunosuppression reduction should be considered in fungal infections. Fluconazole is the drug of choice for *Candida albicans* infection. However, echinocandins are recommended first choice for invasive candidiasis.[35]

Voriconazole is the drug of choice for Aspergillosis followed by amphotericin B. Posaconazole and itraconazole have been shown to be equally efficacious in invasive aspergillosis.[36,37]

Viral Infections

The common opportunistic viral infections are discussed in **Table 7**.

TABLE 6: Fungal biomarkers.

Biomarker	***Sensitivity***	***Specificity***	***PPV***	***NPV***	***Additional information***
1,3 beta-D-glucan *(Candida and Aspergillus)*	75%	65%	17%	96%	False positive with albumin, beta-lactam antibiotics, bacterial infections, intravenous immunoglobulin, or gauze
BAL galactomannan *(Aspergillus)*	85–90%	90–95%			False positive with intravenous immunoglobulins, blood products, beta-lactam antibiotics, and use of plasmaLyte intravenous fluid
Plasma galactomannan *(Aspergillus)*	60–80%	80–95%			False positive with intravenous immunoglobulins, blood products, beta-lactam antibiotics, and use of plasmaLyte intravenous fluid.

(BAL: bronchioalveolar lavage; NPV: negative predictive value; PPV: positive predictive value)

TABLE 7: Viral infections post-liver transplant.

Description	***Diagnosis***	***Treatment***
Cytomegalovirus (CMV): • Most common viral infection after transplant[38] • Infection risk depends on serologic status of both donor and recipient • Immunomodulatory effect, thus, makes patients more prone to infections[39]	Quantitative real-time PCR assays are the first choice for viral detection[40]	• Reduction of immunosuppression • Intravenous (IV) ganciclovir is preferred in severe disease • Valganciclovir is used as a step-down treatment when clinical symptoms have resolved after an initial course with IV ganciclovir[39] • *Induction:* 2–4 weeks (depends on clinical and virologic response) • *Maintenance:* 1–3 months • *If donor-positive/recipient-negative:* 3–6 months prophylaxis • *If recipient positive:* Preemptive therapy or 3 months prophylaxis[39]

Contd...

Contd...

Description	***Diagnosis***	***Treatment***
Epstein–Barr virus (CMV): • Majority of recipients already infected at the time of transplant • Transmitted to recipient from seropositive donor or nonleukoreduced blood products • Can lead to PTLD;[41] Risk factors are:[42] Seronegative recipient age 18 years or older, profound immunosuppression, and the first-year post-transplant • 50% mortality with PTLD	• Quantification of EBV DNA • Histological diagnosis is mandatory before initiating therapy for PTLD	• Immunosuppression reduction, rituximab for CD20-positive PTLD cases, and chemotherapy[43] • Local resection and radiotherapy for localized liver PTLD[42] • Ganciclovir and acyclovir have been used for early PTLD[41]
Varicella zoster virus: Low likelihood of disseminated infection	Clinical	Valacyclovir, acyclovir, and famciclovir are all suitable oral medications, while intravenous acyclovir is used for individuals with complicated or widespread zoster
Herpes simplex virus (HSV): Early infection post-transplant, likely due to reactivation[44]	• Clinical • Serum PCR assay of HSV DNA	Acyclovir or valacyclovir
Human herpesvirus 6 (HHV 6): • By viral activation or transmission from the transplanted allograft or blood products[45] • Infection in first 2–8 weeks post-transplant[45] • Increase risk of CMV infection and acute rejection	• PCR assay • *Gold standard:* Biopsy to show histopathological effects	Ganciclovir, cidofovir, or foscarnet
Adenovirus: • Can be acquired from transplanted organ, de-novo, or by reactivation.[46] • Can cause severe respiratory, gastrointestinal, or conjunctival disease	PCR assay	• Reduction of immunosuppression • IV cidofovir for severe disease[46]
Parvovirus B 19: • Transmitted through respiratory secretions or transplanted organ[47] • Can cause pancytopenia, hepatitis, myocarditis, pneumonitis, vasculitis, and/or neurologic involvement[47]	PCR assay	• Reduction of immunosuppression • IVIg

(IVIg: intravenous immunoglobulins; PCR: polymerase chain reaction; PTLD: post-transplant lymphoproliferative disease)

CONCLUSION

A liver transplant is a complex procedure with far-reaching consequences if comprehensive pretransplant workup, immunization, and stringent infection control practices are not in place. A liver transplant recipient is at high risk of infection, and thus, appropriate prophylactic antimicrobials as per local flora and antibiotic sensitivity pattern must be timely started. Any infection should be identified and diagnosed early along with appropriate treatment to improve overall post-transplant outcome.

REFERENCES

1. Starzl TE, Groth CG, Brettschneider L, Penn I, Fulginiti V, Moon J, et al. Orthotopic homotransplantation of the human liver. Ann Surg. 1968;168(3):392-415.
2. Stepanova M, Wai H, Saab S, Mishra A, Venkatesan C, Younossi ZM. The outcomes of adult liver transplants in the United States from 1987 to 2013. Liver Int. 2015; 35(8):2036-41.
3. Kawecki D, Chmura A, Pacholczyk M, Lagiewska B, Adadynski L, Wasiak D, et al. Bacterial infections in the early period after liver transplantation: Etiological agents and their susceptibility. Med Sci Monit. 2009;15(12):CR628-37.

4. Watt KD, Pedersen RA, Kremers WK, Heimbach JK, Charlton MR. Evolution of causes and risk factors for mortality post-liver transplant: Results of the NIDDK long-term follow-up study. Am J Transplant. 2010;10(6):1420-7.
5. Fishman JA. Infection in solid-organ transplant recipients. N Engl J Med. 2007;357(25):2601-14.
6. Hernandez Mdel P, Martin P, Simkins J. Infectious complications after liver transplantation. Gastroenterol Hepatol (N Y). 2015;11(11):741-53.
7. Anesi JA, Blumberg EA, Abbo LM. Perioperative antibiotic prophylaxis to prevent surgical site infections in solid organ transplantation. Transplantation. 2018;102(1):21-34.
8. Baganate F, Beal EW, Tumin D, Azoulay D, Mumtaz K, Black SM, et al. Early mortality after liver transplantation: Defining the course and the cause. Surgery. 2018;164(4):694-704.
9. Pergam SA. Infection prevention in transplantation. Curr Infect Dis Rep. 2016;18(2):1-10.
10. Martin P, DiMartini A, Feng S, Brown R Jr, Fallon M. Evaluation for liver transplantation in adults: 2013 practice guideline by the American Association for the Study of Liver Diseases and the American Society of Transplantation. Hepatology. 2014;59(3):1144-65.
11. Fagiuoli S, Colli A, Bruno R, Craxì A, Gaeta GB, Grossi P, et al; 2011 AISF Single Topic Group. Management of infections pre- and post-liver transplantation: Report of an AISF consensus conference. J Hepatol. 2014;60(5):1075-89.
12. Molrine DC, Hibberd PL. Vaccines for transplant recipients. Infect Dis Clin North Am. 2001;15(1):273-305, xii.
13. Gangappa S, Kokko KE, Carlson LM, Gourley T, Newell KA, Pearson TC, et al. Immune responsiveness and protective immunity after transplantation. Transpl Int. 2008;21(4):293-303.
14. Danziger-Isakov L, Kumar D; AST ID Community of Practice. Vaccination of solid organ transplant candidates and recipients: Guidelines from the American Society of transplantation infectious diseases community of Practice. Clin Transplant. 2019;33(9):e13563.
15. El-Khoury J, Fishman JA. Linezolid in the treatment of vancomycin-resistant Enterococcus faecium in solid organ transplant recipients: report of a multicenter compassionate-use trial. Transpl Infect Dis. 2003;5(3): 121-5.
16. Taimur S, Pouch SM, Zubizarreta N, Mazumdar M, Rana M, Patel G, et al. Impact of pre-transplant carbapenem-resistant Enterobacterales colonization and/or infection on solid organ transplant outcomes. Clin Transplant. 2021;35(4):e14239.
17. Pérez-Nadales E, Gutiérrez-Gutiérrez B, Natera AM, Abdala E, Reina Magalhães M, Mularoni A, et al.; REIPI/INCREMENT-SOT Investigators. Predictors of mortality in solid organ transplant recipients with bloodstream infections due to carbapenemase-producing Enterobacterales: The impact of cytomegalovirus disease and lymphopenia. Am J Transplant. 2019;20(6):1629-41
18. Johnson K, Boucher HW. Editorial commentary: Imminent challenges: Carbapenem-resistant enterobacteriaceae in transplant recipients and patients with hematologic malignancy. Clin Infect Dis. 2014;58(9):1284-6.
19. Póvoa P, Ramirez P, Blot S. Decolonization strategies against multidrug resistant organisms in the ICU. Intensive Care Med. 2024;50(4):577-9.
20. Pappas PG, Alexander BD, Andes DR, Hadley S, Kauffman CA, Freifeld A, et al. Invasive fungal infections among organ transplant recipients: results of the Transplant-Associated Infection Surveillance Network (TRANSNET). Clin Infect Dis. 2010;50(8):1101-11.
21. Pappas PG, Silveira FP; AST Infectious Diseases Community of Practice. Candida in solid organ transplant recipients. Am J Transplant. 2009;9(Suppl. 4):S173-9.
22. Neofytos D, Fishman JA, Horn D, Anaissie E, Chang CH, Olyaei A, et al. Epidemiology and outcome of invasive fungal infections in solid organ transplant recipients. Transplant Infect Dis. 2010;12(3):220-9.
23. Aslam S, Rotstein C; AST Infectious Disease Community of Practice. Candida infections in solid organ transplantation: Guidelines from the American Society of Transplantation Infectious Diseases Community of Practice. Clin Transplant. 2019;33(9):e13623.
24. Winston DJ, Limaye AP, Pelletier S, Safdar N, Morris MI, Meneses K, et al. Randomized, double-blind trial of anidulafungin versus fluconazole for prophylaxis of invasive fungal infections in high-risk liver transplant recipients. Am J Transplant. 2014;14(12):2758-64.
25. Fortea JI, Cuadrado A, Puente Á, Álvarez Fernández P, Huelin P, Álvarez Tato C, et al. Is routine prophylaxis against *Pneumocystis jirovecii* needed in liver transplantation? A retrospective single-centre experience and current prophylaxis strategies in Spain. J Clin Med. 2020;9(11): 3573.
26. Shi SH, Kong HS, Xu J, Zhang WJ, Jia CK, Wang WL, et al. Multidrug resistant gram-negative bacilli as predominant bacteremic pathogens in liver transplant recipients. Transpl Infect Dis. 2009;11(5):405-12.
27. Trung NT, Thau NS, Bang MH, Song LH. PCR-based Sepsis@Quick test is superior in comparison with blood culture for identification of sepsis-causative pathogens. Sci Rep. 2019;9(1):13663.
28. Falcone M, Daikos GL, Tiseo G, Bassoulis D, Giordano C, Galfo V, et al. Efficacy of Ceftazidime-avibactam plus Aztreonam in patients with bloodstream infections caused by metallo-β-lactamase-Producing Enterobacterales. Clin Infect Dis. 2021;72(11):1871-8.
29. Bocanegra-Ibarias P, Camacho-Ortiz A, Garza-González E, Flores-Treviño S, Kim H, Perez-Alba E. Aztreonam plus ceftazidime-avibactam as treatment of NDM-1-producing Klebsiella pneumoniae bacteraemia in a neutropenic patient: Last resort therapy? J Glob Antimicrob Resist. 2020;23:417-9.

30. Shinde AS, Kapoor D. Infections after liver transplant: Timeline, management and prevention. J Clin Exp Hepatol. 2024;14(3):101316.
31. Khalid M, Neupane R, Anjum H, Surani S. Fungal infections following liver transplantation. World J Hepatol. 2021;13(11):1653-62.
32. Raghuram A, Restrepo A, Safadjou S, Cooley J, Orloff M, Hardy D, et al. Invasive fungal infections following liver transplantation: Incidence, risk factors, survival, and impact of fluconazole-resistant Candida parapsilosis (2003-2007). Liver Transpl. 2012;18(9):1100-9.
33. Vallabhaneni S, Jackson BR, Chiller TM. Candida auris: An emerging antimicrobial resistance threat. Ann Intern Med. 2019;171:432-3.
34. Theodoropoulos NM, Bolstorff B, Bozorgzadeh A, Brandeburg C, Cumming M, et al. Candida auris outbreak involving liver transplant recipients in a surgical intensive care unit. Am J Transplant. 2020;20:3673-9.
35. Pappas PG, Kauffman CA, Andes DR, Clancy CJ, Marr KA, Ostrosky-Zeichner L, et al. Clinical Practice Guideline for the Management of Candidiasis: 2016 Update by the Infectious Diseases Society of America. Clin Infect Dis. 2016;62(4):e1-50.
36. Maertens JA, Raad, Marr KA, Patterson TF, Kontoyiannis DP, Cornely OA, et al: Isavuconazole versus voriconazole for primary treatment of invasive mould disease caused by Aspergillus and other filamentous fungi (SECURE): A phase 3, randomised-controlled, non-inferiority trial. Lancet. 2016;387:760-9.
37. Maertens JA, Rahav G, Lee D G, Ponce-de-León A, Sánchez ICR, Klimko N, et al: Posaconazole versus voriconazole for primary treatment of invasive aspergillosis: A phase 3, randomised, controlled, non-inferiority trial. Lancet. 2021;397:499-509.
38. Razonable RR, Emery VC; 11th Annual Meeting of the IHMF (International Herpes Management Forum). Management of CMV infection and disease in transplant patients. Herpes. 2004;11(3):77-86.
39. Bruminhent J, Razonable RR. Management of cytomegalovirus infection and disease in liver transplant recipients. World J Hepatol. 2014;6(6):370-83.
40. Razonable RR, Hayden RT. Clinical utility of viral load in management of cytomegalovirus infection after solid organ transplantation. Clin Microbiol Rev. 2013;26(4):703-27
41. Allen UD, Preiksaitis JK; AST Infectious Diseases Community of Practice. Epstein-Barr virus and posttransplant lymphoproliferative disorder in solid organ transplantation. Am J Transplant. 2013;13(suppl 4):107-20.
42. Kamdar KY, Rooney CM, Heslop HE. Posttransplant lymphoproliferative disease following liver transplantation. Curr Opin Organ Transplant. 2011;16(3):274-80.
43. Parker A, Bowles K, Bradley JA, Emery V, Featherstone C, Gupte G, et al.; Haemato-oncology Task Force of the British Committee for Standards in Haematology and British Transplantation Society. Management of post-transplant lymphoproliferative disorder in adult solid organ transplant recipients—BCSH and BTS Guidelines. Br J Haematol. 2010;149(5):693-705.
44. Levitsky J, Kalil A, Meza JL, Hurst GE, Freifeld A. Herpes zoster infection after liver transplantation: A case-control study. Liver Transpl. 2005;11(3):320-5.
45. Abdel Massih RC, Razonable RR. Human herpesvirus 6 infections after liver transplantation. World J Gastroenterol. 2009;15(21):2561-9.
46. Florescu DF, Hoffman JA; AST Infectious Diseases Community of Practice. Adenovirus in solid organ transplantation. Am J Transplant. 2013;13(suppl 4):206-11.
47. Eid AJ, Chen SF; AST Infectious Diseases Community of Practice. Human parvovirus B19 in solid organ transplantation. Am J Transplant. 2013;13(suppl 4):201-5.

CHAPTER 13

Rejection Recognition and Treatment in Liver Transplant Setting

Amey Sonavane, Guruprasad Shetty, Amruthraj C

INTRODUCTION

Even after advancements in the understanding of transplant immunology, acute and chronic rejections remain an important clinical entity. Acute T-cell-mediated rejection (TCMR) occurs in 15–25% of liver transplant (LT) recipients who are initiated on tacrolimus-based immunosuppressive regimens. These patients show clinical improvement with pulse corticosteroid treatment. TCMR does not affect long-term patient or graft survival.[1] However, chronic rejection (CR) presents with a difficult clinical situation, which usually does not respond to increased immunosuppression and can carry a grave prognosis. CR often leads to retransplantation or death. It is, hence, imperative to recognize and treat rejection at the earliest time to optimize graft function and patient survival.

TYPES AND DIAGNOSIS OF ALLOGRAFT REJECTION

The following are the types and diagnoses of allograft rejection:

- *Hyperacute rejection* is a rare but severe form of antibody-mediated rejection (AMR) that happens immediately after an ABO-incompatible LT, especially in living donor liver transplant (LDLT) cases, requiring urgent retransplantation. Desensitization strategies, including preoperative rituximab, tacrolimus, and mycophenolate mofetil, have decreased the risk of hyperacute rejection.
- *TCMR* is a more commonly encountered form of rejection in clinical settings, typically occurring within the first few months after liver transplantation (usually within 3 months). Late rejection episodes are sometimes observed due to poor adherence to immunosuppressive medication.[2] The incidence of TCMR is around 10–30% when biopsy is conducted as per clinical judgment but can go up to 65% in protocol-driven surveillance liver biopsies.[3] The use of advanced immunosuppressive drugs has significantly lowered the incidence of TCMR. Histological diagnosis and grading of TCMR follow the Banff Working Group's classification based on three critical histological characteristics.[4] Late TCMR episodes (beyond 3 months after LT) can be more severe and less responsive to pulse steroid therapy.
- *Acute AMR* is uncommon, occurring in <1% of LT recipients. The liver has a remarkable ability to eliminate donor-specific antibodies (DSAs), but very high preformed DSA levels may elevate the risk of AMR. Routine screening for DSAs is not advised except for women with previous pregnancies, retransplantation cases, or when attempting aggressive immunosuppressive minimization. The histological features of AMR are outlined by the Banff Working Group[5] **(Table 1)**.
- *CR* may develop if TCMR episodes happen repeatedly and are treated incompletely and inadequately or after a single severe episode of AMR. CR affects fewer than 5% of adult LT recipients, but the incidence is as high as 15% in pediatric cases. The typical histological changes are detailed by the Banff Working Group.[6] CR is associated with a poor prognosis due to progressive graft fibrosis and eventual graft failure.

BASIC CONCEPTS OF LIVER IMMUNOLOGY IN LIVER TRANSPLANT[3]

The liver is an organ with extreme immune-tolerance.[7] This is due to many resident immune cells that create a protolerance environmental milieu while monitoring for infections, foreign antigens, and cancerous cells as well. In TCMR, the host's lymphocytes detect alloantigens from the transplanted liver. The main molecules involved in TCMR are major histocompatibility complex (MHC) proteins. MHC Class 1 antigens present intracellular

TABLE 1: Histologic criteria for diagnosis and grading of rejection in liver transplant.

Category	*Score and criteria*
T-cell-mediated rejection (TCMR)—Rejection activity index (RAI)	
Inflammatory infiltrate of portal tract	• Predominantly, lymphocytic inflammation affecting, but not significantly enlarging, a small portion of the triads • Widespread expansion of most or all triads due to a mixed infiltrate of lymphocytes, neutrophils, eosinophil, and occasional blasts • Extensive expansion of almost all of the triads with a mixed infiltrate, featuring numerous blasts and eosinophils, and inflammation spilling into the periportal parenchyma
Inflammation of bile duct epithelium	• A small number of ducts are surrounded and infiltrated by inflammatory cells, displaying mild reactive changes such as an increased nuclear-to-cytoplasmic ratio in the epithelial cells • The majority or all of the ducts are infiltrated by inflammatory cells, with some ducts showing degenerative changes such as nuclear pleomorphism, cytoplasmic vacuolization of the epithelium, and disorganized polarity • Similar to previous point, but with most or all ducts exhibiting degenerative changes or focal disruption of the luminal structure
Subendothelial inflammation of hepatic and portal venules	• Lymphocytic infiltration of the subendothelium that involves some of the portal and/or hepatic venules • Lymphocytic infiltration of the subendothelium that involves most or all of the portal and/or hepatic venules, with or without areas of hepatocyte necrosis or dropout affecting a small portion of the perivenular regions • Similar to previous point, but here, perivenular inflammation is moderate to severe, extending into the surrounding parenchyma, accompanied by perivenular hepatocyte necrosis
A mild grade of rejection is indicated by an RAI score of <4, a moderate grade by an RAI score between 4 and 6, and a severe grade by an RAI score of 7 or higher. Early TCMR episodes (within 90 days post-liver transplant) typically show more pronounced bile duct damage and variable portal inflammation, with minimal interface activity. In contrast, late TCMR episodes (beyond 90 days posttransplant) are marked by fewer blastic lymphocytes, reduced venous subendothelial inflammation, and more prominent interface and lobular inflammatory activity.	

Category	*Early chronic rejection (at least 2 findings)*	*Late chronic rejection (at least 2 findings)*
Chronic rejection		
Small bile ducts (<60 μm)	Senescence-related changes, such as bile duct atrophy and pyknosis, affecting the majority of ducts, with bile duct loss occurring in <50% of the portal tracts	Loss of bile ducts in 50% or more of the portal tracts, with degenerative changes observed in the remaining bile ducts
Portal tract hepatic arterioles	Occasional loss affecting <25% of the portal tracts	Loss affecting <25% of the portal tracts
Terminal hepatic venules and zone 3 hepatocytes	Mononuclear inflammation in the perivenular area, along with lytic zone 3 necrosis and inflammation, and mild perivenular fibrosis	Variable inflammation, with areas of focal obliteration and moderate-to-severe bridging fibrosis
Large perihilar bile ducts	Inflammatory damage accompanied by focal deposition of foam cells	Mural fibrosis
Large perihilar hepatic artery branches	Intimal inflammation and localized foam cell deposition, with no compromise to the lumen or artery	The narrowing of lumen due to subintimal foam cell accumulation and fibrointimal proliferation
Other features	"Transition" hepatitis characterized by scattered hepatocyte necrosis	Accumulation of foam cells in the sinusoids, accompanied by cholestasis
Antibody-mediated rejection		
Findings	• Hypertrophy of portal microvascular endothelial cells, capillary dilation, and mixed portal microvasculitis • Portal edema, ductular reaction, and characteristic microvascular C4d deposition, either focal or diffuse	

Source: Adapted from Banff Working Group on Liver Allograft Pathology.[5]

epitopes to CD8+ cytotoxic T cells, while MHC Class 2 antigens present extracellular epitopes to CD4+ helper T cells. Rejection occurs when antigen-presenting cells (APCs) present alloantigens to T cells. During LT, donor APCs are transferred to the recipient, initiating different pathways of allorecognition in the host's lymph nodes: Direct recognition [host T-cell receptors interacting with human leukocyte antigen (HLA) on donor APCs], indirect recognition (presentation of donor alloantigens by recipient APCs), and semi-direct recognition (membrane trafficking or extracellular vesicles between host and donor cells). Effective allorecognition requires three signals: T-cell activation (signal 1), costimulatory receptor binding (signal 2), and cytokine stimulation (signal 3) leading to T-cell proliferation and liver graft damage.

Acute AMR can occur due to DSAs, which are either preformed or developed after the transplant. AMRs are explained by the "two-hit" hypothesis. The first injury (such as ischemia or TCMR) increases HLA Class 2 expression, promoting DSA binding and complement activation. DSAs can also cause cellular toxicity, leading to significant graft damage.

CLINICAL FEATURES AND DIAGNOSIS OF T-CELL-MEDIATED REJECTION, ANTIBODY-MEDIATED REJECTION, AND CHRONIC REJECTION

T-cell-mediated rejection is suspected when liver enzymes (serum aminotransferases, alkaline phosphatase, and gamma-glutamyl transpeptidase) are elevated, but these abnormalities are not specific to TCMR and may have various causes. Clinical symptoms are often mild, including malaise, fever, fatigue, and abdominal pain. A liver biopsy is essential for a definitive diagnosis, with TCMR characterized by subendothelial inflammation of portal veins or hepatic venules, inflammation of the epithelium of bile duct, bile duct inflammation, and infiltration of the portal tract with mixed cells of lymphocytes, eosinophils, plasma cells, and neutrophils. These features are scored and summed to create a rejection activity index (RAI). However, RAI does not have any direct correlation with response to steroids. Differential diagnoses include other causes of liver dysfunction, such as sepsis and opportunistic viral and fungal infection, vascular issues, ischemic-reperfusion injury, biliary duct issue, and recurrence of de-novo disease.

Late-onset TCMR happens 6 months post-transplant when immunosuppression is reduced, although the timeline is not universally defined.[8] This is a grave problem and can lead to CR, graft loss, and reduced patient survival. Diagnosis is made by histopathological findings. Specific histological features include perivenular inflammation with confluent perivenular hepatocyte dropout and central bridging necrosis in the severe form. Female sex, persistent low immunosuppression, and autoimmune etiology of transplant act as risk factors for this kind of rejection. New blood biomarkers, such as micro ribonucleic acids (RNAs), proteomic screens, and donor-derived cell-free deoxyribonucleic acid (DNA),[9] show promise for early TCMR diagnosis, while transient elastography also correlates with TCMR. Along with this, molecular diagnosis of rejection in histopathology samples is evolving and can offer more precision-based diagnostics in future.[10] However, these need further testing in larger studies before becoming standard clinical tools.

Plasma cell-rich rejection is a rare form of TCMR, usually occurring 6 months posttransplant, with possible risk factors including female sex, hepatitis-C treatments, and older donors. It has histological features resembling autoimmune hepatitis, with plasma cell and lymphocytic infiltration in the portal and perivenular areas.

Acute AMR typically occurs in ABO-incompatible LTs and clinically behaves similarly to TCMR. AMR is suspected when graft dysfunction persists despite optimal TCMR treatment. It primarily affects small bile ducts, terminal hepatic venules, hepatocytes in zone 3, portal tracts, hepatic arterioles, and large bile ducts. Diagnosis of AMR relies on histopathological findings, positive DSAs, positive microvascular C4d staining indicating activation of the complement system and antibody deposition, and the exclusion of other graft injury causes. AMR can coexist with TCMR in histopathology sample.

Chronic rejection can develop at any time after transplantation; it may lead to graft failure even within the 1st year of transplant. It typically presents with progressive graft dysfunction, which appears cholestatic in nature and ultimately causes graft loss. The incidence of CR has decreased with advancements in immunosuppression and occurs in about 3–17% of LT recipients. The incidence of CR is lesser in LT than in heart, pancreas, lung, and kidney transplants. Obliterative arteriopathy and ductopenia are characteristic features of CR. It can be further classified as TCMR-related CR (with bile duct loss and foam cell arteriopathy) or AMR-related CR (marked by necroinflammatory activity, fibrosis, C4d staining, and circulating DSAs). However, C4d staining can sometimes be nonspecific, and DSAs may not always have clinical significance.

Risk factors for CR include multiple or severe TCMR episodes, autoimmune liver disease, noncompliance with immunosuppressive therapy, cyclosporine use, retransplantation for rejection, older donor age (>40 years), and donor–recipient gender mismatch. Increased graft loss is associated with greater bile duct and hepatic arteriole loss, elevated bilirubin levels, advanced donor age, foam cell presence, and higher aspartate transaminase levels.

TREATMENT OF T-CELL-MEDIATED REJECTION

Treatment of TCMR is given in **Table 2**.

The treatment of TCMR in LT patients primarily involves the escalation of immunosuppressants and corticosteroid boluses (methylprednisolone as a dose of 500–1,000 mg/day) for 3 consecutive days. TCMR should always be confirmed through histology before starting therapy, and empiric corticosteroid therapy is not recommended. Studies have shown that single-day pulse corticosteroid therapy with gradual taper over the next 6 days is more effective and carries fewer infectious complications as compared to pulse corticosteroid therapy (500–1,000 mg/day) daily for 3 doses.[11] Along with steroid boluses, tacrolimus dose optimization (via drug levels), additional antimetabolites (mycophenolate mofetil or azathioprine), and mammalian target of rapamycin (mTOR) inhibitors can be considered. The duration of enhanced immunosuppression depends on the timing and severity of TCMR, with early cases possibly allowing for reduced immunosuppression after liver function tests normalize, while later TCMR cases may require extended treatment.

Mild TCMR may be managed by increasing the dose of calcineurin inhibitors (CNIs) or using a trial of oral prednisone up to 60 mg/day to assess response. The target tacrolimus trough level should exceed 10 ng/mL. We need to be careful about the side effects of CNIs, such as kidney dysfunction, neurotoxicity, and electrolyte imbalances. Sepsis and infection by hepatotropic viruses should be ruled out before initiating high-dose corticosteroid therapy.

Steroid-resistant rejection, occurring in 4–10% of cases, is identified when liver enzymes do not improve after 3 days of high-dose corticosteroids. Antithymocyte globulin (ATG) or anti-T3 receptor antibody (OKT3) may

TABLE 2: Management strategies for acute and chronic rejection post-liver transplant.

Grade of rejection	*Management strategy*	*Laboratory parameters to be monitored*
Mild TCMR	• Increase maintenance immunosuppression through an increase in tacrolimus dosage • Optimization of adjunctive agents	• Liver enzymes • Bilirubin • Tacrolimus trough levels
Moderate-to-severe TCMR	• Pulse corticosteroid therapy followed by a gradual taper • Increase in maintenance immunosuppression	• Tacrolimus trough levels • Liver enzymes • Blood sugar management
Steroid-resistant TCMR	• Antithymocyte globulin • Should be followed by 3–6 months of prophylaxis against bacterial and viral infections	• Liver enzymes • Leukocyte count • Platelet count
Chronic TCMR/CR	• mTOR inhibitors • Conversion to or optimization of tacrolimus-based regimens • Retransplantation in allograft failure	• Tacrolimus trough levels • mTOR inhibitor through levels • Liver enzymes
Antibody-mediated rejection	Optimize immunosuppressive therapy and pulse corticosteroid therapy	• Tacrolimus trough levels • Blood sugar levels
Antibody-mediated rejection—nonresponsive to modification of immunosuppressive therapy and pulse corticosteroids	Therapeutic plasma exchange, intravenous immunoglobulin therapy, and rituximab	

(CR: chronic rejection; mTOR: mammalian target of rapamycin; TCMR: T-cell-mediated rejection)

be used for steroid-resistant cases.[12] ATG is administered at 1.5–2.5 mg/kg/day for 6–10 days, with close monitoring of CD3 count or absolute lymphocyte count and potential side effects such as fever, leukopenia, thrombocytopenia, and infections. ATG should be discontinued when the total white cell count falls below 2,000 cells/mm^3 or the platelet count goes below 50,000 cells/mm^3. OKT3 is linked to several serious side effects, including cytokine-release syndrome, infections, secondary malignancies, and severe complications such as acute pulmonary edema.

The treatment of AMR in liver transplantation is not universally standardized.[13] AMR is often accompanied by a TCMR component. First-line treatment typically involves steroid boluses, tacrolimus dose adjustment, and plasma exchange. Second-line therapies, such as rituximab, eculizumab, or bortezomib (for B-cell depletion), may be used. AMR is aggressive, with a 30% mortality rate, so medication adherence and early consideration for retransplantation are crucial.

Chronic rejection generally has a poor prognosis and may require retransplantation. However, mTOR inhibitors (sirolimus or everolimus) have shown potential in reversing CR in about 30–40% of cases. Factors such as donor age, bilirubin levels, bile duct and arterial loss, and foam cell clusters help predict poor prognosis in CR.

CONCLUSION

The liver is a privileged organ when it comes to alloreactivity. In the current tacrolimus era, the incidence of rejection has reduced significantly. TCMR, AMR, and CR manifest as graft dysfunction and require a tissue biopsy for confirmation of diagnosis. Early TCMR does not affect overall graft survival if identified and treated promptly. CR may respond to an increase in immunosuppression. CR carries a guarded prognosis and can cause graft failure that may result in mortality in the absence of retransplantation. The exact pathophysiology of AMR and plasma cell rejection is still unclear.

REFERENCES

1. Rodríguez-Perálvarez M, Rico-Juri JM, Tsochatzis E, Burra P, De la Mata M, Lerut J. Biopsy-proven acute cellular rejection as an efficacy endpoint of randomized trials in liver transplantation: A systematic review and critical appraisal. Transpl Int. 2016;29(9):961-73.
2. De Martin E, Londoño MC, Emamaullee J, Lerut J, Potts J, Aluvihare V, et al. The optimal immunosuppression management to prevent early rejection after liver transplantation: A systematic review of the literature and expert panel recommendations. Clin Transplant. 2022; 36(10):e14614.
3. Montano-Loza AJ, Rodríguez-Perálvarez ML, Pageaux GP, Sanchez-Fueyo A, Feng S. Liver transplantation immunology: Immunosuppression, rejection, and immunomodulation. J Hepatol. 2023;78:1199-215.
4. Demetris AJ, Batts KP, Dhillon AP, Ferrell L, Fung J, Geller SA, et al. Banff schema for grading liver allograft rejection: An international consensus document. Hepatology. 1997;25(3):658-63.
5. Demetris AJ, Bellamy C, Hübscher SG, O'Leary J, Randhawa PS, Feng S, et al. 2016 Comprehensive Update of the Banff Working Group on Liver Allograft Pathology: Introduction of antibody-mediated rejection. Am J Transplant. 2016; 16:2816-35.
6. Demetris A, Adams D, Bellamy C, Blakolmer K, Clouston A, Dhillon AP, et al. Update of the International Banff Schema for Liver Allograft Rejection: Working recommendations for the histopathologic staging and reporting of chronic rejection. An International Panel. Hepatology. 2000;31(3): 792-9.
7. Snchezfueyo A, Strom TB. Immunologic basis of graft rejection and tolerance following transplantation of liver or other solid organs. Gastroenterology. 2011;140:51-64.e2.
8. Nacif LS, Pinheiro RS, Pécora RA, Ducatti L, Rocha-Santos V, Andraus W, et al. Late acute rejection in liver transplant: A systematic review. Arq Bras Cir Dig. 2015;28(3):212-5.
9. Levitsky J, Kandpal M, Guo K, Kleiboeker S, Sinha R, Abecassis M. Donor-derived cell-free DNA levels predict graft injury in liver transplant recipients. Am J Transplant. 2022;22:532-40.
10. Madill-Thomsen K, Abouljoud M, Bhati C, Ciszek M, Durlik M, Feng S, et al. The molecular diagnosis of rejection in liver transplant biopsies: First results of the INTERLIVER study. Am J Transplant. 2020;20(8):2156-72.
11. Volpin R, Angeli P, Galioto A, Fasolato S, Neri D, Barbazza F, et al. Comparison between two high-dose methylprednisolone schedules in the treatment of acute hepatic cellular rejection in liver transplant recipients: A controlled clinical trial. Liver Transplant. 2002;8(6):527-34.
12. Lu XJ, Chen YH, Ma Y, Zhu XF, He XS. [Strategies in clinical diagnosis and treatment of steroid-resistant acute rejection after orthotopic liver transplantation]. Zhonghua Gan Zang Bing Za Zhi. 2016;24(4):297-301.
13. Lee BT, Fiel MI, Schiano TD. Antibody-mediated rejection of the liver allograft: An update and a clinico-pathological perspective. J Hepatol. 2021;75(5):1203-16.

CHAPTER 14

Role of Imaging in Post-Liver Transplant: An Evaluation of Vascular Complications

Prabha Ranjana

Liver transplant complications can present with mild, nonspecific clinical symptoms. Diagnostic and grading of these are aided by medical imaging, particularly Doppler ultrasonography. 7 days, the 1st, and 3rd months following transplantation are usually when color Doppler ultrasound examinations are conducted, usually between 24 and 48 hours **(Figs. 1A and B)**. Multidetector computed tomography (MDCT) and magnetic resonance (MR) images are obtained, even in the absence of aberrant liver function, based on the results of the Doppler ultrasound (DUS). Experienced professionals should do DUS since vascular problems often manifest early after surgery. Angiography for diagnostic purposes is rarely used. The following illustrate the primary imaging findings of vascular complications in liver transplant patients: Hepatic veins, portal vein abnormalities (such as occlusion and stenosis), and hepatic artery complications (such as thrombosis, stenosis of the anastomosis, and pseudoaneurysms).

HIGHLIGHTS

- Emphasize the significance of promptly identifying vascular problems following liver transplantation.
- Highlight the primary color Doppler ultrasound (DUS) results as the first imaging test.
- Examine the results of the venous and arterial problems from the CT and MR imaging.

INTRODUCTION

Liver transplantation is currently the first-line treatment for both acute and chronic patients with terminal liver disease.

Liver transplants from living donors have been used more recently, particularly for pediatric patients. It reduces the waiting time for a transplant from a deceased donor as well as the transplanted organ's ischemic period.[1]

Following transplantation, vascular problems are rare. For cadaveric donor liver transplants, their

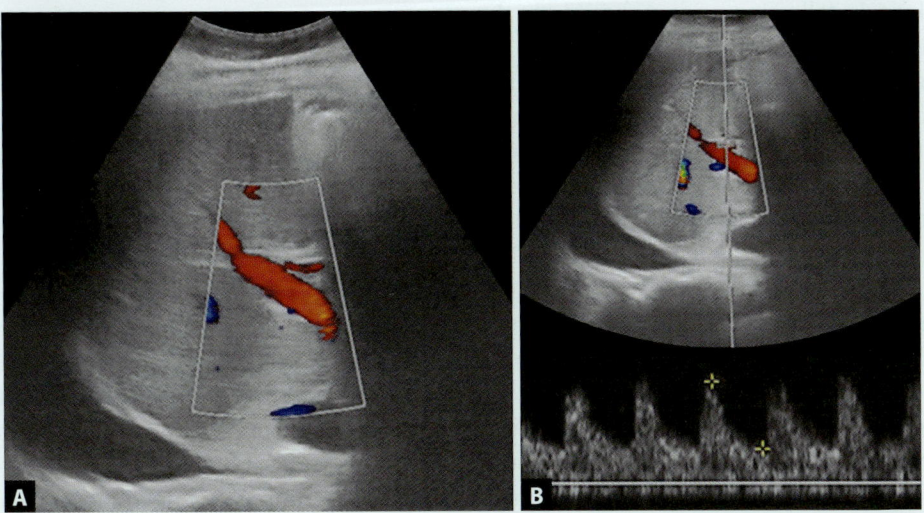

Figs. 1A and B: After surgery, postoperative color Doppler ultrasound (CDUS) is done 24 hours, 48 hours, 1 day, and 7 days later. (A) Normal hepatic artery and (B) portal flow.

reported incidence is approximately 7%, while for living donor liver transplants, they are approximately 13%.[2] Regretfully, vascular anomalies have a high rate of graft loss and mortality and may manifest early after surgery.[3] Because vascular injury symptoms are nonspecific, early radiological testing is crucial to making an early diagnosis and determining the most appropriate course of treatment. Early imaging tests are especially significant since there is a correlation between early endovascular treatment and liver transplantation salvage.[4]

The most suitable imaging test is color Doppler ultrasound (CDUS), which enables accurate assessment of the patency of the graft vasculature and early patient evaluation, even in the recovery unit following surgery.[5] When CDUS shows a vascular abnormality, the surgical anatomy is unclear, or the patient's clinical status is deteriorating, contrast-enhanced computed tomography (CT) or MR imaging must be added to the examination.[6,7]

Although endovascular treatments are now positioned as first options, surgery is regarded as the definitive management, therefore, surgery is only used in circumstances when interventional radiology is ineffective or limited.[8,9] Therefore, when assessing these patients, abdominal radiologists ought to encourage interventional therapy.

Hepatic intraoperative ultrasonography is a relatively novel technology that has been developed in recent years. Before abdominal closure, it enables prompt therapy and real-time assessment of the anastomosis.[10]

Perihepatic hematoma, periportal edema, ascites, and right-sided pleural effusion are typical post-transplantation signs. The initial weeks following surgery should see the resolution of all of them.[11]

Color Doppler ultrasound should be used to evaluate biliary and vascular anastomoses. Since anastomoses are the sites where problems arise most commonly, radiologists should be well-versed in the postoperative anatomy of each individual patient. Furthermore, both in the donor and the recipient, anatomic variants should be recognized.[12]

Nowadays, orthotopic liver transplantation is the most popular surgical procedure in which the native liver is removed and the graft is positioned anatomically in the right upper quadrant.[13] The bile duct, recipient inferior vena cava to donor hepatic veins, hepatic artery, and portal vein anastomoses should all be carefully examined.

The most frequently affected anastomosis is the hepatic artery.[14] The two most frequent sites for this anastomosis are in the hairpin that joins the recipient's left and right hepatic arteries or at the outlet of the gastroduodenal artery, while there are other possible sites.[15]

COMPLICATIONS

Hepatic Artery Complications

Depending on when they initially manifest, hepatic artery issues can be categorized as either early (occurring during the 1st month) or late (occurring beyond 1 month). Early issues are the most important for the patient's prognosis because they are associated with graft loss and a high risk of death.

Thrombosis

Thrombosis is shown in **Figures. 2 and 3.**

Arterial thrombosis is the most serious adverse consequence of orthotopic liver transplantation, occurring in 4–12% of cases.[16] The main reason why liver transplants do not work is thrombosis, which is responsible for almost half of all vascular issues. Although it typically occurs early, it can occur up to 4 months after a transplant.

When assessing the degree of stenosis and flow characteristics at the intrahepatic branches as well as the hepatic artery, pulsed and power CDUS provide a good sensitivity and specificity for thrombus detection. Relevant characteristics to consider are the hepatic artery resistance index, the hepatic artery peak systolic velocity, and the hepatic artery diameter. Intraoperative ultrasound examination has a good sensitivity and specificity for early detection of these anomalies.[17] For CDUS to precisely measure the flow velocity inside the stenosis, the right angle must be used. If the transducer was placed at an angle parallel to or perpendicular to the artery whose speed was to be measured, the measured speeds would be lower than the real ones.

It is frequently difficult to establish the proper angle due to the limited sonographic window and impaired anatomy. On the other hand, because they are not affected by angle, resistance index and spectral curve morphology are easier to study.

Several factors, such as inadequate cardiac output or sluggish flow because of vasospasm, should be considered when CDUS is unable to detect blood flow. In addition, many of these patients have a poor sonographic window due to the surgical dressing materials. In these situations, the use of a contrast agent contrast-enhanced ultrasound (CEUS) can almost completely improve the US diagnostic performance.[18]

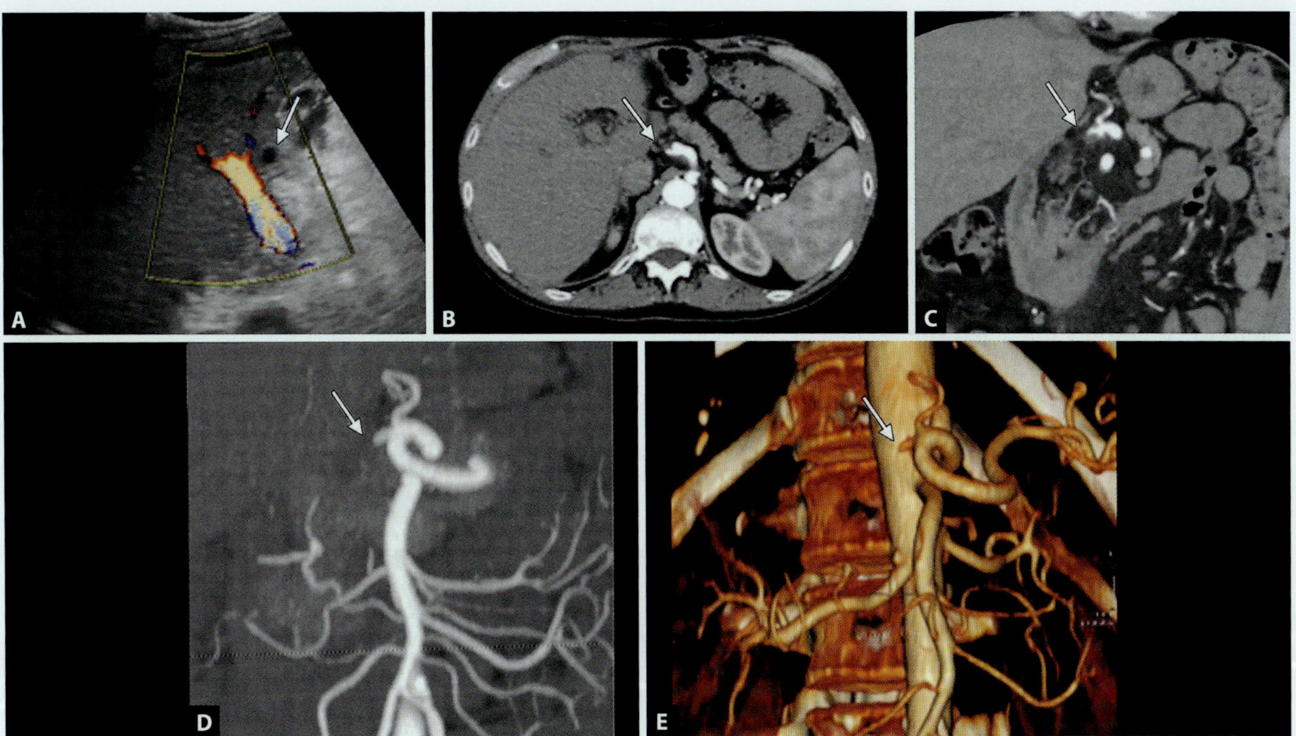

Figs. 2A to E: Thrombosis caused by anastomosis. The most dangerous side effect of orthotopic liver transplantation is artery thrombosis; (A) in a Doppler ultrasound examination, it might be shown as a lack of flow; (B) both the thrombus and the lack of distal flow can be seen on CT; (C to E) to guarantee diagnosis, multiplanar reconstructions and volume rendering pictures may be helpful.

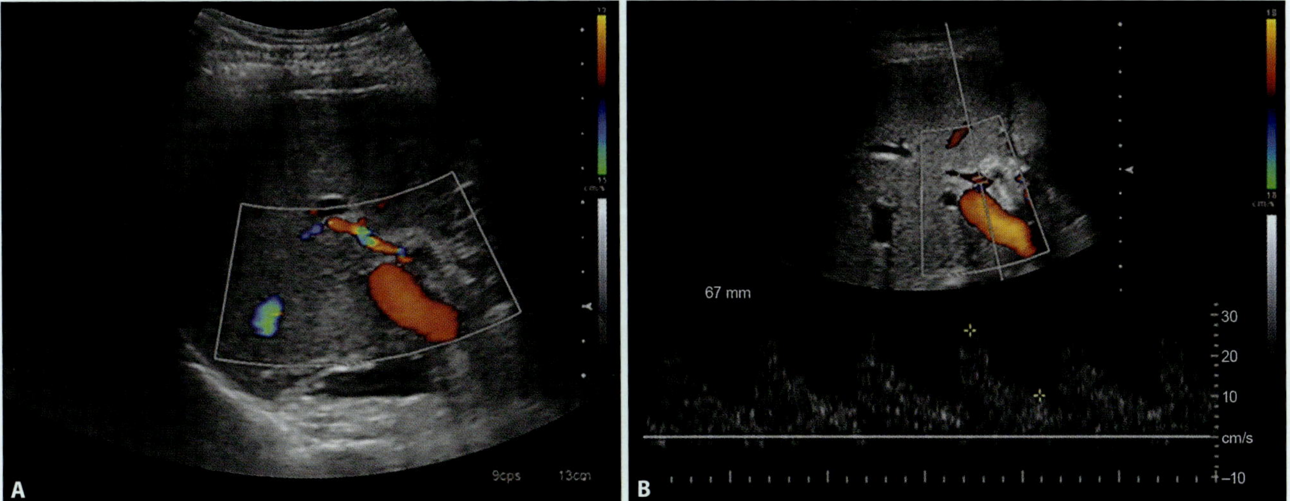

Figs. 3A and B: Doppler image following thrombolysis and angiography (There is normal arterial flow. Normal values for the resistive index (0.6) are displayed).

Because of its great accuracy, quick examination time, and ability to be used even in circumstances where the patient is not in optimal health, CT angiography is the best method for evaluating complex cases.[19] Ultrasonography and magnetic resonance imaging (MRI) have been shown to have comparable diagnostic accuracy,[20,21] with CT angiography showing even greater accuracy.[6]

A diagnostic arteriography can diagnose thrombosis and help determine the best course of treatment if one is suspected. These patients can receive a variety of endovascular therapies, including stent implantation, percutaneous transluminal angioplasty (PTA), and intra-arterial thrombolysis (IAT).[8] If treatment fails, transplantation should be considered as quickly as possible. Studies have shown that retransplantation has a greater survival rate than endovascular treatment.[3] However, because endovascular treatments are less intrusive, they should be used as the initial course of treatment.

Stenosis is shown in **Figs. 4 to 6**. The anastomosis is the most commonly impacted site (2–13% of patients).[22] Thus, this area has to be thoroughly assessed.

Thrombosis can develop from stenosis. Thus, thrombosis and stenosis belong to the same category of vascular problems that might arise after liver donation.

Splenic steal artery syndrome may result from stenosis.[23]

The first 3 months are when it occurs most frequently (median time to diagnosis: 90–120 days).[24,25] This period of time, however, varies from patient to patient and can even happen years after surgery.

As with thrombosis, the best method to detect this problem is DUS. It shows a characteristic pattern, depending on the segment examined and how it relates to stenosis. Power Doppler is also helpful for studying spectral curves and measuring blood flow.[26]

- The prestenotic section has poor flow and an elevated resistance index (>0.8).

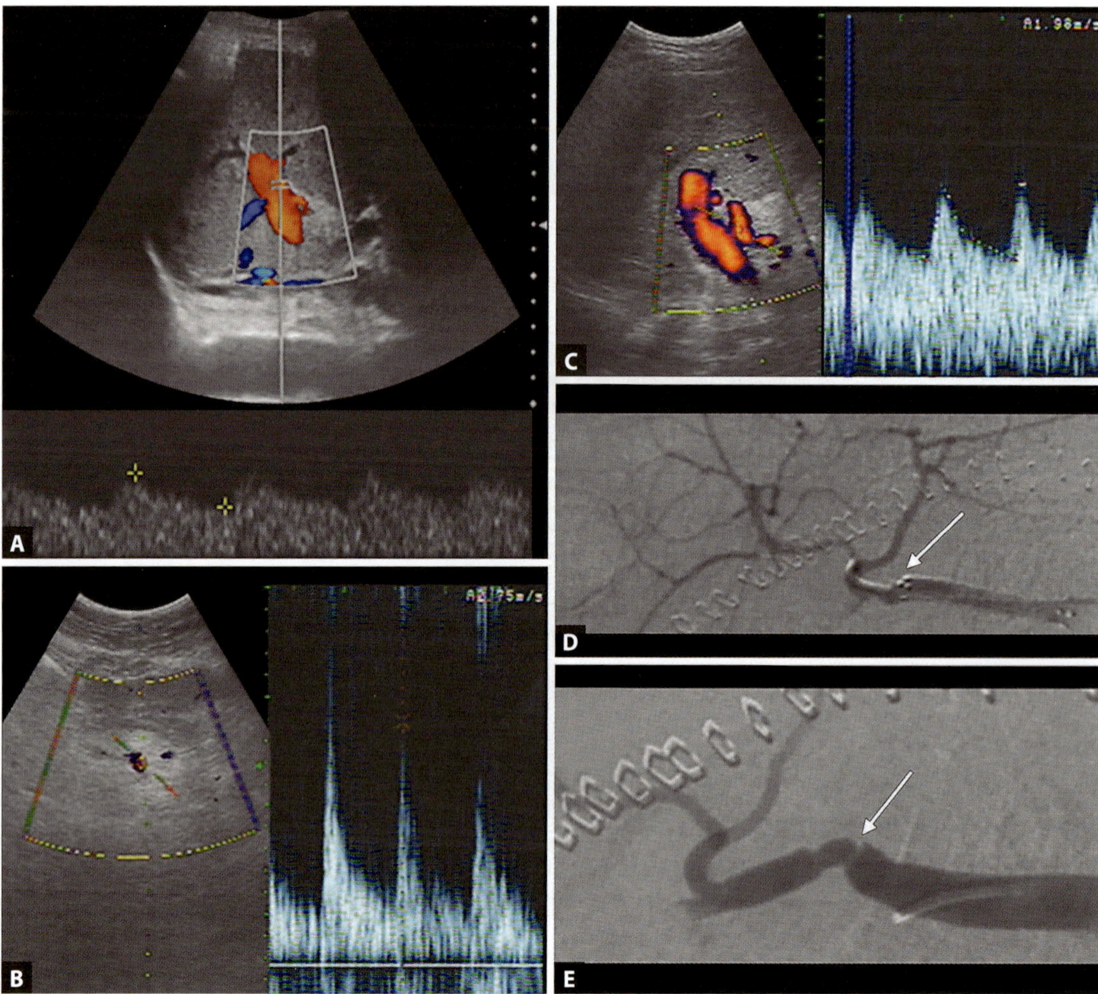

Figs. 4A to E: How well spectral curves work for evaluating hepatic artery stenosis. (A) Spectral curves ought to be acquired even in situations when the color Doppler test is normal. Both before and after the stenosis, they have a distinctive pattern. (B) We may observe strong peaks and an enhanced resistance index in the prestenotic region. (C) A low resistance index and a parvus et tardus pulse are visible in the poststenotic region. (D)Angiography can be used to carry out the treatment and (E) confirm the diagnosis.

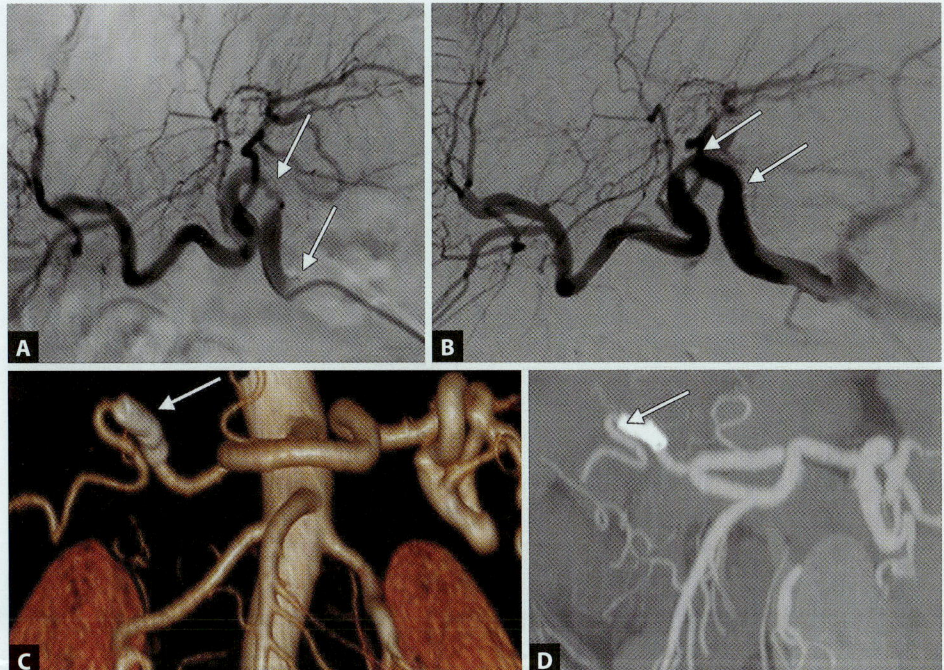

Figs. 5A to D: Multifocal stenosis. There may be several stenotic points in the hepatic artery. Each one should be handled independently in these situations. (A and B) Angiography in this instance revealed two stenotic. For treatment, two stents were implanted. Stent placement was confirmed by control CT, and distal artery flow was observed in both by (C) the volume rendering reconstruction and (D) the MIP reconstruction. (CT: computed tomography; MIP: maximum intensity projection)

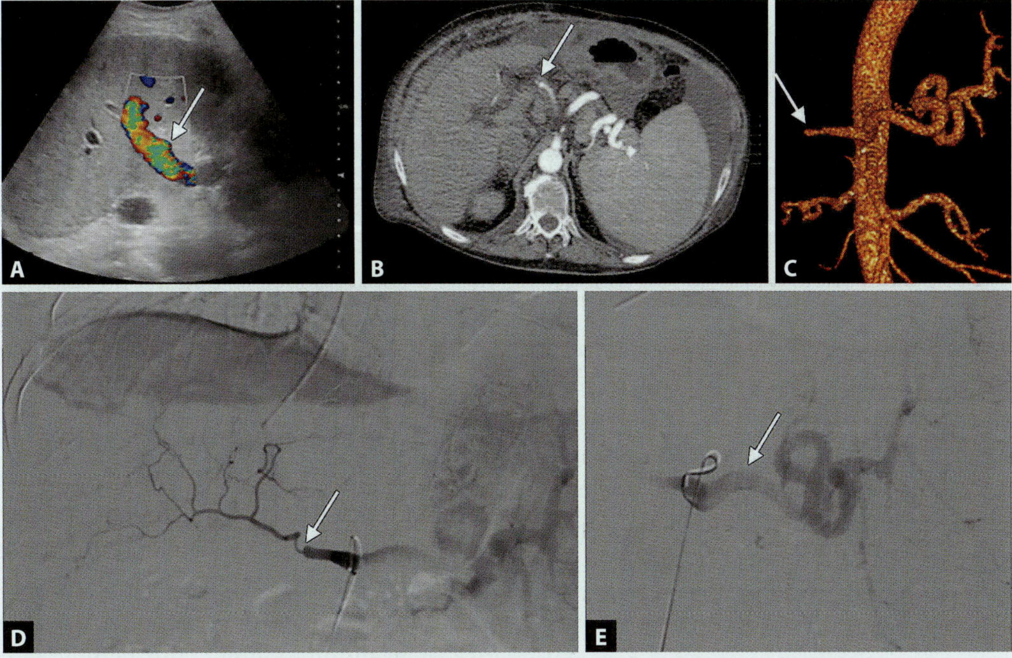

Figs. 6A to E: Splenic artery steal syndrome due to hepatic artery stenosis. The hepatic vein's turbulent flow is visible on the postoperative ultrasound (US). It is difficult to identify the hepatic artery (A). An arterial phase computed tomography (CT) scan reveals filiform enhancement of the hepatic artery's branches and severe localized stenosis of the artery (B and C). It is also important to observe the enlarged splenic artery. The increased turbulent portal flow can be explained by increased splenic artery blood flow. Both the enlarged splenic artery and the stenosis of the hepatic artery are confirmed by angiography (D and E). The splenic artery was distally embolized as a therapeutic procedure.

- Because of the turbulent flow, the stenotic segment exhibits an extremely high flow rate and aliasing artifact. <200 cm/s is the blood's systolic peak.
- The poststenotic section has a long systolic acceleration time (greater than 0.08 s), a parvus et tardus morphology of the spectral curves, and a low resistance index (<0.5). Its flow is tumultuous as well.

An essential factor to take into account: Importantly, in the first 3 days after liver transplantation, approximately 50% of patients had an increased hepatic artery resistance index (>0.8).[27]

If found, it should be monitored until it stabilizes, which is often the 4th day after transplantation.[28]

Ultrasonography is not a good technique to measure the stenosis; CT angiography is the preferred way, even though there is a correlation between the degree of stenosis and the severity of the reported anomalies.[29] Additionally, CT allows for precise evaluation of patients with a limited sonographic window. Multiplanar and three-dimensional curved reformatting are useful for measuring the vessel's lumen.

Due to a high percentage of false positives, MRI angiography is a limiting technique.[20] Early intervention is necessary for hepatic artery stenosis. It is best to perform an angiography and an angioplasty first. Surgery is necessary if this method does not work. Retransplantation, once again, yields superior results; however, it is best used as a last resort in the event that endovascular therapy becomes ineffective.[3]

False Aneurysm or Pseudoaneurysm

False aneurysm or pseudoaneurysm is shown in **Figs. 7 and 8**.

The features of pseudoaneurysm of the hepatic artery and its branches are comparable to those observed in other parts of the body, in contrast to other vascular issues associated with liver transplantation. In this case, it can affect not only the anastomosis point but any branch.

It is an uncommon side effect that occurs in 2.5% of liver transplant cases. According to color Doppler, pseudoechoic structures with turbulent blood flow within are seen on ultrasonography.

Usually, the yin-yang sign may be seen because of the swirl created by the blood outflow and inlet.[30]

When CT angiography is used, it often shows an arterial enhancement that is comparable to that of the other arterial vessels and eventually has an equal wash out.

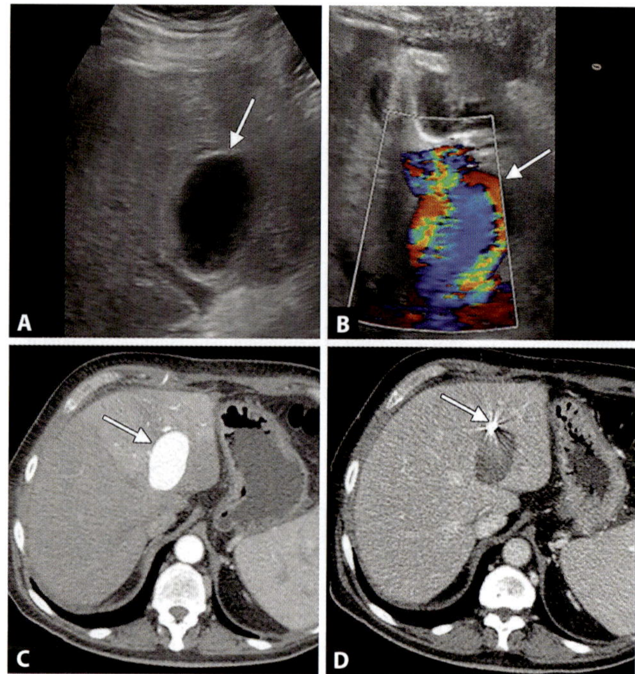

Figs. 7A to D: Hepatic artery pseudoaneurysm. (A) Pseudoaneurysms can be discovered using ultrasound; (B) it shows a characteristic appearance in Doppler ultrasound, due to the turbulent forward and backward flow; (C) arterial phase computed tomography (CT) shows arterial enhancement of the pseudoaneurysm; (D) a coil is placed to block entering the blood and to prevent rupture.

They are divided into two categories based on where they are found: extrahepatic and intrahepatic.

Extrahepatic pseudoaneurysms: The most common site is the artery anastomosis, and they can occur spontaneously or as a consequence of treating an underlying stenosis. Research has shown that a bacterial or fungal infection isolated from the pseudoaneurysm wall or peritoneal fluid may be present in up to 81% of cases.[31]

Intrahepatic pseudoaneurysms: Although bile duct infections may be the secondary cause, it is usually a side effect of percutaneous liver biopsy.[5] The development of a biliary fistula or portal could occur if these aneurysms rupture. When percutaneous liver biopsies are performed in the first few days or weeks after transplantation, the risk of pseudonystagmus and fistulas is considerably increased. Indeed, according to some articles, the risk of developing an arterioportal fistula drops from around 50% in the first week after surgery to 10% if the biopsies are performed about a month later.[29]

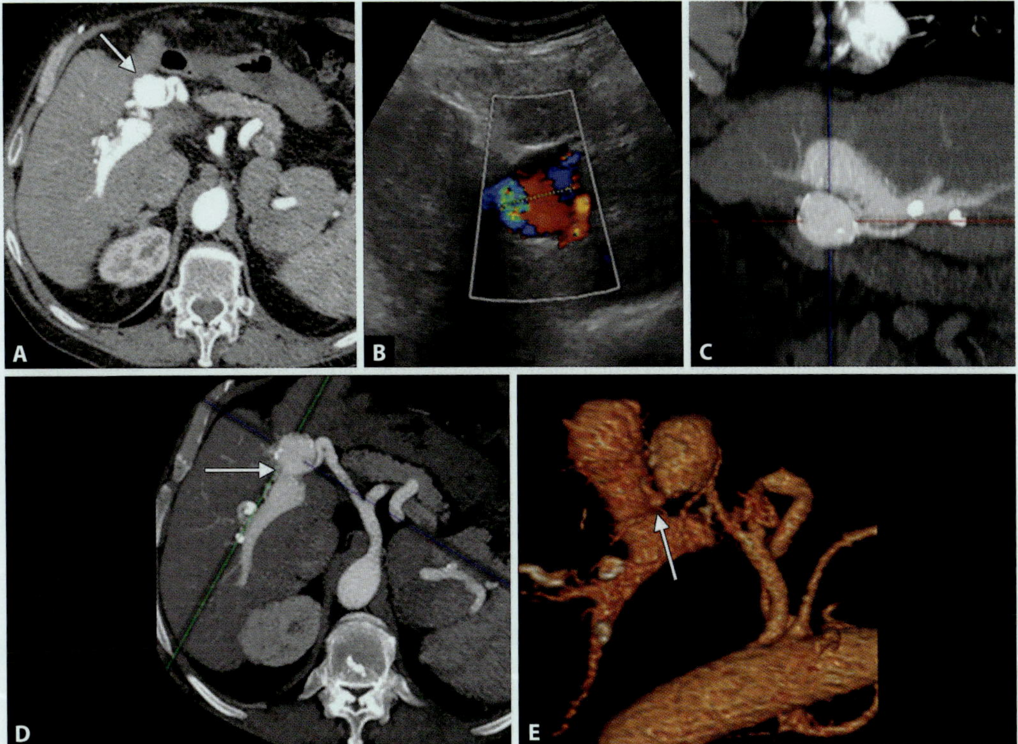

Figs. 8A to E: Portal fistula complicates an intrahepatic artery pseudoaneurysm. An intrahepatic fake aneurysm can be seen. (A) It displays vascular enhancement on computed tomography (CT) and (B)turbulent flow on color Doppler test . The formation of portal or biliary fistulas is one of the potential side effects of this condition. A porta fistula is visible in this instance (portal branches exhibit arterial augmentation). The precise site of the fistula is determined with the aid of multiplanar and volumetric reconstructions (C to E).

Coil embolization and stent implantation are the methods of treatment used in both situations to stop blood flow to the pseudoaneurysm. Surgical resection is an option if the outcomes of this treatment are not acceptable.[32]

Ischemia/Liver Infarction

Since the liver is a highly vascularized organ that receives blood via the portal vein and the hepatic artery, hepatic infarction is quite uncommon in healthy individuals. There are several anastomotic arteries and collateral branches inside the liver.

Hepatic infarction, however, is significantly more likely in liver transplant patients because anastomoses are blocked. In 85% of instances, arterial occlusion is the usual cause; portal vein occlusion is rarely linked to it.[29] Because the bile ducts get all of their blood supply from the hepatic artery, they are particularly vulnerable to impairments in arterial blood flow.[33]

These three hepatic artery alterations—thrombosis, stenosis, and pseudoaneurysm—can all result in ischemia and liver infarction.

Complications of Portal Vein

Complications from portal veins are rare. <2% of liver transplants are affected by them.[34]

The most common surgical technique involves directly joining the donor's portal vein to the recipient's.

Sometimes, this is not feasible because of a portal thrombus that blocks direct anastomosis. In these situations, a bypass and removal of the thrombus-occupied portion are required. Usually, the bypass is made using a donor iliac vein.[35]

It is crucial to understand the location of the anastomosis because problems with the portal vein typically impact it.

This section will discuss the most typical portal vein issues.

Thrombosis

Portal vein thrombosis **(Figs. 9A to C)** is a rare problem. It typically occurs at the extrahepatic portal vein's anastomosis location. A filling shortfall or contrast-enhanced MRI or CT scan without Doppler flow can be used to illustrate it.

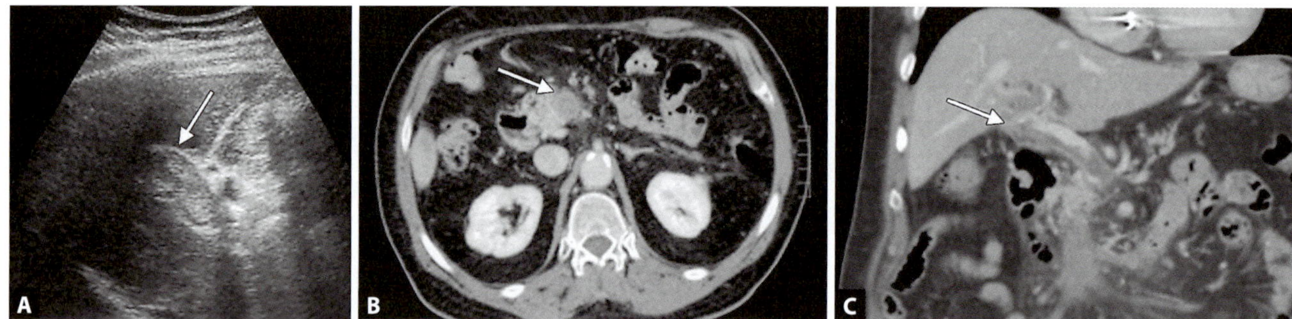

Figs. 9A to C: Portal vein thrombosis. (A) Echogenic material is observed on ultrasound examination; (B) this finding is confirmed in axial computed tomography (CT); and (C) multiplanar reconstructions help in the assessment of the extension.

According to certain research, contrast-enhanced ultrasonography is a potentially useful method for locating thrombosis cases that other imaging methods are unable to detect.[36]

An surgical revision of the anastomosis should be performed if thrombosis is observed within the first 72 hours following surgery. Afterwards, percutaneous thrombolysis, angioplasty, stenting, or, in the event that these less intrusive methods are not possible, surgery are used to treat the condition.

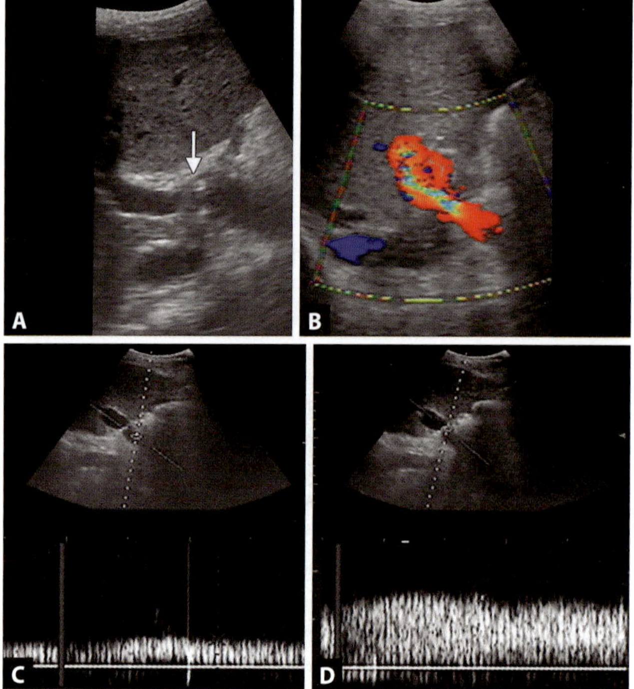

Figs. 10A to D: Spectral curves' utility in evaluating portal vein stenosis. (A) An ultrasound examination reveals several stenotic. (B) Turbulent flow is seen by color Doppler. (C) A distinctive pattern may be seen in the spectral curves both before and at the stenosis. A low flow may be seen in the prestenotic region. (D) High-speed flow (peak velocity above 125 cm/s) is observed in the stenotic segment. The stenotic/prestenotic ratio is a practical metric. The outcome in this instance is obviously greater than three.

Stenosis

Portal stenosis is shown in **Figs. 10 and 11**.

The anastomosis is the location that is most commonly affected. The following are the typical findings for each imaging technique:

- According to Doppler ultrasound, the portal blood flow velocity is typically greater than 125 cm/s at the anastomosis point or three times higher at the stenosis site than in the prestenotic segment.[37] As was previously said for arterial velocity, Doppler measurements need the use of an appropriate angle, which is not always possible due to patient's circumstances. Thus, a more accurate metric is the stenotic/prestenotic ratio.
- Turbulent flow can also create an aliasing artifact to show up in the stenotic segment. This may also be a typical finding in the initial postoperative phase. Thus, anastomosis in turbulent flow cases needs to be assessed for comparison in subsequent controls.[5]
- The degree of stenosis can be seen and measured using CT or MR angiography.

It is important to distinguish stenosis from a physiological mild reduction in vessel caliber at the anastomotic location. If the donor and recipient portal veins differ in size, then this observation is much more noteworthy. The focused constriction in this instance is not associated with stenosis and is a normal finding. Having an understanding of the preoperative anatomy and graft evaluation will aid in the differential diagnosis. However, since this result increases the risk of developing a stenosis, it should be investigated further.[35] Surgical excision is the last resort in the event that previous methods fail. Other treatments include angioplasty and stenting.

Issues with Inferior Vena Cava

Complications involving the inferior vena cava are infrequent. <2% of liver transplants are affected by them.[34]

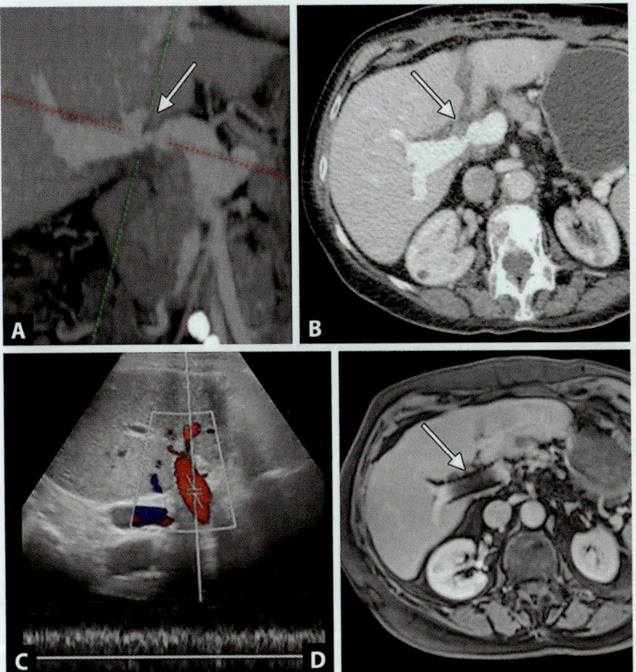

Figs. 11A to D: Stenosis of the portal vein. On computed tomography (CT), portal vein stenosis can be seen in (A) multiplanar reconstructions as well as (B) axial images; (C) a control ultrasonography is conducted following stent implantation; (D) it demonstrates how the portal flow has normalized. The stent's metallic artifact is visible in the control magnetic resonance imaging (MRI). Both proximal and distal to the stent, normal contrast enhancement is observed.

In particular, coronal reconstructions are helpful for determining the thrombus's extent.

Thrombosis

Inferior vena cava thrombosis is shown in **(Figs. 12A and B)**

They typically results from a surgical procedure or a hypercoagulable condition. It can be diagnosed and treated similarly to portal vein thrombosis.

Stenosis

Stenosis is shown in **Figs. 13A and B**.

Similar to the other vessels, the anastomosis is the most common site. Furthermore, hematomas, abscesses, graft edema, or fluid collections can all result in extrinsic compressive stenosis. The diagnostic and therapeutic approaches are similar to those described in the portal vein.

Hepatic Vein Complications

Adverse consequences such as hepatic vein complications **(Figs. 14A and B)** are rare. Thrombosis (Budd-Chiari syndrome) and stenosis are the usual consequences in this situation.

In living donor transplant instances, knowledge of the surgical anatomy is essential. The right hepatic vein is usually preserved in the right lobe of the graft, while the middle hepatic vein is usually left intact for the donor's safety. Postoperative control should assess the middle hepatic vein since it is sometimes absorbed into the graft.[38]

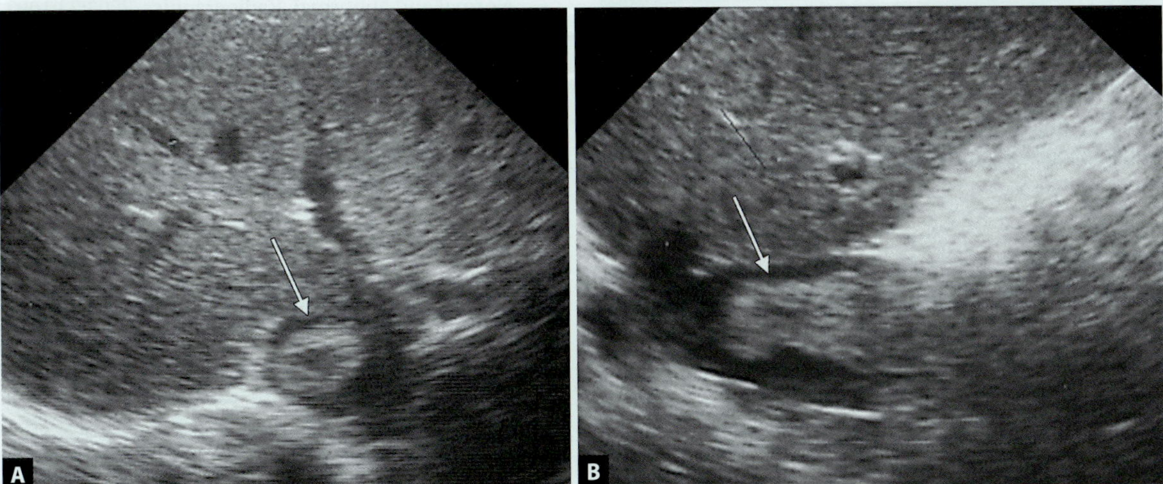

Figs. 12A and B: Inferior vena cava thrombosis. An axial ultrasonography test revealed inferior vena cava thrombosis. Assessing its extension is aided by sagittal inspection.

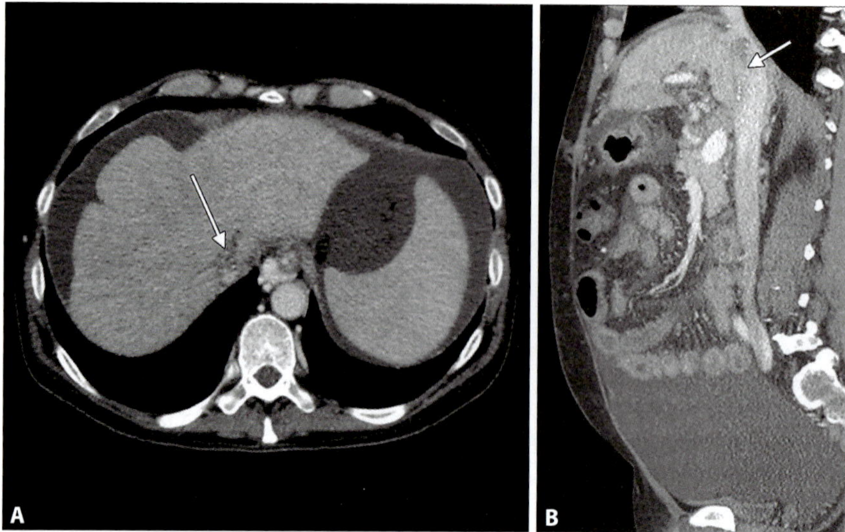

Figs. 13A and B: The inferior vena cava is stenotic. The axial and sagittal scans show stenosis of the inferior vena cava. Hepatic vein confluence is impacted. Ascites is caused by venous drainage issues. Percutaneous angioplasty is used as a therapeutic procedure.

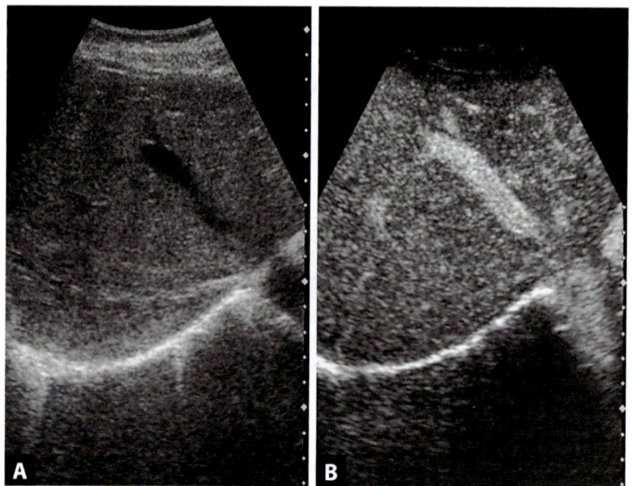

Figs. 14A and B: Right hepatic vein thrombosis. Compared to the middle hepatic vein, the right suprahepatic vein is more echogenic. The middle hepatic vein is enhanced and exhibits normal flow following contrast injection. Due to thrombosis, the right hepatic vein does not enlarge.

CONCLUSION

Effective treatment must be established as soon as vascular issues from liver transplantation are identified. This affects both the transplant's efficacy and the mortality and morbidity of the patients.

Doppler ultrasound is the initial imaging test. It is recommended to use other methods (contrast-enhanced ultrasonography, CT, and MRI) if it is unable to provide a definitive diagnosis.

REFERENCES

1. Monti L, Soglia G, Tomà P. Imaging in pediatric liver transplantation. Radiol Med. 2016;121:378-90.
2. Khalaf H. Vascular complications after deceased and living donor liver transplantation: A single-center experience. Transplant Proc. 2010:42:865-70.
3. Duffy JP, Hong JC, Farmer DG, Ghobrial RM, Yersiz H, Hiatt JR, et al Vascular complications of orthotopic liver transplantation: Experience in more than 4,200 patients. J Am Coll Surg. 2009;208:896-903; discussion 903-5.
4. Singhal A, Stokes K, Sebastian A, Wright HI, Kohli V. Endovascular treatment of hepatic artery thrombosis following liver transplantation. Transpl Int. 2010;23:245-56.
5. Crossin JD, Muradali D, Wilson SR. US of liver transplants: Normal and abnormal. Radiographics. 2003;23:1093-114.
6. Katyal S, Oliver JH 3rd, Buck DG, Federle MP. Detection of vascular complications after liver transplantation. Am J Roentgenol. 2000;175:1735-9.
7. Boraschi P, Della Pina MC, Donati F. Graft complications following orthotopic liver transplantation: Role of non-invasive cross-sectional imaging techniques. Eur J Radiol. 2016;85:1271-83.
8. Chen J, Weinstein J, Black S, Spain J, Brady PS, Dowell JD. Surgical and endovascular treatment of hepatic arterial complications following liver transplant. Clin Transplant. 2014;28:1305-12.
9. Pareja E, Cortes M, Navarro R, Sanjuan F, López R, Mir J. Vascular complications after orthotopic liver transplantation: Hepatic artery thrombosis. Transplant Proc. 2010;42:2970-2.
10. Stanescu AL, Kamps SE, Dick AAS, Parisi MT, Phillips GS. Intraoperative Doppler sonogram in pediatric liver transplants: a pictorial review of intraoperative

and early postoperative complications. Pediatr Radiol. 2018;48:401-10.

11. Ito K, Siegelman ES, Stolpen AH, Mitchell DG. MR imaging of complications after liver transplantation. Am J Roentgenol. 2000;175:1145-9.
12. Girometti R, Pancot M, Como G, Zuiani C. Imaging of liver transplantation. Eur J Radiol. 2017;93:295-307.
13. Lladó L, Figueras J. Techniques of orthotopic liver transplantation. HPB (Oxford). 2004;6:69-75.
14. Girometti R, Como G, Bazzocchi M, Zuiani C. Post-operative imaging in liver transplantation: State-of-the-art and future perspectives. World J Gastroenterol. 1014;20:6180-200.
15. Itri JN, Heller MT, Tublin ME. Hepatic transplantation: Postoperative complications. Abdom Imaging. 2013;38: 1300-33.
16. Wozney P, Zajko A, Bron K, Point S, Starzl T. Vascular complications after liver transplantation: a 5-year experience. Am J Roentgenol. 1986;147:657-63.
17. Gu LH, Fang H, Li FH, Li P, Zhu CX, Zhu JJ, et al. Prediction of early hepatic artery thrombosis by intraoperative color Doppler ultrasound in pediatric segmental liver transplantation. Clin Transplant. 2012;26:571-6.
18. Hom BK, Shrestha R, Palmer SL, Katz MD, Selby RR, Asatryan Z, et al. Prospective evaluation of vascular complications after liver transplantation: Comparison of conventional and microbubble contrast-enhanced US. Radiology. 2006;241:267-74.
19. Kim SY, Kim KW, Kim MJ, Shin YM, Lee MG, Lee SG. Multidetector row CT of various hepatic artery complications after living donor liver transplantation. Abdom Imaging. 2007;32:635-43.
20. Glockner JF, Forauer AR, Solomon H, Varma CR, Perman WH. Three-dimensional gadolinium-enhanced MR angiography of vascular complications after liver transplantation. AJR Am J Roentgenol. 2000;174:1447-53.
21. Legmann P, Costes V, Tudoret L, Girardot C, Hazebroucq V, Uzan E, et al. Hepatic artery thrombosis after liver transplantation: diagnosis with spiral CT. AJR Am J Roentgenol. 1995;164:97-101.
22. Piardi T, Lhuaire M, Bruno O, Memeo R, Pessaux P, Kianmanesh R, et al. Vascular complications following liver transplantation: A literature review of advances in 2015. World J Hepatol. 2016;8:36-57.
23. Sanyal R, Shah SN. Role of imaging in the management of splenic artery steal syndrome. J Ultrasound Med. 2009;28:471-7.
24. Abbasoglu O, Levy MF, Vodapally MS, Goldstein RM, Husberg BS, Gonwa TA, et al. Hepatic artery stenosis after liver transplantation--incidence, presentation, treatment, and long term outcome. Transplantation. 1997;63:250-5.
25. Denys AL, Qanadli SD, Durand F, Vilgrain V, Farges O, Belghiti J, et al Feasibility and effectiveness of using coronary stents in the treatment of hepatic artery stenoses after orthotopic liver transplantation: preliminary report. AJR Am J Roentgenol. 2002;178:1175-9.
26. Uzochukwu LN, Bluth EI, Smetherman DH, Troxclair LA, Loss GE Jr, Cohen A, et al. Early postoperative hepatic sonography as a predictor of vascular and biliary complications in adult orthotopic liver transplant patients. AJR Am J Roentgenol. 2005;185:1558-70.
27. García-Criado A, Gilabert R, Salmerón JM, Nicolau C, Vilana R, Bianchi L, et al. Significance of and contributing factors for a high resistive index on Doppler sonography of the hepatic artery immediately after surgery: Prognostic implications for liver transplant recipients. AJR Am J Roentgenol. 2003;181:831-8.
28. Caiado AH, Blasbalg R, Marcelino AS, da Cunha Pinho M, Chammas MC, da Costa Leite C, et al. Complications of liver transplantation: multimodality imaging approach. Radiographics 2007;27:1401-17.
29. Quiroga S, Sebastià MC, Margarit C, Castells L, Boyé R, Alvarez-Castells A. Complications of orthotopic liver transplantation: Spectrum of findings with helical CT. Radiographics. 2001;21:1085-102.
30. Lupattelli T. The yin-yang sign. Radiology. 2006;238(3): 1070-1.
31. Volpin E, Pessaux P, Sauvanet A, Sibert A, Kianmanesh R, Durand F, et al. Preservation of the arterial vascularisation after hepatic artery pseudoaneurysm following orthotopic liver transplantation: Long-term results. Ann Transplant. 2014;19:346-52.
32. Nagaraja R, Govindasamy M, Varma V, Yadav A, Mehta N, Kumaran V, et al. Hepatic artery pseudoaneurysms: a single-center experience. Ann Vasc Surg. 2013;27:743-9.
33. Orons PD, Sheng R, Zajko AB. Hepatic artery stenosis in liver transplant recipients: Prevalence and cholangiographic appearance of associated biliary complications. AJR Am J Roentgenol. 1995;165:1145-9.
34. Pérez-Saborido B, Pacheco-Sánchez D, Barrera-Rebollo A, Asensio-Díaz E, Pinto-Fuentes P, Sarmentero-Prieto JC, et al. Incidence, management, and results of vascular complications after liver transplantation. Transplant Proc. 2011432011;43:749-50.
35. Singh AK, Nachiappan AC, Verma HA, Uppot RN, Blake MA, Saini S, B, et al. Postoperative imaging in liver transplantation: What radiologists should know. Radiographics. 2010;30(2):339-51.
36. Rennert J, Dornia C, Georgieva M, Roehrl S, Fellner C, Schleder S, et al. Identification of early complications following liver transplantation using contrast enhanced ultrasound (CEUS). First results. J Gastrointestin Liver Dis. 2012;21(4):407-12.
37. Chong WK, Beland JC, Weeks SM. Sonographic evaluation of venous obstruction in liver transplants. AJR Am J Roentgenol. 2007;188(6):W515-21.
38. Yu PF, Wu J, Zheng SS. Management of the middle hepatic vein and its tributaries in right lobe living donor liver transplantation. Hepatobiliary Pancreat Dis Int. 2007;6(4):358-63.

CHAPTER 15

Hepatopulmonary Syndrome: Perioperative Challenges and Management During Liver Transplantation

Tushar Parmar, Suvadeep Sen

INTRODUCTION

Hepatopulmonary syndrome (HPS) is a constellation of features present mostly in end-stage liver disease (ESLD) with portal hypertension and characterized by intrapulmonary vascular dilatation (IPVD) causing arteriovenous shunt, diffusion restriction, and ventilation-perfusion ($\dot{V}/\dot{Q}$) mismatch with a result of chronic hypoxia and features of orthodeoxia. The syndrome is associated with high mortality among patients with ESLD. An orthotopic liver transplant (OLT) is the only definitive treatment for this condition. The condition is prevalent among almost 10–30% of patients being evaluated for liver transplantation (LT).[1] However, most of the patients remain clinically asymptomatic, hence, careful screening of patients in preoperative evaluation is important. It is also imperative to understand that HPS is associated with higher post-transplant mortality and morbidity compared to patients with cirrhosis of the same model for end-stage liver disease (MELD).

DEFINITION AND SEVERITY CLASSIFICATION

Hepatopulmonary syndrome is defined as a triad of chronic liver disease, arterial hypoxemia, and evidence of IPVD. The current diagnostic criteria are based on the European Respiratory Society (ERS) Task Force recommendation and the International Liver Transplant Society (ILTS) Practice Guidelines[2] published in 2016 **(Table 1)**.

PATHOBIOLOGY OF HEPATOPULMONARY SYNDROME

Impaired gas exchange in HPS results from three mechanisms related to changes in the alveolar microcirculation causing dilatation of vessels in capillary and precapillary levels up to 100 µm (normal diameter is 8–15 µm). This alteration in the pulmonary microvascular system results in $\dot{V}/\dot{Q}$ mismatch, diffusion limitation, and anatomic shunting from direct arteriovenous (AV) communications. $\dot{V}/\dot{Q}$ mismatch occurs due to increased pulmonary blood flow from microvascular alterations while ventilation remains unaffected. Diffusion limitation arises as oxygen travels a greater distance due to vascular dilation. Direct AV communications bypass the alveolar microcirculation, leading to venous-arterial blood mixing. These circulatory changes, driven by cirrhosis and portal hypertension, disrupt the balance between vasodilation and vasoconstriction, contributing to the development of HPS.

The pathobiology of hepatopulmonary syndrome is given in **Figure 1**.

TABLE 1: Diagnostic and severity criteria of hepatopulmonary syndrome.

Diagnostic	
Abnormal oxygenation	Partial pressure of oxygen (PaO_2) <80 mm Hg in room air in sitting position or alveolar-arterial oxygen gradient [$P(A-a)O_2$ gradient] ≥15 mm Hg (or ≥20 in case of ≥65 years of age)
Evidence of intrapulmonary vascular dilation (IPVD)	Confirmed by contrast-enhanced transthoracic echocardiography (CE-TTE) or Technetium-99m macroaggregated albumin (Tc-MAA) lung perfusion scanning showing brain shunt fraction >6%
Liver disease	Advanced liver disease (most common), portal hypertension, and congenital portosystemic shunts (CPSSs)
Severity classification	
Stages	*Partial pressure of oxygen in room air*
Mild	≥80 mm Hg with presence of $P(A-a)O_2$ ≥15 mm Hg
Moderate	60–79 mm Hg
Severe	50–59 mm Hg
Very severe	<50 mm Hg or <300 mm Hg while breathing on 100% oxygen

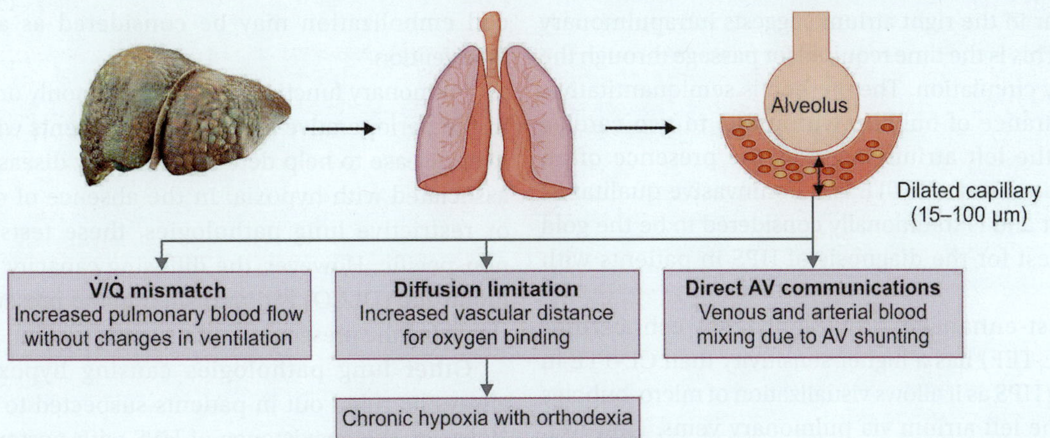

Fig. 1: Pathobiology of hepatopulmonary syndrome.

Two distinct types of HPS have been described based on the location of dilated pulmonary vessels:

1. *Type I:* This is characterized by dilatation of vessels at the precapillary level near the gas exchange regions of the lungs; this is more diffused in pattern and more severe in the basal part of the lung. In this type, supplemental oxygen improves PaO_2.
2. *Type II:* This is less common and involves more significant vessel dilatation, leading to AV shunts that are more focal in nature. Supplemental oxygen does not offer benefits in this type. Computed tomography (CT) pulmonary angiography may help to identify focal AV malformations. This type of shunt may be more responsive to embolotherapy in case of severe hypoxia.

WHEN DO WE SUSPECT THE PRESENCE OF HEPATOPULMONARY SYNDROME DURING PERIOPERATIVE EVALUATION, AND HOW DO WE DIAGNOSE IT?

Any patients with ESLD with the following clinical features should be suspected and screened for the presence of HPS:

- Exertional or resting dyspnea
- Platypnea (shortness of breath that is relieved when lying down and worsens when sitting or standing upright)
- Presence of cyanosis and digital clubbing
- *Diffuse telangiectasia:* Features like spider naevi are more commonly seen in patients with HPS

Initial screening should be done with oxygen saturation (SaO_2), measured by pulse oximetry in the room air. A cutoff of <96%, in the absence of other obvious lung diseases warrants further screening and diagnostics. However, it is to be noted that pulse oximetry has poor sensitivity (18–28%) and specificity (89.8%) as the sole screening tool for HPS when a cutoff of 96% is used.[3]

The presence of hypoxia is confirmed with an arterial blood gas (ABG) analysis at room air, which is mandatory in all such cases. Hypoxia is documented as the PaO_2 <60 mm Hg in room air or elevated alveolar-arterial oxygen [$P(A\text{-}a)\ O_2$] gradient ≥15 mm Hg. The $P(A\text{-}a)O_2$ gradient is calculated as:

$$[(Patm - PH_2O) \times 0.21] - [(PaCO_2/0.8) - PaO_2]$$, where H_2O pressure = 47 mm Hg.

The presence of orthodexia is determined by a drop in PaO_2 in arterial blood by ≥4 mm Hg (0.5 kPa) or by ≥5% when the patient moves from supine to upright. This is found in almost one-fourth of patients with HPS and is very specific for HPS in the presence of ESLD.

The chest radiograph is often normal-appearing in HPS. High-resolution computed tomography (HRCT) chest may show nonspecific changes or a mild interstitial pattern in the lower lungs, indicating diffuse pulmonary vascular dilation in the lower lobe.

The diagnosis is confirmed with evidence of IPVD, using bubble contrast echocardiography and technetium-99m macroaggregated albumin lung perfusion scan.

In bubble contrast-enhanced transthoracic echocardiography (CE-TTE), 10 mL of normal saline (0.9%) is agitated to create microbubbles larger than 10 µm in diameter and is injected into a peripheral vein. The apical four-chamber view is obtained during TTE, which allows visualization of both the right and left side of the heart. Under normal conditions, these bubbles are too large to pass through the pulmonary capillary bed (which has a diameter of 8–15 µm) and are restricted to the right side of the heart. The appearance of microbubbles in the left atrium within three to six cardiac cycles after they appear in the right atrium suggests intrapulmonary shunting. This is the time required for passage through the pulmonary circulation. The method is semiquantitative. The appearance of bubbles within one to two cardiac cycles in the left atrium suggests the presence of an intracardiac shunt. CE-TTE is a noninvasive qualitative assessment and is traditionally considered to be the gold standard test for the diagnosis of HPS in patients with cirrhosis.

Contrast-enhanced transesophageal echocardiography (CE-TEE) has a higher sensitivity than CE-TTE in diagnosing HPS as it allows visualization of micro-bubbles entering the left atrium via pulmonary veins. However, this is invasive and carries inherent risk in the presence of esophageal varices, and it is usually not used routinely as a part of diagnosis and preoperative assessment.

Technetium-99m macroaggregated albumin lung perfusion scan is an alternative method for documenting IPVDs. Under normal conditions, the injected particles (>20 μm in diameter) are trapped in the pulmonary capillaries. However, in the presence of intracardiac or intrapulmonary shunts, these aggregates reach systemic circulation and accumulate in the brain, kidneys, and spleen. By using quantitative imaging to assess the distribution of MAA particles in the brain and lungs, shunt fraction can be determined, which provides a quantitative estimation of the anatomic severity of IPVD in HPS. Brain shunt fraction >6% is considered to be significant.

However, MAA scan does not distinguish intrapulmonary from intracardiac shunt. The test lacks proper standardization and has lesser sensitivity to diagnose mild-to-moderate HPS in adults compared to CE-TTE.[4] MAA scan is usually used as a complementary tool to CE-TTE in two specific situations. First, in patients who have concomitant HPS and intrinsic lung pathology with hypoxemia (PaO_2 <60 mm Hg), an elevated MAA shunt (>6%) suggests that HPS is the primary cause of hypoxemia. Second, calculation of the MAA shunt fraction, which may have a prognostic significance, a positive brain uptake ≥20% in patients with very severe HPS (PaO_2 <50 mm Hg) has been linked to increased mortality following LT.[5]

High-resolution computed tomography (HRCT) chest and CT pulmonary angiography are often done in patients with unexplained hypoxia to rule out intrinsic lung pathology and evidence of AV malformations. CT pulmonary angiography also helps to identify type II communications in HPS, which have been observed to persist after liver LT and may pose a risk for paradoxical embolism and cerebral abscesses. In such cases, coil embolization may be considered as a potential intervention.[1]

Pulmonary function tests are commonly ordered tests in the perioperative evaluation of patients with chronic liver disease to help detect pulmonary diseases that are associated with hypoxia. In the absence of obstructive or restrictive lung pathologies, these tests are often nonspecific. However, the diffusing capacity for carbon monoxide (DLCO) is diminished in the presence of HPS signifying the presence of diffusion restriction.

Other lung pathologies causing hypoxia should always be ruled out in patients suspected to have HPS. However, the coexistence of HPS with portopulmonary hypertension (POPH) and other pulmonary diseases such as obstructive airway diseases and asthma and pulmonary fibrosis may also be observed.[2] MAA scan is helpful to diagnose concomitant shunt physiology in the presence of obvious lung diseases and plays an important role in prognostication.

Common differentials for hypoxia in end-stage liver diseases are given in **Table 2**.

TABLE 2: Common differentials for hypoxia in end-stage liver diseases.

Differentials	*Characteristics*
Hepatic hydrothorax	Presence of pleural effusion in chest radiogram
Intrinsic lung parenchymal lesions	• Basal atelectasis from large ascites and postoperative setting • Infective etiologies such as bacterial and viral infections • Obstructive airway diseases • Restrictive lung diseases from ascites, poor neuromuscular function, pulmonary fibrosis, etc. • High-resolution computed tomography (HRCT) chest and pulmonary function tests usually provide clues
Portopulmonary hypertension	Right heart catheterization and estimation of pulmonary hemodynamics provide valuable information on pulmonary vascular pressures and reversibility
Pulmonary arteriovenous (AV) malformations	Computed tomography (CT) pulmonary angiography provides clues to such large AV malformations
Pulmonary embolism	Diagnosed with CT pulmonary angiography
Intrinsic cardiac shunt	Contrast-enhanced transesophageal echocardiography (TEE) reveals a defect in the interatrial septum

IMPLICATION OF HEPATOPULMONARY SYNDROME IN PERIOPERATIVE OUTCOME IN CIRRHOTICS

Liver transplantation is the only definitive treatment for patients with HPS. A retrospective case-control analysis from the Mayo Clinic analyzed long-term survival in HPS patients, finding that those who underwent orthotopic liver transplantation (OLT) had significantly better 5-year survival (76%) compared to nontransplant patients (23%).[6] In the absence of OLT, hypoxia worsens with a decline in PaO_2 <5.2 + 2.3 mm Hg per year, as per the earlier-mentioned study. The degree of hypoxia in HPS is unrelated to Child–Pugh severity of liver disease. Hence, a diagnosis of hepatopulmonary syndrome with a PaO_2 below 60 mm Hg warrants a need for LT, and such patients are prioritized for OLT with standard MELD exception points. Post-liver transplant hypoxia gradually resolves within a period of 6–12 months in 95% of cases.[1] The time of resolution again depends on the pretransplant severity of HPS.

Hepatopulmonary syndrome is an independent risk factor of perioperative mortality in patients with ESLD admitted for elective liver transplant. The strongest predictors of postoperative mortality are preoperative PaO_2 <50 mm Hg (very severe HPS) and MAA scan showing brain uptake >20%.[7] Perioperative surgical, infectious, and cardiac complications are also found to be higher in a retrospective case-control study on 71 patient populations with HPS when compared to patients without HPS.[8] Hypoxemia is considered the primary factor contributing to the increased rate of complications in patients with HPS. It is a well-established risk factor for cardiovascular issues. It has well-documented negative impacts on immune function, including reduced resistance to bacterial infections, impaired wound healing, and a higher risk of anastomotic leaks and strictures. A retrospective analysis of 1,152 HPS patients from the United Network for Organ Sharing (UNOS) registry, published in 2021, found that post-transplant mortality was highest in patients with preoperative PaO_2 values <45 mm Hg.[9] However, the median survival in this category of patients was 11.5 years, with an increased mortality risk observed after 2.6 years post-liver transplantation (OLT). This report supports the potential benefits of OLT even in the sickest cohort of patients with HPS, given the high probability for reversibility of the condition following transplantation.

PERIOPERATIVE OPTIMIZATION

The perioperative evaluation and optimization of patients with HPS admitted for OLT is more or less similar to those without HPS. However, it is important to evaluate the severity of hypoxia in all cases and assess the degree of improvement with supplemental oxygen. Most patients with severe HPS show improvement in PaO_2 with 100% oxygen. The two strongest predictors of severe postoperative hypoxia are (1) intrapulmonary shunt fraction >20% and (2) DLCO <40%.

The intraoperative ventilation strategy follows lung-protective ventilation with (positive end-expiratory pressure) PEEP as per requirement. Supine position in the operating room (OR) favors oxygenation in HPS patients. It is important to monitor mixed venous oxygen saturation (SvO_2) in the intraoperative period, and if it falls to <65% despite maximum oxygen support, venovenous bypass may be considered.

POSTOPERATIVE MANAGEMENT OF HEPATOPULMONARY SYNDROME AFTER LIVER TRANSPLANT

Orthotopic liver transplant is challenging in patients with HPS as the patients often undergo a stormy postoperative course. Hypoxia commonly worsens in the postoperative setting for several reasons.

- Concomitant atelectasis and lung parenchymal pathology (infection, volume overload, or acute lung injury from any reason) that occur commonly in postoperative settings
- Effect of sedation or pain from subcostal incision causing restricted chest excursion
- V/Q mismatch exacerbates due to impaired hypoxic pulmonary vasoconstriction (HPV) in the dilated pulmonary vessels, leading to disproportionate constriction of normal pulmonary vessels.
- The practical disadvantage of continuous Trendelenburg position in the postoperative setting

Oxygen administration is the most common method to treat hypoxia in postoperative settings in these patients. It can be administered by nasal cannula, face mask, high flow nasal cannula, or noninvasive ventilation strategy depending on the patient's need. Mechanical ventilation is often prolonged in patients with HPS after liver transplantation surgery. However, early extubation should be attempted in all cases with the provision of supplemental oxygen. Target >85%. Fluid therapy should

Flowchart 1: Stepwise approach for management of post-transplant hypoxia in patients with hepatopulmonary syndrome (HPS).

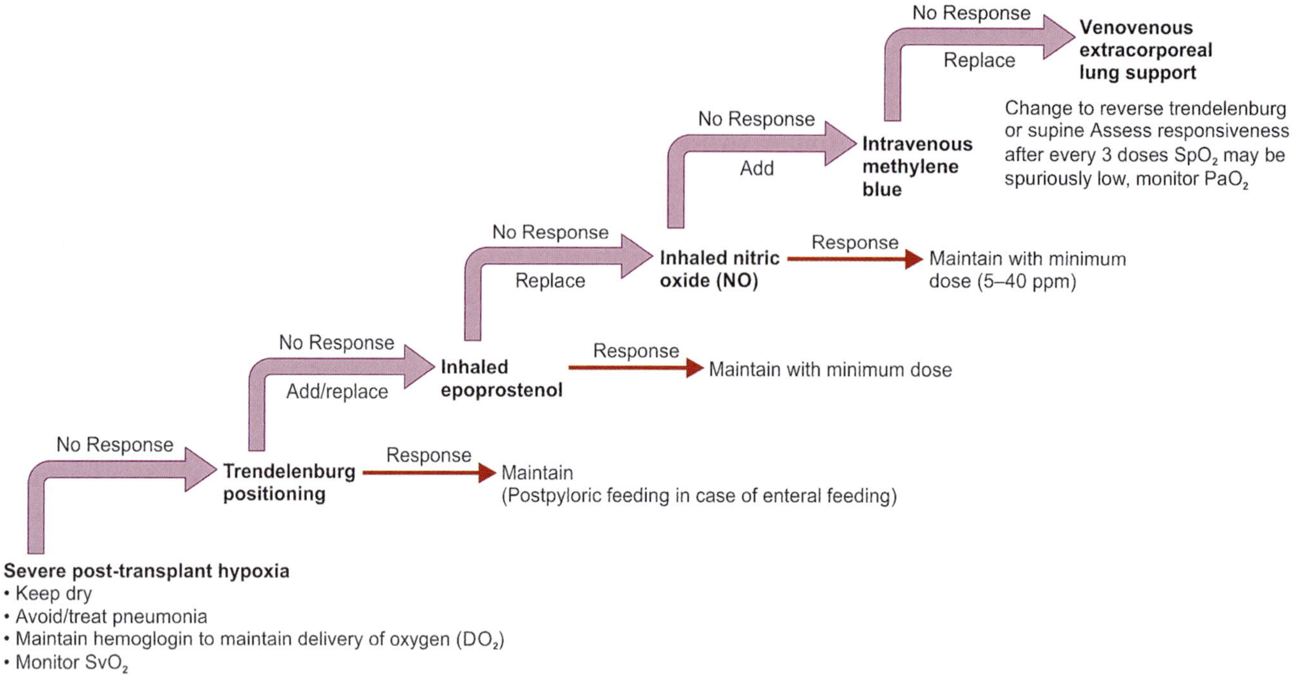

Severe post-transplant hypoxia
- Keep dry
- Avoid/treat pneumonia
- Maintain hemoglogin to maintain delivery of oxygen (DO_2)
- Monitor SvO_2

No Response → **Trendelenburg positioning** — Response → Maintain (Postpyloric feeding in case of enteral feeding)

No Response, Add/replace → **Inhaled epoprostenol** — Response → Maintain with minimum dose

No Response, Replace → **Inhaled nitric oxide (NO)** — Response → Maintain with minimum dose (5–40 ppm)

No Response, Add → **Intravenous methylene blue** — Change to reverse trendelenburg or supine Assess responsiveness after every 3 doses SpO_2 may be spuriously low, monitor PaO_2

No Response, Replace → **Venovenous extracorporeal lung support**

be judicious with a goal-directed approach. Standard infection control measures to prevent lung infection are necessary.

Apart from oxygen administration, several strategies can be adopted to counteract the pathophysiology of HPS in perioperative settings. Experts recommend continuing all initially effective therapies and sequentially adding additional treatments if recurrent hypoxemia occurs.

Severe post-transplant hypoxemia, characterized by the need for 100% fraction of inspired oxygen (FiO_2) to maintain SpO_2 above 85%, occurs in 6–21% of patients with HPS and is associated with a peritransplant mortality rate of 45%.[10] Severe post-transplant hypoxia should be managed as a stepwise algorithm, with different interventions **(Flowchart 1)**. A response is defined as a 20% improvement in the PaO_2/FiO_2 (P/F) ratio, while deterioration is indicated by a 20% decrease in the P/F ratio.[11] These changes are measured at 30 minutes for all interventions, except for methylene blue (MB), where the assessment is made at 5 hours. While MB may show an early response as soon as 30 minutes, its peak effect is typically observed at 5 hours.

Trendelenburg Positioning

In HPS, intrapulmonary vascular dilatations are primarily localized in the basal lung regions. Trendelenburg positioning works by inducing a gravitational redistribution of pulmonary blood flow toward the upper and mid-lung zones, thereby reducing perfusion through the dilated vessels in the lung bases and potentially improving overall oxygenation.

Inhaled Nitric Oxide

Inhaled nitric oxide (iNO) is widely recognized as an effective therapeutic agent for managing severe post-transplant hypoxemia in patients with HPS. iNO selectively dilates blood vessels in the mid and upper lung zones through two basic mechanisms. First, the vessels in the basal lung regions, which are already maximally dilated due to chronic remodeling in longstanding HPS, exhibit reduced responsiveness to further vasodilation by nitric oxide (NO). Second, iNO is preferentially distributed to well-ventilated areas of the lung, while the lung bases, typically poorly ventilated in the postoperative setting due to atelectasis, receive less of the gas. Additionally, iNO may help alleviate postoperative pulmonary vasoconstriction in normal pulmonary vessels.

Inhaled NO is considered safe and highly selective for pulmonary circulation, with minimal systemic effects, including no significant impact on systemic hemodynamics at recommended doses. The effects of iNO are also rapidly reversible, with a half-life of approximately

111–130 milliseconds. It is administered concurrently with existing oxygen delivery devices with a dose of up to 40 ppm for a duration of 2–14 days.

Inhaled Epoprostenol

Inhaled epoprostenol likely exerts its effects through a mechanism akin to that of iNO. It shares similar pharmacokinetic properties, being fast-acting with a short duration of action, as evidenced by its approximate half-life of 5 minutes. Inhaled epoprostenol is selective for pulmonary circulation, with minimal systemic side effects, making it a well-tolerated therapeutic option.

Intravenous Methylene Blue

Methylene blue is a potent vasoconstrictor that exerts its effects through the inhibition of the cyclic guanosine monophosphate (GMP) pathway. In patients with cirrhosis, impaired hypoxic pulmonary vasoconstriction and corresponding V/Q mismatch are most prominent in the lung bases, where the majority of IPVDs are located. Additionally, microatelectasis in the basal regions contributes to regional ventilation impairment. MB may induce vasoconstriction in these dilated basilar pulmonary arterioles, where nonremodeled vessels may still retain some capacity for vasoconstriction, thus potentially improving $\dot{V}/\dot{Q}$ matching. While MB may also cause vasoconstriction in normal pulmonary vessels, the dilated basilar arterioles, which receive a disproportionate share of pulmonary blood flow, are more likely to experience a significant effect, especially at higher total doses.

To optimize basilar delivery, it is recommended that the patient be positioned in reverse Trendelenburg, as gravity will preferentially direct blood flow to the lung bases. Close hemodynamic monitoring is essential during the administration of MB, as it can potentially reduce cardiac output by systemic vasoconstriction. However, this may be compensated by an improvement in oxygen saturation, resulting in a net increase in tissue oxygen delivery.

Methylene blue is usually given in a dose of 3 mg/Kg every 2 hours in 50–100 mL normal saline IV over 15 min. The maximum recommended duration of treatment is 24–48 hours.

Although the effects of large cumulative doses of MB remain poorly understood, case reports suggest that the recommended doses are safe and effective. The drug has also been shown to be safe post-LT, where it has been utilized for its potential anti-inflammatory effects.

There are case reports of combining MB with inhaled vasodilators in the postoperative management of HPS. This combination strategy is considered potentially synergistic and low-risk. Inhaled vasodilators preferentially dilate vessels in well-ventilated areas, while MB targets vasoconstriction in poorly ventilated regions where HPS-induced vascular dilation occurs due to impaired hypoxic vasoconstriction. The combination may reduce the potential vasoconstrictive effects of MB on well-ventilated pulmonary vessels, enhancing the heterogeneity of its effect and redistributing blood flow away from dilated HPS vessels. Inhaled epoprostenol, which acts through cyclic adenosine monophosphate (AMP) rather than cyclic GMP, is less likely to be inhibited by MB and may therefore be more effective than iNO in achieving this desired effect. Combining iNO with MB, however, has not been found to improve gas exchange and hypoxemia.[10]

EMBOLIZATION OF LOWER LOBAR PULMONARY VESSELS

Embolotherapy for diffuse IPVDs can theoretically improve oxygenation in HPS, likely by redistributing pulmonary blood flow. This is supported by similar findings in patients with hereditary hemorrhagic telangiectasia, who also have diffuse, basilar-predominant IPVDs resembling those in HPS. However, this is not a regular practice in most of the transplant centers.

EXTRACORPOREAL LIFE SUPPORT

The use of venovenous extracorporeal lung support (ECLS) in adult patients with HPS remains controversial. There are case reports of successful use of venovenous extracorporeal membrane oxygenation (VV-ECMO) for severe post-transplant hypoxemia demonstrating its potential efficacy.[12]

Extracorporeal lung support serves as a bridge to recovery, and its use is theoretically well-suited to HPS patients, as LT typically results in nearly complete resolution of intrapulmonary shunting and improved gas exchange. Early initiation of ECLS is preferable to reduce ventilation requirements and mitigate organ hypoxia, given the complications associated with prolonged mechanical ventilation, such as ventilator-associated pneumonia and lung injury.

However, the timing of improvement in HPS-related hypoxemia is highly variable and difficult to predict, and prolonged ECLS use carries significant risks, including complications and mortality. Therefore, ECLS should be viewed as a "last resort" therapeutic option in this population.

EXTENDED POSTOPERATIVE CARE

These patients usually require prolonged intensive care unit (ICU) and hospital stay post-LT. Supplemental oxygen is usually required for a few months till complete resolution of IPVD. The time frame for resolution is temporally correlated with the pretransplant severity of HPS. Oxygen may be discontinued when patients maintain SpO_2 >88% in rest, exertion, and sleep.

CONCLUSION

Hepatopulmonary syndrome is an under-recognized condition that is increasingly linked to a higher incidence of postoperative complications following LT. Given its significant impact on post-transplant outcomes, cirrhotic patients should be routinely and systematically screened for HPS to facilitate timely referral to LT centers. Post-transplant care for these patients requires heightened vigilance to ensure optimal oxygen delivery and early detection of complications in the immediate postoperative period. A systematic, stepwise approach is essential to manage and mitigate post-operative hypoxia in HPS patients, thereby improving overall transplant outcomes.

REFERENCES

1. Raevens S, Boret M, Fallon MB. Hepatopulmonary syndrome. JHEP Rep. 2022;4(9):100527.
2. Krowka MJ, Fallon MB, Kawut SM, Fuhrmann V, Heimbach JK, Ramsay MA, et al. International liver transplant society practice guidelines: Diagnosis and management of hepatopulmonary syndrome and portopulmonary hypertension. Transplantation. 2016;100(7):1440-52.
3. Forde KA, Fallon MB, Krowka MJ, Sprys M, Goldberg DS, Krok KL, et al. Pulse oximetry is insensitive for detection of hepatopulmonary syndrome in patients evaluated for liver transplantation. Hepatology. 2019;69(1):270-81.
4. Grilo I, Pascasio JM, Tirado JL, López-Pardo FJ, Ortega-Ruiz F, Sousa JM, et al. The utility of the macro-aggregated albumin lung perfusion scan in the diagnosis and prognosis of hepatopulmonary syndrome in cirrhotic patients candidates for liver transplantation. Rev Esp Enferm Dig. 2017;109:335-43.
5. Machicao VI, Balakrishnan M, Fallon MB. Pulmonary complications in chronic liver disease. Hepatology. 2014;59(4):1627-37.
6. Swanson KL, Wiesner RH, Krowka MJ. Natural history of hepatopulmonary syndrome: Impact of liver transplantation. Hepatology. 2005;41(5):1122-9.
7. Rodríguez-Roisin R, Krowka MJ. Hepatopulmonary Syndrome: A liver-induced lung vascular disorder. N Engl J Med. 2008;358:2378-87.
8. Morvan A, Gazon M, Duperret S, Schmitt Z, Pradat P, Mohkam K, et al. Hepatopulmonary syndrome and post-liver transplantation complications: A case-control study. Int J Organ Transplant Med. 2020;11(4):166-75.
9. Kadry Z, Schaefer E, Krok K, Faust A, Stine JG, Schreibman IR, et al. Excellent outcomes with liver transplantation in hepatopulmonary syndrome across pre-transplant PaO_2 spectrum. JHEP Rep. 2021;3(5):100351.
10. Nayyar D, Jeffrey Man HS, Granton J, Gupta S. Defining and characterizing severe hypoxemia after liver transplantation in hepatopulmonary syndrome. Liver Transplant 2014;20(2):182-90.
11. Nayyar D, Man HS, Granton J, Gupta S. Proposed management algorithm for severe hypoxemia after liver transplantation in the hepatopulmonary syndrome. Am J Transplant. 2015;15(4):903-13.
12. Auzinger G, Willars C, Loveridge R, Best T, Vercueil A, Prachalias A, et al. Extracorporeal membrane oxygenation for refractory hypoxemia after liver transplantation in severe hepatopulmonary syndrome: A solution with pitfalls. Liver Transplant. 2014;20:1141-4.

CHAPTER

16

Extracorporeal Blood Purification in Patients with Liver Failure in Intensive Care Unit

Abdul S Ansari, Suvadeep Sen

INTRODUCTION

Liver failure occurs when significant loss of functional liver tissue reaches a critical threshold, impairing its ability to perform essential functions such as detoxification, biotransformation, excretion, and secretion of both endogenous and exogenous substances. Although its clinical presentation can vary, it typically involves jaundice, coagulopathy, hepatic encephalopathy (HE), increased susceptibility to infections, hemodynamic instability, and eventual multiorgan failure, often leading to death. This is commonly seen in two settings: (1) Acute liver failure (ALF) when there is no preexisting liver dysfunction and (2) acute-on-chronic liver failure (ACLF) when there is preexisting chronic liver disease. The definitions and clinical characteristics of these two entities were described in separate chapters.

Extracorporeal liver support (ECLS) is a system that replicates the liver's key functions by filtering and detoxifying blood through an external device, aiming to reduce mortality or serve as a bridge to liver transplantation. ACLF is associated with dysfunctional albumin in blood and accumulation of damage- and pathogen-associated molecular patterns (DAMPs and PAMPs) that promote severe forms of systemic inflammation. Extracorporeal liver assist devices (ELADs) have been designed to serve two basic purposes: (1) Adsorption of endotoxins from blood, mitigating the effect of systemic inflammation, and (2) aiding the removal of various water-soluble and albumin-bound toxins from blood till regeneration hepatocytes to a functional level **(Fig. 1)**.

The main indications for ECLS include hemodynamic instability, HE, cerebral edema, and renal dysfunction or hepatorenal syndrome (HRS) that does not respond to medical treatment, especially when organ transplantation is not immediately available.

Extracorporeal therapies always remained a key focus in managing liver failure and multiorgan failure as a bridging strategy. ECLS has demonstrated significant improvements in biochemical parameters such as serum bilirubin, bile acids, and urea levels. However, early clinical trials have not shown that these biochemical improvements translate into increased survival. Despite no evident mortality benefit in clinical trials, enthusiasm for these therapies remained unwavering and they continued to be used as per institutional protocol in sick liver failure patients all across the world. A systematic review and meta-analysis, published recently covering 25 randomized controlled trials (RCTs) including 1,796 patients, provided substantial evidence that ECLS has significant association in reducing all-cause mortality, with a number needed to treat (NNT) of 22 in patients with ALF and 16 in patients with ACLF.[1] Ongoing research is focused on continuously upgrading the existing system to more closely replicate hepatic physiology, enhance its effectiveness, and to expand its clinical utility.

There are five basic forms of ECLS **(Flowchart 1)**:

1. *Conventional renal replacement therapies (RRTs):* Diffusion and convection system
2. *Albumin dialysis:* To remove toxins that are bound to albumin
3. Adsorption modalities with or without the process of plasma separation

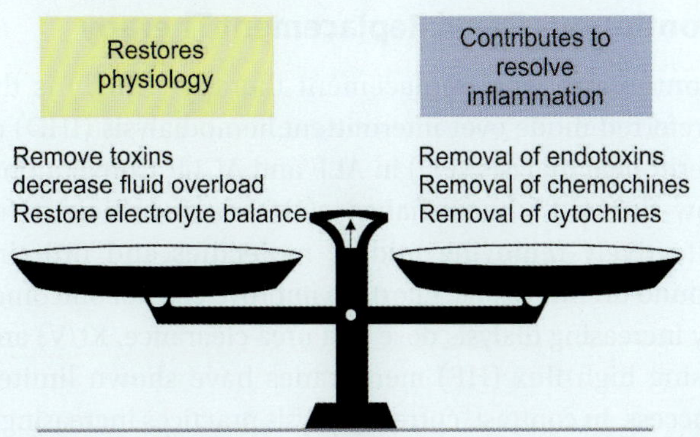

Fig. 1: Benefits of extracorporeal therapies in liver failure.

Flowchart 1: Different forms of extracorporeal liver support (ECLS).

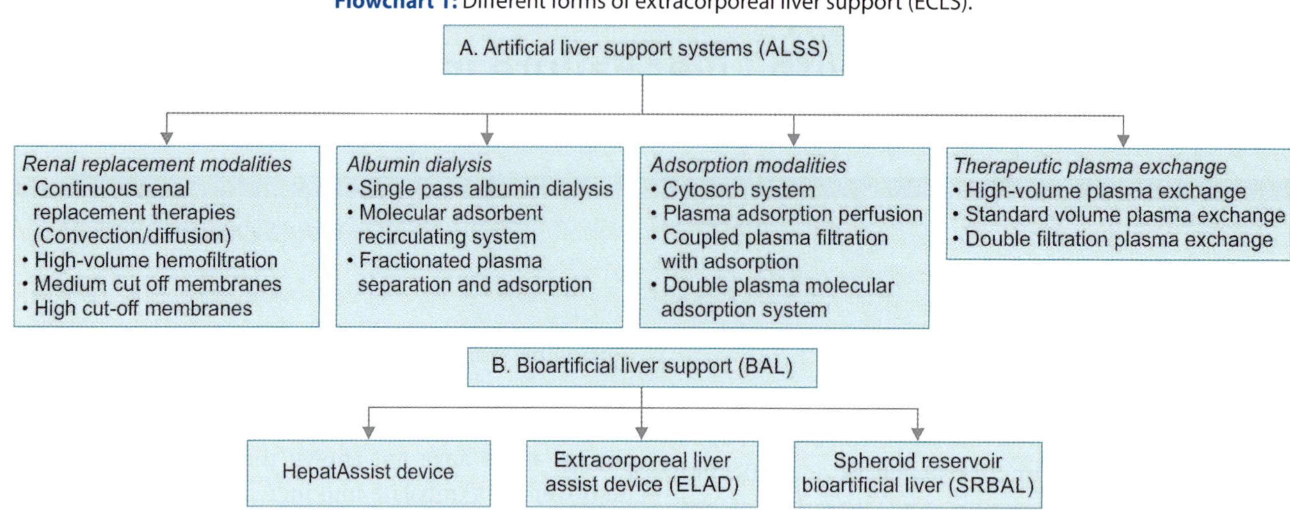

4. Therapeutic plasma exchange (TPE)
5. Bioartificial liver (BAL) support systems

RENAL REPLACEMENT THERAPIES

Conventional RRTs are the most frequent form of extracorporeal blood purification used in the setting of liver dysfunction. They are indicated in patients with liver failure for both renal and nonrenal indications.

- *Patients with ALF or ACLF with concomitant acute kidney injury (AKI):* Standard indications such as acidosis, volume overload, and refractory hyperkalemia
- In patients with ALF, if there is a progressive encephalopathy along with rising ammonia levels, that correlates with raised intracranial pressure (ICP) and cerebral edema.
- In the presence of vasodilatory systemic inflammation, to counteract the effects of proinflammatory cytokines.

Continuous Renal Replacement Therapy

Continuous renal replacement therapy (CRRT) is the preferred mode over intermittent hemodialysis (IHD) or peritoneal dialysis (PD) in ALF and ACLF. Conventional low-flux (LF) hemodialysis (HD) is insufficient for effectively removing middle molecules and protein-bound uremic toxins. Efforts to improve clinical outcomes by increasing dialysis dose (via urea clearance, Kt/V) and using high-flux (HF) membranes have shown limited success. In contrast, current dialysis practices increasingly incorporate convective therapies and highly permeable membranes to enhance middle molecule removal. High-volume hemodiafiltration (HDF) is more efficient in clearing these toxins and may reduce the risk of all-cause and cardiovascular mortality compared to LF- and HF-HD.

Continuous renal replacement therapy has the following advantages in this group of patients:

- CRRT is tolerated better in the presence of hemodynamic instability and extreme volume shifts.
- It has a more favorable safety profile in terms of shifts of solutes and changes in osmolality in the presence of brain edema. It does not cause rapid fluxes of fluid and electrolytes, which in turn diminishes the risk of disequilibrium syndrome and its complications.
- Control of fluid and metabolic and electrolyte balance is more than intermittent IHD, especially in patients with third-space fluid loss. CRRT allows more gradual correction of sodium in oliguric patients.
- CRRT with standard M100 dialyzer extracts middle molecules such as cytokines nonselectively along with water-soluble, small-, and medium-sized molecules (urea, creatinine, phosphorus, and ammonia). However, it does not remove albumin-bound molecules in the standard doses. High-volume hemofiltration (HVHF) is another adoption of CRRT in patients who are extremely vasodilated from cytokine storm of any reason.

Disadvantage of CRRT:

- Anticoagulation management is challenging in patients with ALF and coagulopathy.

- The dialysis efficacy is much inferior to sustained low-efficiency dialysis (SLED) or IHD in the case of CRRT.

High-Volume Hemofiltration

This is termed when continuous venovenous hemofiltration (CVVH) is continued with a higher effluent rate than standard 25–35 mL/kg/h. In HVHF, effluent dose is kept as high as 50–70 mL/kg/h. This technique is more effective in convective clearance of water-soluble middle molecules like cytokines (ranging from molecular weights, from 5 to 60 kDa). This allows some degree of adsorption as well as targeting substances with molecular weight beyond the threshold of the filter. These techniques are often adopted in sick ALF/ACLF patients during the initiation of CRRT. However, albumin-bound uremic toxins are less well removed in this technique.

High-volume hemofiltration is associated with a greater degree of loss of nutrients, electrolytes, and drugs such as antibiotics. It exacerbates negative nitrogen balance in a highly catabolic patients. Hence, careful drug dose monitoring and adjustments need to be contemplated.

High Cut-off Membranes

High cut-off (HCO) membranes have revolutionized RRT by enhancing the clearance of middle-molecular-weight substances and cytokines. These membranes have the same membrane surface and material as in any standard HF dialyzer but have a higher pore size (a median pore size of approximately 0.01 μm), corresponding to a molecular weight cut-off (MWCO) of 50–60 KDa, similar to the filtration capabilities of healthy glomeruli. This design allows for more effective removal of uremic toxins, especially those that are protein-bound or fall within the middle molecular weight range. However, this also leads to the unintended loss of albumin during treatment. In addition to removing uremic toxins, HCO membranes are particularly efficient at diffusive removal of various cytokines, including interleukin (IL)-8, IL-6, and tumor necrosis factor-α (TNF-α).[2]

Medium Cut-off Membranes

This is a novel addition to the armamentarium, with an aim to remove of large middle molecules while preventing albumin loss that happens with HCO membranes. However, their clinical application at present in patients with ALF and ACLF is investigational.

TREATMENTS ON THE PRINCIPLE OF ALBUMIN DIALYSIS

Conventional RRTs are primarily designed to remove small, water-soluble molecules that are minimally bound to plasma proteins. As a result, they are of limited effectiveness in clearing the common toxins associated with liver failure, which are predominantly hydrophobic and bound to albumin. Therapies based on convection technologies can remove middle molecules to a limited extent. As a result, it is not surprising that these therapies do not have any survival benefit in liver failure patients. Consequently, significant efforts have been focused on developing therapies that more closely mimic the liver's natural detoxification processes—systems capable of removing lipophilic substances such as bile acids, bilirubin, medium-chain fatty acids, and aromatic amino acids, as well as other protein-bound toxins. Since albumin is the primary plasma protein carrier for these toxins and waste products, it is targeted by two purification strategies—(1) Albumin-based clearance techniques and (2) total plasma exchange. Along with this, a third strategy of hemoperfusion or hemoadsorption utilizes adsorption membranes for purification of whole blood without the need for plasma separation.

Single-Pass Albumin Dialysis

Single-pass albumin dialysis (SPAD) is a specialized extracorporeal therapy used for removing toxins from the blood in patients with liver failure.

Single-pass albumin dialysis utilizes albumin, a major plasma protein that has a high binding affinity for a variety of toxins, including bilirubin, bile acids, ammonia, drugs, and other metabolic waste products. The mechanism of action involves the use of a single-pass dialyzer system, where blood is filtered through a circuit that uses a solution of albumin to bind and remove these toxins. Unlike conventional dialysis, which uses an electrolyte-based solution (dialysate), the albumin in SPAD specifically binds toxins that the liver would normally process. These modalities are adapted to integrate the addition of albumin to the dialysate, turning it into a molecular adsorber for removing toxins from the bloodstream **(Fig. 2)**.

Single-pass albumin dialysis is often performed using CRRT machines, typically through CVVHD (continuous venovenous hemodialysis) or CVVHDF (continuous venovenous hemodiafiltration) circuits. Albumin is added to a standard bicarbonate-based dialysate in

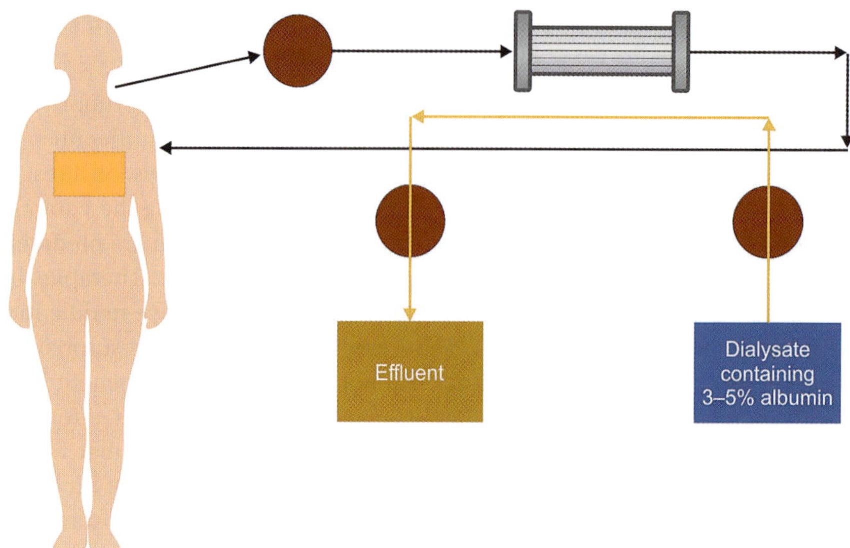

Fig. 2: Schematic diagram of single pass albumin dialysis system (SPAD).

concentrations ranging from 1 to 5% (10 to 50 g/L). The albumin-containing dialysate flows counter-current to the blood in the filter, drawing hydrophobic substances from the saturated albumin in the blood into the dialysate, which is then discarded.

The term "single-pass" refers to the fact that blood only passes through the dialysis system once (without being recirculated). After it interacts with the albumin solution, the blood is returned directly to the patient.

The treatment time typically ranges from 6 to 8 hours, although this may vary depending on the patient's condition and response to the therapy.

Advantages of Single-Pass Albumin Dialysis

- *Targeted toxin removal:* The use of albumin enables the removal of specific toxins (such as ammonia and bile acids), and can provide temporary liver support.
- *Nonrecirculating process:* SPAD's single-pass design avoids the risk of complications associated with recirculating systems, such as clotting, infection, and hemodynamic instability.
- No requirement of anticoagulation as the treatment duration is relatively shorter.

Limitations and Challenges

- It is not a comprehensive replacement for liver function. Its effectiveness is best in cases where the toxins are albumin-bound or liver-metabolized substances. SPAD can significantly lower serum bilirubin levels, but its efficacy to remove cytokines is not established.
- There is a significant decrease in fibrinogen and platelet count seen with the treatment.
- The need for concentrated albumin solutions and specialized equipment makes SPAD resource intensive.
- Ready-made albumin-containing CRRT fluids are not provided by companies. Due to the potential for contamination, the addition of albumin to the dialysate should always be performed under sterile conditions, often in a laminar flow hood.
- The need to add albumin to each dialysis fluid increases the workload for medical staff.
- Being a single-pass mechanism, the all of the albumin used in dialysis system are discarded in the effluent. This increases the cost and makes system resource intensive.
- Adding albumin to the dialysate can cause changes in the final electrolyte concentrations. Physicians need to be meticulous about monitoring of the systemic electrolytes.
- The flow rate for the dialysate is not universally standardized and often varies based on local practice, economic factors, and logistical constraints. To reduce costs and preserve albumin stores, some centers use lower concentrations of albumin (e.g., 1%) in the dialysate or opt for CVVHDF with albumin-containing dialysate at lower flow rates (1 L/h).

Molecular Adsorbent Recirculating System

Molecular adsorbent recirculating system (MARS) shares similarities with SPAD in that both utilize a dialysis-like process with albumin as the molecular adsorber. However, unlike SPAD, in MARS, the spent albumin used in the process is recycled rather than discarded. This allows for a continuous detoxification procedure without needing to replace the albumin after each pass through the system. The system removes both albumin-bound and water-soluble toxins and decreases the plasma concentrations of bilirubin, ammonia, creatinine, urea, and cytokines in patients with liver failure.

The MARS detoxification procedure involves a specialized system consisting of two coupled circuits that work in tandem to cleanse the patient's blood of toxins **(Fig. 3)**.

First circuit—dialysis with albumin: In the first circuit, the patient's blood is passed through a HF dialysis membrane (MARS® FLUX2.1 filter), with a molecular cutoff of 50 kDa at a blood flow of 200 mL/min. The dialysate used here contains 20% human serum albumin, which serves as the molecular adsorber for removal of toxins from the blood. The albumin dialysate creates a favorable concentration gradient that enhances the removal of toxins from the patient's blood.

Purification of spent albumin-dialysate: After the initial contact with the patient's blood, the spent albumin-enhanced dialysate (now containing toxins) is processed in a multi-step cleansing process to remove the bound toxins: The spent dialysate first undergoes dialysis using a HF filter (diaFLUX1.8 filter), which removes water-soluble toxins from the solution. Next, the dialysate passes through two sequential adsorbent columns:

1. The first column contains activated charcoal (diaMARS AC250), which adsorbs organic, lipophilic toxins.
2. The second column contains an anion exchange resin (diaMARS IE250), which helps remove charged toxins from the solution.

This purification process cleanses the dialysate of toxins, effectively regenerating the spent albumin solution.

Recirculation of purified albumin dialysate: After the adsorptive purification, the cleaned albumin-dialysate solution is recirculated back through the first filter, where it again serves as "fresh" dialysate, continuing the detoxification process. This recycling of the albumin solution enables the system to work efficiently over extended periods without requiring fresh albumin to be added constantly.

Limitations of MARS:

- This is not a definite treatment. It acts as a bridge to liver regeneration or liver transplant.
- Resource-intensive therapy, requiring specialized equipment and human serum albumin. MARS requires skilled operators and careful monitoring.

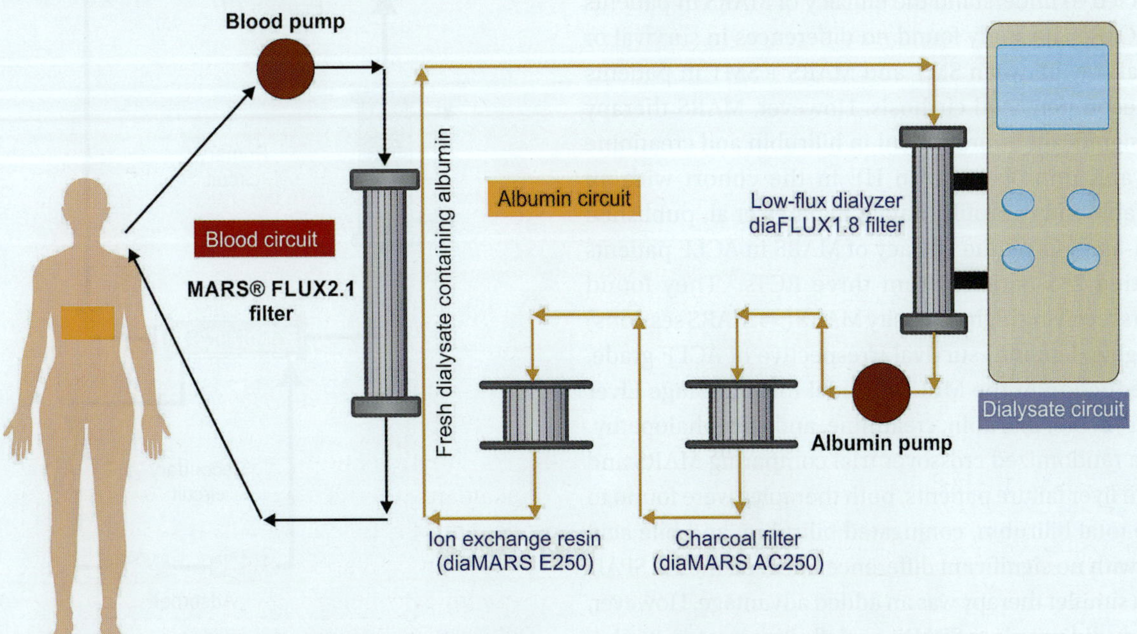

Fig. 3: Schematic diagram of molecular adsorbent recirculating system (MARS).

- Anticoagulation is necessary in the circuit, which raises the risk of bleeding, particularly in patients with coagulopathy. As a result, anticoagulation protocols in MARS are crucial, with unfractionated heparin being the most commonly used anticoagulant.
- Many systemically administered drugs like antibiotics get cleared by the MARS system, hence careful dose adjustments and therapeutic drug monitoring are required.
- Increased risk of fungal and bacterial infections

Hard clinical evidence with MARS in liver failure is not robust as in most of the data are from retrospective uncontrolled trials and case series. The modality is used in the sickest group of patients, making interpretation unclear. Most of the benefits are in terms of improvement of hemodynamics and encephalopathy, without any survival advantage.

The FULMAR study was a multicenter RCT that evaluated the effects of the MARS enrolling 102 patients with ALF awaiting a liver transplant.[3] The study found no significant difference in survival outcomes between standard medical therapy (SMT) and SMT + MARS, but transplant-free survival was better in patients receiving >3 MARS sessions. MARS helped reduction of bilirubin, creatinine, and lactate levels, making it valuable for patients not eligible for liver transplantation.

A similar multicentric study (RELIEF study) was conducted to understand the efficacy of MARS in patients with ACLF.[4] The study found no differences in survival or hospital stay between SMT and MARS + SMT in patients with decompensated cirrhosis. However, MARS therapy led to significant improvement in bilirubin and creatinine levels and improvement in HE in the cohort with an acceptable safety profile. Rafael Banares et al. published a meta-analysis on the efficacy of MARS in ACLF patients recruiting 285 patients from three RCTs.[5] They found patients receiving high-intensity MARS (>4 MARS sessions) had higher 1-month survival irrespective of ACLF grade, with reduction in the MELD (Model for End-Stage Liver Disease) score, bilirubin, creatinine, and encephalopathy.

In a randomized crossover trial comparing MARS and SPAD in liver failure patients, both therapies were found to reduce total bilirubin, conjugated bilirubin, and bile acid levels, with no significant difference between them.[6] SPAD being a simpler therapy was an added advantage. However, the study did not place SPAD as a definitive treatment plan in patients with liver failure.

Fractionated Plasma Separation and Adsorption

Fractionated plasma separation and adsorption (FPSA) is an ECLS therapy that combines plasma separation with adsorption techniques.

Working Principle of FPSA System (Fig. 4)

- *Blood filtration through the AlbuFlow® filter:* The patient's blood first passes through an albumin-permeable biocompatible filter called AlbuFlow® AF01 filter, which has a high screening coefficient of 250 kDa. This filter selectively separates albumin-rich plasma fraction from blood. This is the primary circuit in the system.
- *Adsorption of toxins:* The albumin-rich plasma fraction then passes through two key adsorptive columns in the secondary circuit:
    1. *Neutral resin adsorber (Prometh® 01):* This adsorber captures a wide range of lipophilic toxins bound to albumin such as bile acids, aromatic amino acids, and phenols.
    2. *Anion-exchange resin (Prometh® 02):* This allows the absorption of bilirubin, bile acids, ammonia, and other water-soluble substances.

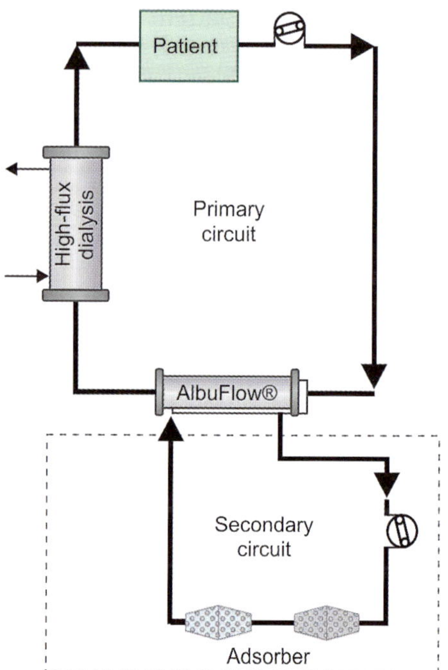

Fig. 4: Simplified schematic diagram of FPSA (Prometheus) system.[7] (FPSA: fractionated plasma separation and adsorption)

These columns effectively remove toxins from the plasma, preparing the albumin-rich fraction for reinfusion.

- *Reconstitution and return to the patient:* After passing through the adsorptive columns, the cleansed plasma fraction is then reinfused into the primary circuit. The reconstituted blood (now enriched with albumin) undergoes HF dialysis using a polysulfone dialyzer. This step helps to remove small, water-soluble toxins, and waste products (e.g., urea and creatinine), similar to conventional HD.

The process is usually continuous (often 6–8 hours per session), with the plasma being treated in cycles until an adequate level of detoxification is achieved. Citrate may be used as an anticoagulation agent in the system.

Clinical Evidence

Prometheus® system has been studied in patients with ACLF and severe HRS as a bridge to transplant. The biochemical clearance rate of bilirubin, bile acids, creatinine, and urea is found to be in the range of 40–68%.[7]

The FPSA systems are superior to MARS in terms of removal of most protein-bound toxins as well as water-soluble substances. The subgroup analysis of the HELIOS trial[8] showed survival benefits in ACLF with MELD >30 and HRS type 1.

A systematic review of 12 trials involving 653 patients evaluated the efficacy and safety of MARS, SPAD, and Prometheus in liver dysfunction.[9] The study found that MARS, SPAD, and Prometheus significantly reduced bilirubin but had no impact on bile acids or ammonia levels compared to SMT. MARS was also linked to improved HE, but none of the therapies showed a significant reduction in mortality or adverse events. Overall, the therapies were equally effective in removing albumin-bound and water-soluble substances.

The result of the use of FPSA system in patients with ALF was published in a retrospective analysis on 101 patients.[10] Although there was no survival benefit, this ECLS allowed a significant extension of waiting time before liver transplant compared to standard therapy.

ADSORPTION MODALITIES

Adsorption modalities are used as standalone modalities to remove albumin-bound toxins and cytokines, with less technical complexities and more cost-effectiveness compared to MARS or FPSA systems. The techniques of hemoperfusion and hemoadsorption involve the placement of an adsorbent, often charcoal or resin-based, in direct contact with blood through an extracorporeal circuit to remove solutes with larger molecular sizes. The main limitation to the use of these devices is their biocompatibility, with thrombocytopenia and an increased bleeding risk being the most significant potential side effects.

CytoSorb

CytoSorb works through a process known as extracorporeal blood purification. The key component of the CytoSorb system is an adsorptive filter cartridge, which is filled with highly porous and crosslinked polystyrene divinyl benzene co-polymer beads with a biocompatible coating that are designed to trap toxins and inflammatory mediators. The filter provides a large active surface area of 45,000 m^2 for adsorption, which helps the removal of midsize hydrophobic molecules up to a size of approximately 60 kDa (10–55 kDa). The system typically works best with blood flow of 150–500 mL/min and mostly remains effective for 12–24 hours of period. This circuit is connected to the patient's bloodlines, and the whole setup is usually integrated with other devices such as dialysis machines or CRRT systems.

A recent retrospective observational study on patients with ACLF found that the use of CytoSorb adsorber resulted in a significant decline in proinflammatory cytokines and bilirubin without no serious complications.[11] Similarly, a prospective evaluation of the use of CytoSorb in 28 patients with ALF suggested providing superior biochemical control and a bridge to transplant or recovery.[12] However, its role in lowering ammonia in critically ill patients with liver failure is doubtful.[13] A comparative analysis of several ECLS systems showed that the CytoSorb system outperformed coupled plasma filtration with adsorption (CPFA), MARS, Prometheus, and plasma adsorption perfusion (PAP) in removing total bilirubin, direct bilirubin, and bile acids in patients with liver failure.[14]

Advantages of CytoSorb

- CytoSorb is effective at removing a wide variety of toxic substances, including proinflammatory cytokines, endotoxins, plasma bilirubin, ammonia, bile acids, and C-reactive protein (CRP) and myoglobin, and other mediators involved in inflammatory and metabolic disturbance.

- By removing inflammatory mediators such as IL-6, TNF-α, and IL-1, CytoSorb can help to reduce the cytokine storm in patients with high levels of proinflammatory cytokines in conditions like ALF. IL-6 has been especially found to be a potential target of cytokines.
- CytoSorb can be easily integrated with existing CRRT and dialysis machines. The system is relatively simple to operate.
- The single cartridge system, the simplicity in configuration, and the lesser need for anticoagulation make this system safer and with lesser risks like bleeding and sepsis.

Limitations of CytoSorb

- *Temporary solution:* It is used as a bridge to allow time for recovery, treatment, or liver regeneration.
- *Cost:* The cartridge is costlier than most of the other available filters used for dialysis which sometimes becomes prohibitive in low- and middle-income countries (LMICs).
- Thrombocytopenia remains one of the most important side effects that need to be observed during the treatment.
- While CytoSorb shows promise as a therapeutic option and may serve as a bridge to transplantation in patients with ALF or ACLF, the available evidence in the form of larger, prospective RCTs in terms of survival advantage is still lacking. The optimal timing for initiation, treatment endpoints, and the number of sessions required remain unclear and vary from center to center at this stage.

Double Plasma Molecular Adsorption System

This is an advanced form of extracorporeal blood purification that combines plasma separation with adsorption techniques to remove a wide range of toxins, inflammatory mediators, and waste products from the blood.

Working Principle

- *Plasma separation:* In a double plasma molecular adsorption system (DPMAS) system, plasma (containing the majority of toxins) is first separated from the cellular components, typically using a centrifugation process or a filtration-based method.
- *Dual adsorption columns:* The separated plasma then passes through two separate hemoperfusion columns placed in tandem, each designed to capture different types of substances. BS330 is composed of anion exchange resin that helps adsorption of lipophilic toxins such as bilirubin, bile acid, ammonia, phenol, and mercaptan, while the HA330-II is a neutral microporous resin that targets water-soluble toxins and proinflammatory cytokines (such as TNF-α, IL-6, IL-1, and endotoxins).
- *Plasma regeneration:* After passing through the adsorptive columns, the cleansed plasma is typically reinfused into the patient's bloodstream. This helps to maintain the patient's plasma volume and ensures that important plasma proteins such as albumin and immunoglobulins are not lost during the treatment. The return line is often integrated with a dialysis machine or a CRRT system.

Depending on the severity of the patient's condition, DPMAS can be performed continuously (e.g., over 6–8 hours) or intermittently (e.g., daily or several times a week). Continuous treatment is often preferred in critically ill patients, as it helps to gradually reduce toxin levels and minimize fluctuations in the patient's condition.

Advantages of Double Plasma Molecular Adsorption System

- The system does not require plasma or fluid replacement during treatment. DPMAS allows for the regeneration and reinfusion of the patient's own plasma, preserving essential proteins such as albumin and immunoglobulins. This also minimizes transfusion-related complications in patients.
- Reduced risk for anaphylactic reactions, which are commonly associated with plasma exchange
- The treatment is usually well tolerated.
- DPMAS is capable of removing a wide variety of toxins, inflammatory mediators, and waste products from the blood, including protein-bound, lipophilic, and water-soluble substances, making it more comprehensive than conventional HD or single-pass dialysis systems.
- The dual adsorption system enhances the overall detoxification capacity by targeting both lipophilic and hydrophilic toxins simultaneously. This makes DPMAS especially useful for patients with complex metabolic disturbances or multiorgan failure.

Limitations of Double Plasma Molecular Adsorption System

- Existing coagulopathy cannot be corrected with DPMAS. To overcome this, DPMAS is sometimes used in conjunction with PLEX.
- DPMAS requires specialized equipment and trained personnel, making it resource-intensive and sometimes unavailable in smaller or less-equipped centers.
- The cost of DPMAS can be high, particularly when long or repeated treatments are required.
- Saturation of the adsorbent columns comes within 6–8 hours.
- Being a newer modality, its full potential, efficacy, and safety profile are still under scrutiny and warrants conduction of a prospective randomized trials.
- Like other forms of artificial liver support systems, DPMAS is also a temporary support in absence of fully functioning liver, rather than a definitive solution.

Plasma Adsorption Perfusion

This is similar in concepts with DPMAS, except a single cartridge made of styrene-divinylbenzene copolymer (BS330) is used instead of two filters.

The advantage is that it does not require coagulation factors and is not as costly as MARS. Secondly, loss of coagulation factors is not as profound.

Coupled Plasma Filtration with Adsorption

This also comes with a similar concept that utilizes a CRRT machine (Amplya) to separate plasma from blood using a high-permeability polyethersulfone filter. The separated plasma is then passed through a styrene-divinylbenzene copolymer cartridge for purification before being reconstituted with blood and returned to the CRRT system, where in the final step, a polyphenylene hemofilter removes water-soluble molecules.

Liver Dialysis Device: DIALIVE Concept

In ALF, three critical aspects play the most significant role in overall survival (OS). The first is the filtration of circulating dysfunctional albumin and water-soluble toxins, the second is the adsorption of endotoxins, and the third is infusion of healthy albumin. DIALIVE is a novel liver dialysis device for the treatment of patients with ACLF.[15] The system has four basic components: (1) a Prismaflex machine, (2) a septeX treatment kit, (3) an

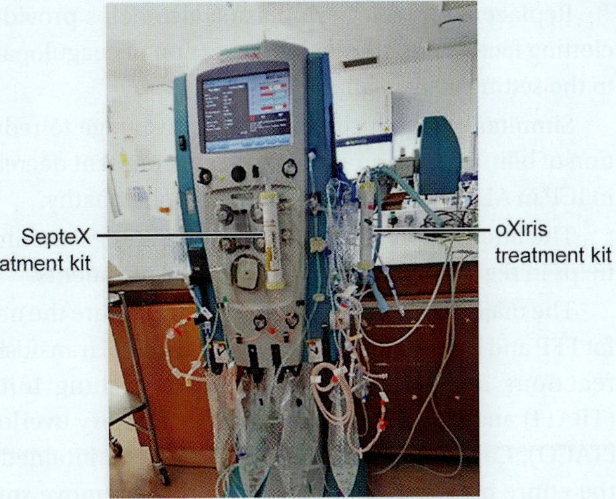

Fig. 5: DIALIVE concept of liver dialysis system.

oXiris treatment kit, (4) connecting tubing **(Fig. 5)**. The septeX, the first filter in the series, helps ultrafiltration of albumin and cytokines, while the next oXiris filter adsorbs PAMPs, such as endotoxins, and DAMPs, such as genomic DNA. Approximately 25–30 g of albumin is lost after 12 hours of treatment, which is replaced by 200 mL of 20% albumin preferably at the end of treatment.

This technology is currently at "technology readiness level" (TRL) 5 and completed phase 2 clinical trials. The first first-in-man study was published in 2023, which was a multicentric, randomized, controlled clinical trial on patients of ACLF[16] and showed a promising effect of this system in rapid resolution of ACLF without any serious adverse event (SAE). Mortality benefit as a secondary endpoint was not different from the standard of care (SOC) in this study.

THERAPEUTIC PLASMA EXCHANGE

This has been used in liver failure patients since the 1960s as a method to remove harmful substances from the blood. The procedure involves separating the patient's plasma—containing immune complexes, antibodies, cytokines, endotoxins, and albumin-bound compounds—and replacing it with a "clean" replacement fluid, usually a combination of albumin and fresh frozen plasma (FFP).

Rationale: The basic advantage of PE in patients with liver failure comes from the immunomodulatory effect of the treatment which plays a major role in attenuating the inflammatory cascades during ALF. It helps to remove cytokines and albumin-bound and water-soluble toxins.

Replacement with fresh plasma also helps providing clotting factors and thus helps correction of coagulopathy in the setting of liver failure.

Simultaneously, it confers added advantage to reduction of bilirubin and ammonia with concomitant decrease in ICP in ALF and improvement of encephalopathy.

The attenuation of systemic inflammation sometimes helps in regaining hemodynamic control in patients.

The major challenges associated with TPE are the need for FFP and blood products that increase risk of transfusion reactions and transfusion-related acute lung injury (TRALI) and transfusion-associated circulatory overload (TACO). Calcium hemostasis needs to be maintained in the entire process. PE does not effectively remove small and medium molecular weight water-soluble molecules, hence in the setting of AKI, simultaneous CRRT is required.

The core of TPE is the separation of plasma from the remaining blood components, which can be achieved by either centrifugation technique, where separation is achieved based on differences in density or filtration, where a HCO hollow fiber filter is used, allowing plasma proteins to pass through while retaining blood cells.

Gravimetric Centrifugation-based Plasma Exchange

The patient's blood is withdrawn into a blood processing machine and spun in a centrifuge to separate the plasma from the cellular components. Plasma is discarded, and the remaining blood cells are mixed with a replacement fluid (usually albumin or FFP) before being returned to the patient.

Advantages

- Higher plasma removal efficiency (PRE), typically 80–85%. PRE is defined as the ratio between the removed plasma and processed plasma.
- Does not require large priming volumes and can be more precise
- The closed circuit minimizes the risk of infection.
- The system can work with lower flow (40–120 mL/min) and may not necessarily require large-bore hemodialysis catheter.

Disadvantages

- Requires specialized equipment and trained personnel
- Citrate anticoagulation increases risk of hypocalcemia.

Filtration-based Plasma Exchange

This technique employs a high-permeability membrane with pores larger than 0.2 µm, enabling the separation of plasma and the removal of medium- and high-molecular-weight molecules, such as immune complexes, antibodies, paraproteins, and lipoproteins.

Advantages

- Simpler and less expensive equipment compared to centrifugal systems
- Widely available, particularly in low-resource settings
- Can be performed using modified standard RRT devices

Disadvantages

- Lower PRE, around 30–35% due to filter limitations and shorter treatment times
- Higher blood flow requirement (100–150 mL/min) necessitating need for HD catheter
- Requires larger priming volumes to prevent clotting
- Potential clogging of filters and more frequent monitoring of the circuit for issues such as clotting or reduced flow
- Thrombocytopenia well-known association with filtration-based TPE

Double Filtration Plasma Exchange

Principle

Here whole blood is first processed to separate plasma from blood cells using a low cut-off filter. The separated plasma passes through an adsorptive filter or HCO filter, removing toxic substances like such as bilirubin, ammonia, and cytokines. The plasma is then replaced with an albumin-based fluid or FFP, and the purified plasma is returned to the patient.

Advantages

- Effective removal of toxins, including protein-bound substances and inflammatory mediators
- This process is particularly useful in state of high systemic inflammation used to treat conditions like ALF.

Disadvantages

- More complex and costly than simple filtration-based TPE
- Requires specialized equipment and may not be available in all centers

High-Volume Therapeutic Plasma Exchange

High-volume therapeutic plasma exchange (HV-TPE) exchanges large volumes of plasma, usually 8–12 liters or more, compared to the typical volume of 1–1.5 times the patient's plasma volume. The rationale for HV-TPE is that the large volumes exchanged help remove toxins from multiple body compartments, leading to improved metabolic parameters, such as reductions in cytokines, endotoxins, and ammonia. Clinical benefits, such as improvements in encephalopathy and tissue perfusion, have been reported, suggesting that HV-TPE may act as a bridge to liver transplantation or recovery.

Disadvantages of High-Volume Therapeutic Plasma Exchange

- Increased risk of complications such as hypocalcemia from citrate anticoagulation, infection, and thrombocytopenia
- More resource-intensive, requiring more fluid replacement and longer treatment times

Clinical Evidence for Therapeutic Plasma Exchange

An open RCT by Larsen et al.[17] in 182 ALF patients showed that high-volume plasma exchange (8–12 L) for 3 days improved liver transplant-free survival ($p = 0.0083$) compared to SMT. Plasma exchange also helps better control over hemodynamic status, improvement in coagulation parameters, reduced bilirubin, ammonium and alanine aminotransferase (ALT), while lowering proinflammatory DAMPs such as TNF-α, IL-16, and IL-18.

The volume of exchange is a matter of debate so far. High-volume plasma exchange requires a higher number of plasma and albumin as replacement volume, which increases the risk of transfusion reactions and may worsen cerebral edema if volume management is not done properly. This also increases the cost of treatment and is highly resource-intensive.

In a study by Maiwall et al., 40 ALF patients showed higher transplant-free survival at 21 days with standard plasma exchange (1–1.5 plasma volumes per PE session), performed using centrifugal apheresis compared to SMT alone.[18]

European Association for the Study of the Liver (EASL) clinical practice guidelines on the management of acute (fulminant) liver failure suggest early initiation of plasma exchange in patients with especially who will not undergo liver transplant with level 1 evidence.[19]

The role of TPE is less well established in ACLF. Clinical evidence data is lacking in patients with ACLF regarding universally adopted initiation threshold and end point of treatment.

A systematic review and meta-analysis of 16 RCTs involving 1,670 ACLF patients compared the effectiveness of SMT, ELAD, MARS, Prometheus, and plasma exchange. The results indicated that plasma exchange is currently the best available support therapy among all other artificial liver support systems in terms of overall and transplant-free survival at 1 and 3 months.[20]

The PALS score[21] helps **(Table 1)** to identify which patients will benefit from TPE-based ALSS therapy (DPMAS plus standard volume plasma exchange) and suggests an appropriate number of sessions. Patients with PALS score 0–2 benefit most with 1–2 sessions of TPE-based ALSS, patients with PALS grade 2, 3–5 sessions of TPE are beneficial. Patients with PALS grade 3 are the sickest and require ≥6 sessions and show high mortality in the absence of a timely transplant.

A study of 103 patients with hyperbilirubinemia from ALF/ACLF compared three therapies (MARS, PAP, and PE), starting treatment when bilirubin >20 mg/dL or increased by >2 mg/dL/day. PE showed the greatest bilirubin reduction (35%), followed by PAP (30%) and MARS (24%). PE was the least expensive, while MARS, though costly, is beneficial for patients with AKI.[22]

TABLE 1: PALS score and grade.

PALS score						PALS grade	
Points	**Liver cirrhosis**	**Total bilirubin (μmol/L)**	**PT-INR**	**Infection**	**Hepatic encephalopathy**	**Grade**	**Score**
0	No	<425	<2.0	No SBP	No	I	0–2
1	Yes	425–650	2.0–2.5	SBP only	I–II	II	3–5
2	–	≥650	≥2.5	SBP plus other site infection	III–IV	III	6–9

(PALS: prognostic acute liver failure score; PT-INR: prothrombin time and international normalized ratio; SBP: spontaneous bacterial peritonitis)

A meta-analysis of 11 RCTs found that DPMAS + plasma exchange significantly improved 90-day survival and lowered bilirubin and ALT levels in patients with ACLF, compared to plasma exchange alone.[23]

BIOARTIFICIAL LIVER

Bioartificial liver systems use living cells, such as porcine hepatocytes (HepatAssist) or human hepatoblastoma (ELAD®), to detoxify blood by running plasma through a hollow-fiber network. Of this, the latter is of particular interests in recent trials. The ELAD cartridge uses the VTL C3A cell line, a subclone of HepG2, which exhibits liver cell-like characteristics and produces important proteins such as albumin, factor V, and α-1-antitrypsin. VTL C3A cells also secrete factors that may modulate inflammatory pathways, including anti-inflammatory molecules such as IL-1Ra and factors promoting hepatocyte regeneration, such as vascular endothelial growth factor (VEGF) and angiopoietin 2. These properties make VTL C3A cells potentially beneficial in treating inflammatory liver diseases. The ELAD cartridge contains thousands of hollow fibers made of semipermeable polysulfone, allowing ultrafiltrate to flow through and interact with VTL C3A cells. These cells metabolize toxins and produce proteins such as albumin, IL-1Ra, VEGF, and ANG2, which diffuse back into the ultrafiltrate for return to the patient.

While BAL systems can mimic liver functions, they are less effective than artificial systems in detoxification.

However, there are few clinical trials supporting their use, and challenges exist in the design, such as ensuring adequate blood and nutrient delivery to hepatocytes. New cryogel-based scaffolding has shown promise in improving hepatocyte viability and perfusion, potentially enhancing BAL system functionality.

An open-label, randomized controlled clinical trial on safety and efficacy of ELAD in patients of ACLF showed ELAD treatment significantly improved transplant-free survival at 28 days and treatment was relatively well tolerated.[24] However, a phase 3 clinical trial on ELAD therapy (VTL-308 trial) in severe alcoholic hepatitis (sAH) failed to show any significant difference in OS between ELAD plus SOC and SOC alone. The study identified high creatinine and INR as predictors of negative outcomes with ELAD, and a new trial is exploring its benefits in younger patients with better renal function and less severe coagulopathy.[25]

CONCLUSION

Extracorporeal liver assist devices are designed to replicate key liver functions, such as detoxification, protein synthesis, and the removal of both hydrophobic toxins (e.g., bile acids, bilirubin) and protein-bound substances, which traditional RRTs cannot effectively address. These devices are primarily used to provide temporary support in patients with ALF, helping to stabilize their condition while awaiting liver recovery or transplantation, with the potential to improve survival in certain cases.

REFERENCES

1. Fuhrmann V, Bauer M, Wilmer A. The persistent potential of extracorporeal therapies in liver failure. Intensive Care Med. 2020;46:528-30.
2. Weidhase L, Haussig E, Haussig S, Kaiser T, de Fallois J, Petros S. Middle molecule clearance with high cut-off dialyzer versus high-flux dialyzer using continuous veno-venous hemodialysis with regional citrate anticoagulation: A prospective randomized controlled trial. PLoS One. 2019;14:e0215823.
3. Saliba F, Camus C, Durand F, Mathurin P, Letierce A, Delafosse B, et al. Albumin dialysis with a noncell artificial liver support device in patients with acute liver failure: a randomized, controlled trial. Ann Intern Med. 2013;159:522-31.
4. Bañares R, Nevens F, Larsen FS, Jalan R, Albillos A, Dollinger M, et al. Extracorporeal albumin dialysis with the molecular adsorbent recirculating system in acute-on-chronic liver failure: the RELIEF trial. Hepatology. 2013;57:1153-62.
5. Bañares R, Ibáñez-Samaniego L, Torner JM, Pavesi M, Olmedo C, Catalina MV, et al. Meta-analysis of individual patient data of albumin dialysis in acute-on-chronic liver failure: focus on treatment intensity. Therap Adv Gastroenterol. 2019;12:1756284819879565.
6. Wallon G, Guth C, Guichon C, Thevenon S, Gazon M, Viale JP, et al. Extracorporeal Albumin Dialysis in Liver Failure with MARS and SPAD: A Randomized Crossover Trial. Blood Purif. 2022;51:243-50.
7. Rifai K. Fractionated plasma separation and adsorption: current practice and future options. Liver Int. 2011;31 Suppl 3:13-5.
8. Rifai K, Kribben A, Gerken G, Haag S, Herget-Rosenthal S, Treichel U, et al. Extracorporeal liver support by fractionated plasma separation and adsorption (prometheus (R)) in patients with acute-on-chronic liver failure (HELIOS study): a prospective randomized controlled multicenter study. J Hepatol. 2010;52:S3.
9. Gadour E, Kaballo MA, Shrwani K, Hassan Z, Kotb A, Aljuraysan A, et al. Safety and efficacy of Single-Pass

Albumin Dialysis (SPAD), Prometheus, and Molecular Adsorbent Recycling System (MARS) liver haemodialysis vs. Standard Medical Therapy (SMT): meta-analysis and systematic review. Prz Gastroenterol. 2024;19:101-11.
10. Kotulski M, Patkowski W, Grodzicki M, Zieniewicz K. Results of treatment of patients with acute liver failure by albumin dialysis using the prometheus system. Transplantation. 2020;104: S493.
11. Haselwanter P, Scheiner B, Balcar L, Semmler G, Riedl-Wewalka M, Schmid M, et al. Use of the CytoSorb adsorber in patients with acute-on-chronic liver failure. Sci Reports. 2024;14:1-12.
12. Tomescu D, Popescu M, David C, Sima R, Dima S. Haemoadsorption by CytoSorb® in patients with acute liver failure: A case series. Int J Artif Organs. 2021;44:560-4.
13. Liebchen U, Paal M, Gräfe C, Zoller M, Scharf C; Cyto-SOLVE Study Group. The cytokine adsorber CytoSorb® does not reduce ammonia concentrations in critically ill patients with liver failure. Intensive Care Med. 2023;49:360-2.
14. Riva I, Marino A, Valetti TM, Marchesi G, Fabretti F. Extracorporeal liver support techniques: a comparison. J Artif Organs. 2024;27:261-8.
15. Aliver. DIALIVE Concept. [online] Available from https://aliver.info/project/dialive-concept/. [Last accessed May, 2025]
16. Agarwal B, Cañizares RB, Saliba F, Ballester MP, Tomescu DR, Martin D, et al. Randomized, controlled clinical trial of the DIALIVE liver dialysis device versus standard of care in patients with acute-on-chronic liver failure. J Hepatol. 2023;79:79-92.
17. Larsen FS, Schmidt LE, Bernsmeier C, Rasmussen A, Isoniemi H, Patel VC, et al. High-volume plasma exchange in patients with acute liver failure: An open randomised controlled trial. J Hepatol. 2016;64:69-78.
18. Maiwall R, Bajpai M, Singh A, Agarwal T, Kumar G, Bharadwaj A, et al. Standard-Volume Plasma Exchange Improves Outcomes in Patients With Acute Liver Failure: A Randomized Controlled Trial. Clin Gastroenterol Hepatol. 2022;20:e831-54.
19. Wendon J, Cordoba J, Dhawan A, Larsen FS, Manns M, Samuel D, et al. EASL Clinical Practical Guidelines on the management of acute (fulminant) liver failure. J Hepatol. 2017;66:1047-81.
20. Ocskay K, Kanjo A, Gede N, Szakács Z, Pár G, Erőss B, et al. Uncertainty in the impact of liver support systems in acute-on-chronic liver failure: a systematic review and network meta-analysis. Ann Intensive Care. 2021;11(1):10.
21. Du L, Ma Y, Zhou S, Chen F, Xu Y, Wang M, et al. A prognostic score for patients with acute-on-chronic liver failure treated with plasma exchange-centered artificial liver support system. Sci Reports. 2021;11(1):1469.
22. Viggiano D, de Pascale E, Marinelli G, Pluvio C. A comparison among three different apheretic techniques for treatment of hyperbilirubinemia. J Artif Organs. 2018;21:1106.
23. Bai W, Yao C, Mao D, Wu J, Wang K, Wei H, et al. The Clinical Efficacy of Double Plasma Molecular Absorption System Combined with Plasma Exchange in the Treatment of Acute-on-Chronic Liver Failure: A Systematic Review and Meta-Analysis. J Healthc Eng. 2022;2022:3139929.
24. Duan Z, Xin S, Zhang J, You S, Chen Y, Liu H, et al. Comparison of extracorporeal cellular therapy (ELAD®) vs standard of care in a randomized controlled clinical trial in treating Chinese subjects with acute-on-chronic liver failure. Hepat Med. 2018;10:139-52.
25. Thompson J, Jones N, Al-Khafaji A, Malik S, Reich D, Munoz S, et al. Extracorporeal cellular therapy (ELAD) in severe alcoholic hepatitis: A multinational, prospective, controlled, randomized trial. Liver Transplant. 2018;24:380-93.

CHAPTER 17

Frailty in Liver Transplant Patients: Problem Statement, Assessment, and Nutritional Rehabilitation in Perioperative Period of Liver Transplantation

Pooja Lakhani, Suvadeep Sen

INTRODUCTION

Frailty is defined as a significant decline in physiological reserve, which increases the risk of adverse health outcomes in response to stressors. In patients with end-stage liver disease (ESLD), frailty often manifests through skeletal muscle wasting, malnutrition, and reduced physical capacity. This condition reflects a progressive deterioration across multiple physiological systems, ultimately impairing the body's ability to cope with stress and leading to heightened vulnerability to complications, increased unplanned hospitalizations, and greater mortality risk. Approximately 50% of individuals with cirrhosis exhibit signs of frailty, regardless of its underlying cause, and it contributes to higher rates of complications and mortality in patients with ESLD.[1,2] Despite its importance, there remains a lack of comprehensive understanding and standardized assessment and treatment approach for frailty in liver cirrhosis, particularly in patients presenting with decompensated symptoms such as ascites and encephalopathy. This chapter delves into the risk factors contributing to frailty, explores various assessment tools used to evaluate frailty in cirrhotic patients, the significance of the identification of frailty in patients with liver diseases in the peritransplant period, and outlines management strategies.

DEFINITION OF FRAILTY

The concepts of frailty, malnutrition, and sarcopenia have close resemblance and are sometimes used interchangeably based on individual experience and institutional protocols.

The American Association for the Study of Liver Diseases (AASLD) 2021 guidelines for management of malnutrition, frailty, and sarcopenia in patients with cirrhosis[3] have described operational definitions of these terms, specifically applicable to patients with cirrhosis.

- *Malnutrition:* An imbalance (deficiency or excess) of nutrients that cause measurable adverse effects on tissue/body form (body shape, size composition) or function and clinical outcome.
- *Frailty:* The phenotypic representation of impaired muscle contractile function. Frailty can be defined as a condition where patients undergo a reduction in their physical capacity to perform daily activities and become more susceptible to health-related challenges, leading to negative health consequences. It is a multifaceted concept involving physical, psychological, social, and environmental factors.
- *Sarcopenia:* The phenotypic representation of gradual and widespread decline of muscle mass and strength.

It is important to acknowledge that these three concepts are interrelated and may often co-exist in an individual patient. For example, a patient with decompensated liver cirrhosis might be assessed to be frail, sarcopenic, and malnourished at the same time, demonstrating poor clinical condition and prognosis.

PREDISPOSING FACTORS FOR FRAILTY IN END-STAGE LIVER DISEASE (FIG. 1 AND TABLE 1)

- *Malnutrition:* Malnutrition in cirrhosis has multiple causative factors, such as suboptimal intake of macronutrients, decreased micronutrient intake, early satiation due to ascites, disturbance in levels of ghrelin and leptin, compromised nutrient uptake and utilization, malabsorption, gut bacterial dysbiosis, and hepatic encephalopathy (HE). Research has demonstrated that malnourished patients have a 3.38 times increased risk of developing frailty as compared to well-nourished patients.[4]
- *Salt restriction:* Salt restriction is a key component in managing ascites, helping prevent sodium overload

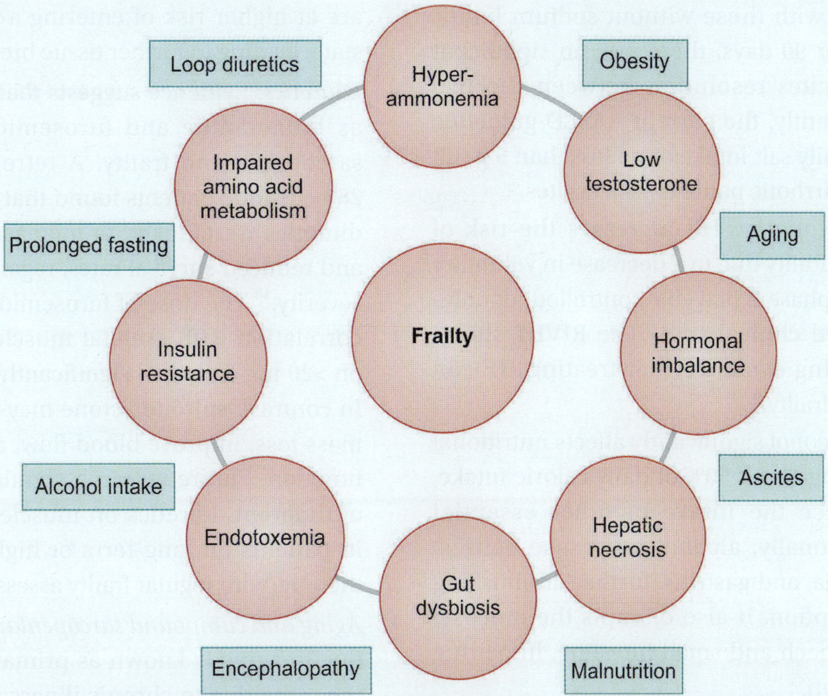

Fig. 1: Predisposing factors for frailty in ESLD. (ESLD: end-stage liver disease)

TABLE 1: Clinical manifestations of predisposing factors for frailty and recommendations for management.

Predisposing factor	***Clinical manifestations***	***Management***
Ascites	Decreased appetite, difficulty in physical activity and performing ADLs, reduced stomach capacity, poor digestion, protein–energy deficiency	Large volume paracentesis with IV albumin infusion, salt intake no less than 5 g per day to preserve palatability of food
Hepatic encephalopathy (HE)	Reduced voluntary food intake, decreased ambulation and physical activity, increased risk of falls	Avoid unnecessary protein restriction, oral nutritional supplementation for low dietary intake, aspiration precautions for EN support, PN if not receiving any other form of nutrition
Alcohol intake	• Difficult diagnosis of frailty • Reduced physical capacity • Increased muscle fat	1.2–1.5 g/kg/day of protein intake with calorie restriction as necessary, personalized exercise program for maintaining muscle mass
Prolonged fasting	• Increased catabolism • Accelerated muscle breakdown	Overnight fasting of no more than 10–12 hours, early morning breakfast, and late evening snacks to shorten fasting around procedures, and small and frequent meals
Loop diuretics	Worsening of muscle mass loss	Periodic frailty assessments, switching to spironolactone wherever feasible
Aging	Organic progression of muscle mass loss	Periodic frailty assessments, nutritional education, and monitoring for preventing compound sarcopenia

(ADLs: activities of daily living; EN: enteral nutrition; PN: parenteral nutrition)

and facilitating fluid mobilization. Studies show that strict sodium intake (<5 g daily) can reduce diuretic needs, hasten ascites resolution, and shorten hospital stays. However, excessive sodium restriction may not always be beneficial. A trial by Gauthier et al.[5] compared cirrhotic patients on strict salt restriction

(1,230 mg daily) with those without sodium limits. Surprisingly, after 90 days, there was no significant difference in ascites resolution between the two groups. Consequently, the current AASLD guideline recommends a daily salt intake of no less than 5 g salt (2 g sodium) for cirrhotic patients with ascites.[3]

- *Hepatic encephalopathy:* HE increases the risk of malnutrition and frailty due to a decrease in voluntary dietary intake. A phase 2 placebo-controlled, double-blind randomized clinical trial (The RIVET study) provides promising evidence that treating HE can positively impact frailty.[6]
- *Alcohol intake:* Alcohol significantly affects nutritional status by providing about 50% of daily caloric intake, which can reduce the intake of other essential nutrients. Additionally, alcohol can cause nausea, vomiting, anorexia, and gastritis, further diminishing nutrient consumption. It also disrupts the mucosal lining of the stomach and small intestine, impairing nutrient absorption.
- *Physical inactivity:* Reduced physical activity and sedentary behavior are often seen in individuals with cirrhosis and are linked with frailty and sarcopenia as well as mortality. There are not enough prospective longitudinal studies assessing the direct role of lack of physical activity on the progression of frailty and/or sarcopenia. However, many trials have shown the benefit of interventions to decrease physical inactivity (in addition to nutritional counseling) on muscle function, muscle mass, and functional capacity.[7]
- *Sarcopenic obesity:* Sarcopenic obesity is a condition associated with low lean muscle mass in a patient with a high body mass index. Sarcopenic visceral obesity (SVO) is measured using CT-based estimation of the skeletal mass index (SMI) and visceral-to-subcutaneous adipose tissue ratio for evaluating adipose tissue distribution in the body. SVO has been found to negatively impact disease progression and mortality in individuals with liver cirrhosis, and also increased post-transplant mortality.[8]
- *Prolonged fasting:* Patients with liver cirrhosis experience a more rapid breakdown of body tissues in response to starvation compared to healthy individuals. After an overnight fast, their metabolic response is similar to that of healthy individuals who have fasted for 2–3 days.[9] This suggests that cirrhotic patients undergoing medical procedures with prolonged fasting are at higher risk of entering a significant catabolic state, leading to further tissue breakdown.
- *Diuretics:* Evidence suggests that loop diuretics, such as bumetanide and furosemide, may exacerbate sarcopenia and frailty. A retrospective analysis of 266 cirrhotic patients found that higher doses of loop diuretics were linked to increased muscle mass loss and reduced survival rates, regardless of liver disease severity.[10] The dose of furosemide showed an inverse correlation with skeletal muscle mass and patients on >20 mg daily had significantly lower survival rates. In contrast, spironolactone may help prevent muscle mass loss, improve blood flow, and enhance muscle function. Future research should explore the effects of different diuretics on muscle health, particularly in patients on long-term or high-dose loop diuretic therapy, with regular frailty assessments.
- *Aging and compound sarcopenia:* Loss of muscle mass due to aging is known as primary sarcopenia, while the same due to chronic illness is termed secondary sarcopenia. A combination of both gives rise to a situation called "compound sarcopenia". Compound sarcopenia has been linked with prolonged length of hospital stay, increased healthcare costs, and detrimental effects on patient survival, in clinical studies with hospitalized cirrhotic patients.

PREVALENCE AND CLINICAL RELEVANCE OF FRAILTY IN END-STAGE LIVER DISEASE

Frailty prevalence among nonhospitalized cirrhosis patients ranges from 17 to 43%.[11] In hospitalized patients, frailty is seen in 38% with HE and 18% without HE. It is often assessed using Activities of Daily Living (ADLs) tool.[11] Frailty prevalence has been reported to be as high as 68% when evaluated as impaired performance status using the Karnofsky Performance Status (KPS) scale. Frailty typically worsens over time in cirrhotic patients. Among those on the liver transplant waitlist in the US, <20% showed stable or improved KPS scores. Worsening of frailty in patients with cirrhosis is associated with a significantly higher rate of decompensation of chronic liver disease and waitlist mortality independent of their baseline model for end-stage liver disease (MELD) score.[12]

Frailty directly affects the outcome after a liver transplant. Patients with a liver frailty index (LFI) ≥4.5 are associated with higher post-transplant complications and mortality as well as prolonged ICU and hospital stay.[13] Pretransplant physical functional status is a strong predictor of robust post-transplant high physical function.[14]

ASSESSMENT OF FRAILTY IN END-STAGE LIVER DISEASE

Accurate and timely estimation of frailty in liver cirrhosis patients is crucial for effective care. Well-compensated cirrhosis patients should be reassessed annually,[3] while those with decompensated cirrhosis or undergoing active frailty management need reassessment every 8–12 weeks. There are multiple tools to assess frailty in clinical practice, each one has its unique methodologies and its limitations. Clinicians need to select the most suitable assessment tool **(Tables 2 and 3)** for a particular patient and interpret results as per its validation standard. The following paragraphs will summarize the three most commonly used frailty assessment tools for cirrhotic patients, highlighting their strengths and limitations.

TABLE 2: Frailty assessment and diagnosis.

	Diagnosis of frailty		
	Clinical questions	***Physical examination findings***	***Objective measures***
Screen for malnutrition and assess for frailty and/or sarcopenia	• Karnofsky performance scale • Clinical frailty scale • Activities of daily living • Royal Free Hospital–Nutrition Prioritizing tool	• Physical examination to identify muscle wasting • Use of a walking aid • Inability to stand up from the chair or get off after the examination independently • Slowness	• CT scan L3 skeletal muscle index • Liver frailty index • Handgrip strength • 6-minute walk test • 4 meter gait speed • Triceps skinfold thickness (pediatric)
Identify factors contributing to frailty and sarcopenia	• Reduced macro- and micronutrient intake • Physical inactivity	• Ascites • Hepatic encephalopathy • Poor dentition • Dysgeusia	• MELD-Na • Child–Pugh score • Testosterone level (men)

(MELD: model for end-stage liver disease)

TABLE 3: Commonly used assessment tools for frailty and sarcopenia.

Frailty indicator	***Components***	***Significance***
Fried frailty index	Unintentional weight loss >4.5 kg in 6 months, self-reported exhaustion, weakness (grip strength), slow gait speed, low physical activity	• 1–2: Prefrail • ≥3: Frail
Clinical frailty scale (CFS)	Level of comorbidity, function, ability to perform daily activities, and need for assistance	A continuous scale from 1 (very fit) to 9 (terminally ill)
Liver frailty index (LFI)	Dominant hand grip strength, time to do 5 chair stands, seconds holding 3-position balance *https://liverfrailtyindex.ucsf.edu*	• <3.2: Robust • 3.2–4.4: Prefrail • ≥4.5: Frail
Karnofsky performance status (KPS)	Activities of daily living, limitations due to chronic diseases, cognitive decline	Scale ranges from 1 to 100. KPS <70 (group B, C, and D) associated with poor outcome
6-minute walk test (6-MWT)	Distance a patient can quickly walk on a flat, hard surface in a period of 6 minutes	<250 m associated with poor outcome
Skeletal muscle index (SMI)	Total muscle area at the 3rd lumbar vertebrae/height^2	SMI <50 cm^2 in males and <39 cm^2 in females associated with worse outcome
SARC-F score	Questionnaire-based screening tool for sarcopenia consisting of five questions: Strength (S), Assistance walking (A), Rising from a chair (R), Climbing stairs (C), and Falls (F) on a scale of 0–2	≥4 associated with mean muscle volume loss in cirrhosis patients

Fried Frailty Index

The fried frailty index (FFI) is a quick and reliable assessment tool that includes both subjective and objective components to measure frailty. It has been shown to predict morbidity and mortality in individuals with liver cirrhosis, with higher scores associated with elevated MELD scores, reduced albumin levels, ascites, and HE. A single-point increase in the FFI is associated with a 50% increase in mortality rates among patients with ESLD while waiting for a transplant. However, the validity of FFI may be questionable in patients with decompensated cirrhosis,[15] especially those with HE, due to difficulties in reporting subjective components and executing objective components such as walking speed and grip strength.

Clinical Frailty Scale

The clinical frailty scale (CFS) is a quick and congruous method utilized for the evaluation of frailty. The scale takes into account—the subjects' level of comorbidity, function, and reliance on others for daily activities. The score ranges from 1 (very fit) to 9 (terminally ill). The score is well validated in the geriatric population (age >65 years) in general. Among outpatient cirrhotics, individuals with CFS >4 have been found to have higher rates of acute hospitalization or mortality.[16] Among hospitalized patients with liver cirrhosis, CFS is associated with acute kidney injury and hepatorenal syndrome. However, the CFS demonstrates only an elementary analysis of the status of frailty and is not precise enough to take into account changes in frailty brought about by therapeutic interventions.[16]

Liver Frailty Index

The LFI is a rapid, three-part assessment that accurately predicts hospital readmission and identifies high-risk transplant candidates in patients with liver disease. Among all the objective tools, LFI has been validated the most in the majority of multicentric large clinical trials in patients with liver cirrhosis. It measures handgrip strength, handgrip strength of the dominant hand, the time taken to perform five chair stands, and the time taken to maintain three different balance positions. It provides a rapid assessment of frailty levels within 3–5 minutes. A higher LFI score indicates greater frailty. A cut-off of >4.62 has been recognized as a specific indicator in the estimation of a potentially higher risk for hospital readmission with decompensation within 30 days among patients with liver cirrhosis.[11] Changes in LFI have significant prognostic value in predicting waitlist mortality when adjusted with other confounders such as MELD-Na score and HE. Compared to the KPS scale, which focuses on a single dimension of frailty, the LFI provides a more comprehensive and accurate assessment of mortality risk by accounting for multiple facets of frailty. Pretransplant frailty is also associated with post-transplant hospital length of stay and mortality and also impaired 1-year post-transplant quality of life.[14] However, LFI cannot be measured in patients with sick acute-on-chronic liver failure (ACLF) as this tool requires patient participation.

Importantly, in patients with compensated cirrhosis, annual frailty assessment may be sufficient, while in patients with decompensated cirrhosis, more frequent assessments (once in 3 or 6 months) may be required. In addition to this, given the strong and consistent association between muscle mass and clinical outcomes in both adults and children with cirrhosis, objective measures of muscle loss should be included for the assessment of risk for poor outcomes in cirrhotics. Skeletal muscle index (total muscle area at the 3rd lumbar vertebrae/height^2) as assessed by CT image analysis is recommended as one of the most consistent and reproducible methods to quantify muscle mass and assess sarcopenia in patients with cirrhosis.[3] Skeletal muscle index is important in individuals in whom assessment of muscle contractile function is not practical or feasible for example, in acutely ill patients or very young children.[3]

MANAGEMENT OF FRAILTY IN END-STAGE LIVER DISEASE

Management of frailty in individuals with liver cirrhosis requires an incessant process, that involves various interventions and periodic reassessments of the patients to monitor the progress and plan follow-up steps. In this chapter, we will discuss in detail the interventions for the treatment of frailty in cirrhosis, as depicted in **Table 4**.

Exercise

For improving physical frailty and quality of life in patients with cirrhosis, a personalized care plan including both aerobic and resistance exercise programs is required for a minimum of 12 weeks.[17] A scientific nutrition care plan should also be formulated at the same time. Both these plans should be tailored to the individual's degree of frailty, dividing patients into mild, moderate, or severe

TABLE 4: Overview of frailty diagnosis and management.

Patients with cirrhosis	*Primary prevention*	*Secondary prevention*	*Tertiary prevention*	*Prevent the occurrence of undesirable health outcomes*
Aim	• Prevent development • Delay onset	• Early diagnosis • Prompt initiation of treatment • Slow progression	• Rehabilitate • Reverse	*Frailty diagnosis*
Assessment	• Malnutrition screening • Assessment of muscle dysfunction	• Evaluate for etiologic risk factors • Explore dietary preferences and barriers to exercise	Periodic reassessment for progression of frailty, malnutrition, and sarcopenia	
Action	• Educate patient and caregivers • Encourage positive health behaviors • Empower patients with specific skills	• Symptomatic medical management • Co-management with a registered dietitian and certified exercise therapist/physical therapist	• Refer to a registered dietitian, certified exercise therapist/ physical therapist for co-management • Consider center-based rehabilitation, enteral nutrition therapy	*Management of frailty*

categories. For severe frailty, an inpatient rehabilitation program is recommended for accurate monitoring and to prevent complications. Individuals with moderate frailty may benefit from regular home-based exercises focusing on amplification of ADLs. Mild or no frailty allows for moderate-intensity exercise for at least 150 minutes per week. Periodic reassessment of frailty status is crucial and is of utmost importance in all ESLD patients to tailor nutrition and exercise interventions periodically.

Nutritional Management

There is ample evidence to demonstrate that interventions aimed at improving nutritional status—such as nutrition education, protein-energy supplementation, and enteral nutritional therapy—can significantly help alleviate frailty. The AASLD recommends creating tailored nutrition plans for all cirrhosis patients, taking their current nutritional status into account.

Energy Intake

Studies indicate that individuals with liver cirrhosis typically have an energy expenditure ranging from 28 to 38 kcal/kg/day.[18] Consequently, recent nutrition guidelines suggest that patients with chronic liver disease or cirrhosis should consume a daily caloric intake of at least 35 kcal/kg/day. For patients experiencing edema and ascites, their dry weight can be estimated by either using the postparacentesis weight or adjusting based on the level of fluid retention—5% for mild, 10% for moderate, and 15% for severe cases. An additional 5% reduction is recommended for patients with bilateral pedal edema extending to the knees. For those with obesity, the AASLD advises considering both weight and BMI when planning nutritional care. The caloric intake guidelines based on BMI are 25–35 kcal/kg/day for patients with a BMI between 30 and 40 kg/m^2 and 20–25 kcal/kg/day for those with a BMI of 40 kg/m^2 or higher.[3]

Protein Intake

Patients with cirrhosis have increased protein requirements. A positive protein balance can be achieved with a protein intake of at least 1.2 g/kg/day; European Association for the Study of the Liver (EASL) and AASLD guidelines recommend a daily protein intake of 1.2–1.5 g/kg/day for adult patients with liver cirrhosis due to its safety, lack of negative effects on HE, and reduced protein loss compared to protein restriction. While there is no consensus on the weight measurement (measured, dry, or ideal body weight) for calculating protein targets, the AASLD recommends using ideal body weight (based on height) for practical purposes.[3,19]

There is limited data regarding the use of branched-chain amino acid (BCAA) supplementation (leucine, isoleucine, and valine) for treating complications associated with cirrhosis, particularly HE. As per a recent review, in adult patients with advanced liver disease, the administration of BCAAs is worth considering. BCAA supplementation has been shown to improve muscle mass, muscle strength and albumin levels in patients with sarcopenia. A minimum dose of 12 g per day has been shown to be more effective than lower doses. However, high quality data such as RCTs in this regard is still lacking.[20]

The evaluation of multiple other amino acid-based treatments for nutritional management in frail cirrhotic patients remains inconclusive. Although compounds like β-hydroxy-β-methylbutyrate, acetyl-L-carnitine, and L-ornithine L-aspartate have been studied for their potential benefits—such as reducing blood ammonia levels, current evidence[21] does not robustly support their routine use in clinical practice. Further research is needed to clarify their effectiveness and practicality in managing the nutritional needs of this patient population.

Frequency of Nutritional Intake

Patients with cirrhosis should eat small, frequent meals and snacks every 3–4 hours to manage their nutritional status. Patients should avoid prolonged fasting and consume small, frequent meals and snacks every 3–4 hours, including an early morning breakfast and a late evening snack. A landmark RCT showed that nighttime supplemental nutrition of 710 kcal per day with various carbohydrate and protein composition increased total body protein and fat-free mass in patients with cirrhosis.[22] While snack options vary in calorie content and composition, personal habits and preferences influence snack choices. The AASLD recommends creating customized care plans to guide patients on timing and composition of additional snacks.[23]

Route of Nutritional Intake

Based on current clinical data, enteral nutrition should only be considered for cirrhotic patients who have not succeeded with oral supplementation. Additionally, the placement of percutaneous feeding devices in cirrhotic patients, particularly those with ascites, is generally advised against. A retrospective study involving 75 patients with cirrhosis and known esophageal varices indicated that 15% experienced gastrointestinal bleeding within 48 hours of feeding tube placement. Notably, a higher MELD-Na score was identified as a significant predictor of this bleeding.

Based on available clinical data, enteral nutrition should be considered only in cirrhotics who have failed attempts of oral supplementation; on the other hand, placement of percutaneous feeding devices in cirrhotics, specifically for the ones with ascites, should be avoided. A retrospective study of 75 patients with cirrhosis and known esophageal varices, who were subjected to placement of feeding tube, showed that 15% of patients had a gastrointestinal bleed within 48 hours of placement.[24] Furthermore, a higher MELD-Na score was a strong predictor of gastrointestinal bleeding. However, for patients at risk of protein energy malnutrition (PEM) where oral intake is not adequate, pretransplant medical enteral nutritional intervention plan should be in place.

Nutritional Management in Hospitalized Patients with Cirrhosis

Hospitalized patients with cirrhosis are at a higher risk of developing cumulative calorie and protein deficits due to increased duration of fasting for procedures, lower palatability of hospital food, reduced appetite in acute decompensation, contraindications to oral and enteral feeding such as variceal or lower GI bleed, severe ascites, and HE. Attempts should be made to initiate enteral nutrition therapy as soon as the clinical conditions are favorable. Palatable options of meals and snacks along with oral nutritional supplements should be provided to prevent higher calorie and protein deficits.

In critically ill patients, the availability of cirrhosis-specific data to guide energy targets is lacking. Indirect calorimetry (IC) continues to be the gold standard for the measurement of total calorie requirements. Yet given the unavailability of IC in many clinical settings, predictive or weight-based equations for the calculation of energy requirements may be utilized, considering the potential gap in the estimation of calorie targets given the spontaneous changes in metabolic requirements and excess fluid retention in acutely ill cirrhotics. For critically ill patients, higher protein goals such as 1.2–2.0 g/kg/day are generally recommended.[3] Noteworthy to mention in this context, ideal body weight is recommended for practical purposes.[3]

Enteral nutrition should be considered for hospitalized cirrhotics who cannot meet energy targets through oral intake alone and for critically ill patients within 24–48 hours of ICU admission. Parenteral nutrition (PN) has mixed evidence regarding its effectiveness in patients with cirrhosis. PN is associated with a higher risk of hyperglycemia and sepsis, and higher mortality rates compared to those receiving enteral nutrition in critically ill patients. PN should be considered a second-line option for patients who cannot achieve their nutritional goals through oral intake alone and is preferred over no nutritional supplementation in hospitalized patients who are diagnosed positive for frailty and/or sarcopenia.[25]

Prehabilitation

Prehabilitation refers to a range of interventions before a medical procedure, intending to alleviate and prevent complications. In liver transplantation, prehabilitation focuses on identifying high-risk patients early and improving their physical capacity. This can be accomplished through various interventions including exercise, nutrition, and psychological stress management. A recent systematic review showed that prehabilitation can enhance aerobic capacity in liver transplant candidates and is a safe and pragmatic approach that helps to attain notable advancement in several aspects including VO_2 peak, 6-minute walking capacity, hand grip strength, LFI, and quality of life.[26] A dedicated focused home-based or institutional prehabilitation plan should be a mandatory part of the preoperative optimization of liver transplant candidates at all centers.

CONCLUSION

Frailty and sarcopenia are common and often detrimental complications of ESLD. Accurate identification and management is not only chellenging but is often overlooked. A continued approach including serial assessments of frailty, sarcopenia and nutritional status should be implemented in all centres providing care for patients with ESLD.

Patients diagnosed with moderate to severe frailty and/or moderate to severe malnutrition should receive detailed prescription and guidance including management of nutritional intake, need for additional nutrient supplementation and regular physical activity.

Education on implications of frailty, sarcopenia and diminished nutritional status to healthcare practitioners, care providers, patients and families by skilled and trained dietitians plays a crucial role in implementing aforementioned standards of care.

While current standards and recommendations for management of frailty and sarcopenia in patients with ESLD, show promising results, further scope for research includes identification of predominant drivers of frailty, explore the potential interplay between gut health, nutrient absorption and utilisation. In addition to this, research regarding increased precision in management of nutritional intake, and dosing of nutrient supplements, currently observed to have potential benefits and possible link between structured physical activity programs and improvement in frailty related outcomes, may be needed.

REFERENCES

1. Karakousis N, Chrysavgis L, Chatzigeorgiou A, Papatheodoridis G, Cholongitas E. Frailty in metabolic syndrome, focusing on nonalcoholic fatty liver disease. Ann Gastroenterol. 2022;35(3):234-42.
2. Siramolpiwat S, Kiattikunrat K, Soontararatpong R, Pornthisarn B, Vilaichone RK, Chonprasertsuk S, et al. Frailty, as tested by the Liver Frailty Index, is associated with decompensation and unplanned hospitalization in patients with compensated cirrhosis. Scand J Gastroenterol. 2021;56(10):1210-9.
3. Lai JC, Tandon P, Bernal W, Tapper EB, Ekong U, Dasarathy S, et al. Malnutrition, Frailty, and Sarcopenia in Patients With Cirrhosis: 2021 Practice Guidance by the American Association for the Study of Liver Diseases. Hepatology. 2021;74(3):1611-44.
4. Traub J, Reiss L, Aliwa B, Stadlbauer V. Malnutrition in Patients with Liver Cirrhosis. Nutrients. 2021;13(2):540.
5. Gauthier A, Levy VG, Quinton A, Michel H, Rueff B, Descos L, et al. Salt or no salt in the treatment of cirrhotic ascites: a randomised study. Gut. 1986;27(6):705-9.
6. Bajaj JS, Fagan A, Gavis EA, Mousel T, Gallagher ML, Puri P, et al. The RIVET RCT: Rifamycin SV MMX improves muscle mass, physical function, and ammonia in cirrhosis and minimal encephalopathy. Hepatol Commun. 2024; 8(2):e0384.
7. Vuille-Lessard É, Berzigotti A. Exercise Interventions for Cirrhosis. Curr Treat Options Gastroenterol. 2022;20:336-50.
8. Ha NB, Montano-Loza AJ, Carey EJ, Lin S, Shui AM, Huang CY, et al. Sarcopenic visceral obesity is associated with increased post-liver transplant mortality in acutely ill patients with cirrhosis. Am J Transplant. 2022; 22(9):2195-202.
9. Owen OE, Trapp VE, Reichard GA, Mozzoli MA, Moctezuma J, Paul P, et al. Nature and quantity of fuels consumed in patients with alcoholic cirrhosis. J Clin Invest. 1983;72(5):1821-32.
10. Hanai T, Shiraki M, Miwa T, Watanabe S, Imai K, Suetsugu A, et al. Effect of loop diuretics on skeletal muscle depletion in patients with liver cirrhosis. Hepatol Res. 2018;49(1):82-95.

11. Lai JC, Covinsky KE, Dodge JL, Boscardin WJ, Segev DL, Roberts JP, et al. Development of a novel frailty index to predict mortality in patients with end-stage liver disease. Hepatology. 2017;66(2):564-74.
12. Lai JC, Dodge JL, Kappus MR, Dunn MA, Volk ML, Duarte-Rojo A, et al.; Multi-Center Functional Assessment in Liver Transplantation (FrAILT) Study. Changes in frailty are associated with waitlist mortality in patients with cirrhosis. J Hepatol. 2020;73(3):575-81.
13. Lai JC, Shui AM, Duarte-Rojo A, Ganger DR, Rahimi RS, Huang CY, et al; from the Multi-Center Functional Assessment in Liver Transplantation (FrAILT) Study. Frailty, mortality, and health care utilization after liver transplantation: From the Multicenter Functional Assessment in Liver Transplantation (FrAILT) Study. Hepatology. 2022;75(6):1471-9.
14. Tandon P, Zanetto A, Piano S, Heimbach JK, Dasarathy S. Liver transplantation in the patient with physical frailty. J Hepatol. 2023;78(6):1105-17.
15. Sinclair M, Poltavskiy E, Dodge JL, Lai JC. Frailty is independently associated with increased hospitalisation days in patients on the liver transplant waitlist. World J Gastroenterol. 2017;23(5):899.
16. Tandon P, Tangri N, Thomas L, Zenith L, Shaikh T, Carbonneau M, et al. A Rapid Bedside Screen to Predict Unplanned Hospitalization and Death in Outpatients With Cirrhosis: A Prospective Evaluation of the Clinical Frailty Scale. Am J Gastroenterol. 2016;111(12):1759-67.
17. Williams FR, Berzigotti A, Lord JM, Lai JC, Armstrong MJ. Review article: impact of exercise on physical frailty in patients with chronic liver disease. Aliment Pharmacol Therap. 2019;50(9):988-1000.
18. Guglielmi F, Panella C, Buda A, Budillion G, Caregaro L, Clerici C, et al. Nutritional state and energy balance in cirrhotic patients with or without hypermetabolism. Multicentre prospective study by the 'Nutritional Problems in Gastroenterology' Section of the Italian Society of Gastroenterology (SIGE). Dig Liver Dis. 2005;37(9):681-8.
19. European Association for the Study of the Liver. EASL Clinical Practice Guidelines on nutrition in chronic liver disease. J Hepatol. 2019;70(1):172-93.
20. Marrone G, Serra A, Miele L, Biolato M, Liguori A, Grieco A, et al. Branched chain amino acids in hepatic encephalopathy and sarcopenia in liver cirrhosis: Evidence and uncertainties. World J Gastroenterol. 2023;29(19):2905-15.
21. Goh E, Stokes C, Sidhu S, Vilstrup H, Gluud L, Morgan M. L-ornithine L-aspartate for prevention and treatment of hepatic encephalopathy in people with cirrhosis. Cochrane Database Syst Rev. 2018;5(5):CD012410.
22. Plank LD, Gane EJ, Peng S, Muthu C, Mathur S, Gillanders L, et al. Nocturnal nutritional supplementation improves total body protein status of patients with liver cirrhosis: a randomized 12-month trial. Hepatology. 2008;48(2):557-66.
23. Tsien CD, McCullough AJ, Dasarathy S. Late evening snack: Exploiting a period of anabolic opportunity in cirrhosis. J Gastroenterol Hepatol. 2012;27(3):430-41.
24. Al-Obaid LN, Bazarbashi AN, Cohen ME, Kim J, Lei Y, Axelrad JE, et al. Enteric tube placement in patients with esophageal varices: Risks and predictors of postinsertion gastrointestinal bleeding. JGH Open. 2020;4(2):256-9.
25. McClave S, Taylor B, Martindale R, Warren M, Johnson D, Braunschweig C, et al. Guidelines for the Provision and Assessment of Nutrition Support Therapy in the Adult Critically Ill Patient. JPEN. 2016;40(2):159-211.
26. Jetten WD, Hogenbirk RNM, Van Meeteren NLU, Cuperus FJC, Klaase JM, De Jong R. Physical Effects, Safety and Feasibility of Prehabilitation in Patients Awaiting Orthotopic Liver Transplantation, a Systematic Review. Transpl Int. 2022;35:10330.

CHAPTER 18

Simultaneous Liver–Kidney Transplant

Guruprasad Shetty, Amit C Langote, Suvadeep Sen

INTRODUCTION

A simultaneous liver-kidney transplant (SLKT) is a surgical procedure where a patient receives both a liver and a kidney transplant (KT) at the same time. This is typically performed in patients who have both liver failure and kidney failure, often due to end-stage organ disease, and are in need of both organs simultaneously. In the majority of cases, SLKT involves transplanting both the liver and kidney from a single deceased donor in one procedure. The Sequential liver-kidney transplantation or kidney after liver transplantation (KALT) occurs in two separate stages: the liver (or kidney) is transplanted first, followed by the second organ (either kidney or liver) at a later time, which may come from either the same living donor or different deceased donors.

Simultaneous liver-kidney transplant represents about 10% of all liver transplants (LTs) and is the most commonly performed type of multivisceral transplant in the United States.[1] This dual organ transplantation was first performed by Margreiter et al.[2] to address both end-stage liver and renal disease, and the procedure has become more common after the Model for End-Stage Liver Disease (MELD) scoring system was introduced in 2002.

RATIONALE AND BENEFIT OF DUAL ORGAN TRANSPLANT

Decompensated cirrhosis is commonly associated with chronic kidney disease (CKD) due to multiple reasons, such as hepatorenal syndrome (HRS), hypovolemia, parenchymal renal damage due to glomerulonephritis, systemic diseases such as diabetes mellitus and hypertension, and drug-induced renal failure, all of which are linked to lower survival rates with single organ transplants.

Several factors should be considered when evaluating patients with liver failure and concurrent kidney dysfunction, including the following:

- In patients with liver failure, serum creatinine-based estimated glomerular filtration rate (GFR) can often overestimate true kidney function due to their typically low muscle mass. Alternative methods, such as measuring cystatin C levels or performing a nuclear GFR scan, can provide a more accurate assessment of kidney function. However, these techniques may not be easily accessible at all medical centers.
- The presence of proteinuria or albuminuria, along with radiologic signs such as increased kidney echogenicity and small kidney size, suggests CKD. However, the absence of proteinuria/albuminuria, along with normal echogenicity and kidney size, does not definitively exclude the possibility of CKD.
- A kidney biopsy can assist in detecting chronic pathological alterations, including glomerulosclerosis, interstitial fibrosis, and tubular atrophy. However, this procedure may pose an elevated risk of bleeding, as patients with liver failure are prone to coagulopathy.

The outcome of LT alone in patients with end-stage liver disease (ESLD) and concomitant CKD had a poorer outcome in terms of long-term graft function. One retrospective validation analysis of patients from the Organ Procurement and Transplant Network (OPTN) and United Network for Organ Sharing (UNOS) registry revealed that the incidence of 1-year post-transplant graft loss is 35% higher in patients receiving LTs alone than in patients who required SLKTs.[3] The requirement of post-transplant dialysis is an independent risk factor for graft loss. Patients undergoing SLKT have better outcomes in terms of 5-year survival rate as well when compared to LT alone.[4]

Overall, the potential benefits of combined liver–kidney transplants are:

- *Improved survival:* Patients who receive both organs at the same time tend to have better survival outcomes than those who receive one transplant first and the other later.

- *Reduced risk of organ rejection:* By transplanting both organs together, the risk of rejection is reduced because both the liver and kidney may be considered "new" organs to the immune system at the same time.
- *Faster recovery:* Since the liver and kidney are transplanted together, the patient may recover more quickly than if they had to wait for one transplant to "take" before undergoing the other.

INDICATIONS FOR SIMULTANEOUS LIVER–KIDNEY TRANSPLANT

Simultaneous liver–kidney transplant is generally recommended in the following group of patients:

- *End-stage liver disease* with CKD due to glomerulonephritis, diabetic and hypertensive nephropathy, interstitial renal disease, polycystic disease, and calcineurin inhibitors (CNIs) toxicity
- *End-stage kidney disease:* Has associated cirrhosis of the liver
- *Multisystem organ failure:* Where the liver and kidney dysfunction are intertwined, making separate transplants less effective, e.g., conditions such as primary hyperoxaluria I, α-1-antitrypsin deficiency, glycogen storage disease type I, sickle cell disease, amyloidosis, hemolytic uremic syndrome, and methylmalonic acidemia.

It is important to note that there are many indications for SLKT in the pediatric age group. A detailed discussion of all these pediatric indications is beyond the scope of this chapter.

The decision of whether to proceed with SLKT can be complex. For patients needing a LT who also have kidney dysfunction, the rationale for choosing SLKT is that it offers a survival benefit over liver-alone transplantation. The challenge lies in distinguishing between acute, reversible kidney dysfunction, where SLKT may be unnecessary, and CKD, where the simultaneous transplant is potentially beneficial. A recently published study by Cheng et al. demonstrated that SLKT provides a survival benefit over liver-alone transplantation only for patients with end-stage kidney disease, suggesting that a more selective SLKT strategy may be advantageous at the national policy level.[5]

CRITERIA FOR SELECTION

The medical eligibility criteria for listing patients on SLKT were implemented by OPTN in 2017. Patients considered for SLKT must meet certain criteria, which are given in **Table 1**.

Patients who do not meet the criteria for SLKT may still be prioritized for a "safety-net" deceased donor KT if their GFR remains ≤20 mL/min or if they are dialysis-dependent for 60–365 days following orthotopic liver transplantation (OLT).

The implementation of the OPTN policy has standardized the SLKT listing process and reassured clinicians that a backup KT option will be available for patients who experience persistent kidney dysfunction

TABLE 1: Indication of simultaneous liver–kidney transplant.

Condition	*Criteria*
• Patients with primary liver disease developing kidney diseases • Patients with ESLD (cirrhosis and liver failure) listed for liver, who have renal disease	• *AKI setting:* ESLD patients with AKI • Duration of AKI >6 weeks with persistent GFR ≤25 mL/min documented every 7 days • Dialysis dependence for >6 weeks[6]
	• CKD setting due to any reason with regular requirement for dialysis • GFR ≤60 mL/min for ≥3 months and subsequent drop to GFR ≤30 mL/min at the time of registration
Metabolic diseases	• Primary hyperoxaluria type 1 • Atypical hemolytic uremic syndrome (HUS) from mutations in factor H or I • Familial non-neuropathic systemic amyloidosis • Methylmalonic aciduria
Patients with ESRD listed for kidney and have liver disease	• Polycystic kidney diseases causing CKD associated with polycystic liver diseases • CKD with associated cirrhosis due to any cause

(AKI: acute kidney injury; CKD: chronic kidney disease; ESLD: end-stage liver disease; ESRD: end-stage renal disease; GFR: glomerular filtration rate)

after OLT. This policy aims to reduce unnecessary SLKT listings by distinguishing between patients with potentially reversible kidney dysfunction.

SURGICAL TECHNIQUE

- The traditional method of SLKT involves the implantation of the liver and kidney separately. As a usual practice, SLKT is conducted using two separate incisions: a subcostal incision for the liver allograft and an incision in the lower abdomen for the KT. However, both graft implantations can be performed with a single subcostal incision, with comparable outcomes and shorter surgical times, as per a single-centric retrospective cohort analysis from the USA.[7]
- The en bloc technique for SLKT involves recovering both organs together and connecting the donor renal artery to the splenic artery, allowing for simultaneous reperfusion. This approach is particularly beneficial for recipients with extensive iliac artery disease, morbid obesity, or those with renal failure driving a high MELD score. A comparison of en bloc versus traditional SLKT showed that en bloc has shorter kidney ischemia and operative times, with similar graft survival and kidney function outcomes, making it a safe and feasible alternative.[8]
- In pediatric patients, the outcome of SLKT has been compared for the grafts taken from a deceased donor and a living donor (partial liver and kidney). The results were equivalent, highlighting that both can be safe and effective.[9]

RISKS AND COMPLICATIONS

The simultaneous implantation of both liver and kidney comes with its inherent challenges.

Graft Function Post-Simultaneous Liver–Kidney Transplant

The major issue of SLKT is delayed graft function (DGF) for transplanted kidney. The following parameters influence post-SLKT graft function following SLKT:[1]

- Hemodynamic status of patients post-SLKT
- Kidney donor profile index (KDPI) or kidney donor risk index (KDRI) of transplanted kidney for kidney allograft quality
- Cold ischemia time (CIT)
- Human leukocyte antigen (HLA)-matched and cross-matched negative kidney allografts
- Timing KT in SLKT
- MELD score for recipient
- Age of recipient. Some centers avoid SLKT for patients beyond 65 years
- Recipient hyperlipidemia
- Etiology of acute renal failure. Acute tubular necrosis (ATN) has a worse outcome than HRS[10]
- Pretransplant dialysis duration in AKI setting

Liver transplantation recipients are often sick and vasodilated. The presence of coagulopathy and portal hypertension increases the risk of bleeding during the transplant. The hemodynamic instability of recipients in immediate post-transplant is suboptimal for the newly implanted kidney allograft.

After liver engraftment, postreperfusion syndrome (PRS) leads to cytokine release and microcirculatory dysfunction, which further triggers kidney injury.

Elevated bilirubin levels in LT recipients can lead to bilirubin crystallization in the kidney tubules, raising the risk of acute kidney injury (AKI) and further renal dysfunction in the kidney allograft.

A retrospective single-center study analyzing the outcome of 145 patients requiring SLKT demonstrated a 20.7% incidence of renal allograft futility (RAF—patient death or need for renal replacement therapy at 3 months) among the cohort.[11]

Studies from the UNOS database of analysis of more than thirty thousand patients suggested that SLKT improved 1-year survival only in low MELD score (16–20) recipients with renal dysfunction, while it did not benefit survival in high MELD recipients.[12]

Ekser et al. described the "Indiana Approach" in SLKT, which involves delaying kidney graft implantation for 2–3 days after LT.[13] This technique was described in the deceased donor setting, where the kidney graft is preserved using a hypothermic pulsatile perfusion machine. A delayed KT allows for hemodynamic stabilization, coagulopathy correction, and varices decompression, and has been shown to improve kidney allograft outcomes, even with prolonged CITs greater than 48 hours.

A sequential KT with a different donor at a later date post-LT (KALT) is another approach adopted by many centers. However, we should remember that the requirement of post-transplant renal replacement therapy (RRT) is an independent risk factor for liver graft loss at 1 year. A single-center experience from a Korean institute revealed that in case of dual organ need, a living donor liver transplant (LDLT) followed by a KT either from a deceased donor or a living donor at a later date is a rising trend.[14] In some centers, sequential organ transplants have been shown to provide better outcomes compared to SLKTs.[15]

Lee et al. explored the "en bloc" SLKT as an alternative approach, where both the liver and the right kidney are procured together, with the renal vein attached to the inferior vena cava.[8] This technique allows a single incision for the LT and reduces CIT for the kidney, potentially shortening the overall operative time. However, the method has limitations: The use of the left kidney is challenging, and the right kidney with multiple arteries or a liver with aberrant arteries requires complicated reconstruction. Another concern is the risk of thrombosis or stenosis affecting both allografts. Despite these issues, the en bloc approach may be beneficial in centers without perfusion machines for delayed kidney transplantation or when different teams handle liver and KTs. Lee et al. reported a 23% delayed graft function (DGF) rate for both traditional and en bloc simultaneous transplants.

One promising technique is liver double kidney transplantation (LDKT), where both kidneys from the same donor are transplanted alongside the liver. This is particularly helpful in extended donor criteria kidneys for patients requiring SLKT. A case-control study involving four LDKT cases showed outcomes similar to 11 SLKT.[16] The decision to use a kidney for SLKT or LDKT was guided by the Remuzzi score from the donor kidney biopsy. However, with a mean MELD score of only 22 in this study, more data is needed, particularly for patients with higher MELD scores, before this approach can be recommended as standard practice.

Immunological Aspects of Simultaneous Liver–Kidney Transplant

In general, LT in SLKT provides immune protection to kidney grafts, reducing the incidence of acute rejection and improving kidney allograft survival, especially in the presence of preformed donor-specific anti-HLA antibodies. The proposed mechanisms of these immune protections are like the adsorption of preformed donor-specific antibody (DSA) by Kupffer cells and the production of soluble HLA class I antigens that neutralize DSA and cytotoxic T-lymphocytes.

The choice of induction therapy and maintenance immunosuppressive regimens for SLKT is a subject of ongoing debate, mainly due to the increased antigen load from both organs. A study by AbdulRahim et al. analyzed data from the UNOS database and found that rabbit antithymocyte globulin (r-ATG) induction increased mortality risk compared to no induction in SLKT recipients.[17] However, Ekser et al. reported favorable outcomes in their cohort using r-ATG.[18] The choice of induction therapy with interleukin-2 receptor antagonists or r-ATG or induction only with steroids depends on the institution protocol. Recent studies suggest that SLKT recipients experience lower rates of both T-cell-mediated and antibody-mediated kidney rejection compared to KT alone patients, likely due to the protective effect of the liver allograft. Taner et al. further demonstrated that SLKT helps reduce inflammation and T-cell activation in kidney biopsies, especially in cross-match positive recipients.[19] Another study indicated that delaying kidney transplantation for 2–3 days after LT in cross-match positive SLKTs led to a reduction in DSAs, likely because the liver absorbs these antibodies before the kidney transplant, improving clinical outcomes. Overall, SLKT appears to offer immunological advantages for kidney allografts, including reduced rejection and lower DSA levels.

OUTCOMES

Simultaneous liver–kidney transplant had poor outcomes, with a 20–30% mortality rate in the 1st year in the pre-MELD era. However, the outcome improved significantly in subsequent years as allocation policy had become streamlined and surgical and immunosuppressant strategies improved. While it is a complex procedure, many patients experience significant improvements in quality of life, as well as better survival rates compared to patients who undergo single organ transplants in cases of combined liver and kidney failure.

Multiple analyses of national US transplant registry data and single-center studies have reported 5-year patient survival rates after SLKT ranging from 64 to 76%.[4]

In the United States, the UNOS and other organizations use specific criteria to determine the allocation of organs for these types of transplants, ensuring that those most in need receive appropriate care.

United States SLKT study (US-SLKT) retrospectively analyzed data of 572 SLKT recipients across six US centers from 2002 to 2017.[20] The study found a significant improvement in 1-year survival from 89% in 2002 to 96% in 2017. Key factors influencing 1-year survival included hemodialysis at listing and delayed kidney function, while overall mortality was driven by factors such as acute kidney dysfunction, body mass index (BMI), and donor quality.

CONCLUSION

Simultaneous liver–kidney transplantation has greatly benefited patients with dual-organ disease. Over the past two decades, both the total number of SLKTs and the proportion of SLKT recipients among LT patients have steadily increased. The decision to pursue SLKT in patients with liver failure and kidney dysfunction requires careful evaluation of kidney dysfunction's acuity and reversibility, with input from a multidisciplinary team of specialists. The transplanted liver, in general, provides some immunological protection to the new kidney graft. However, delayed kidney graft function and 1-year graft loss remain the main concern to date in the entire process. Careful patient selection and technique and timing of the transplant are the most important factors in the overall outcome.

REFERENCES

1. Ekser B, Contreras AG, Andraus W, Taner T. Current status of combined liver-kidney transplantation. Int J Surg. 2020;82:149-54.
2. Margreiter R, Kramar R, Huber C, Steiner E, Niederwieser D, Judmaier G, et al. Combined liver and kidney transplantation. Lancet. 1984;323:1077-8.
3. Nagai S, Safwan M, Collins K, Schilke RE, Rizzari M, Moonka D, et al. Liver alone or simultaneous liver-kidney transplant? Pretransplant chronic kidney disease and post-transplant outcome - a retrospective study. Transpl Int. 2018;31:1028-40.
4. Prudhomme T, Mesnard B, Branchereau J, Roumiguié M, Maulat C, Muscari F, et al. Simultaneous liver-kidney transplantation: future perspective. World J Urol. 2024;42:489.
5. Cheng XS, McElroy LM, Sanoff SL, Kwong AJ. One size does not fit all: Differential benefits of simultaneous liver-kidney transplantation by eligibility criteria. Liver Transpl. 2023;29:1208-15.
6. Formica RN, Aeder M, Boyle G, Kucheryavaya A, Stewart D, Hirose R, et al. Simultaneous Liver–Kidney Allocation Policy: A Proposal to Optimize Appropriate Utilization of Scarce Resources. Am J Transplant. 2016;16:758-66.
7. Imai D, Sambommatsu Y, Sharma A, Kumaran V, Cotterell AH, Khan AA, et al. Single incision simultaneous liver kidney transplantation: Feasibility and outcomes. Clin Transplant. 2023;37(1):e14849.
8. Lee TC, Cortez AR, Kassam AF, Morris MC, Winer LK, Silski LS, et al. Outcomes of en bloc simultaneous liver-kidney transplantation compared to the traditional technique. Am J Transplant. 2020;20:1181-7.
9. Gautier S, Monakhov A, Tsiroulnikova O, Voskanov M, Miloserdov I, Dzhanbekov T, et al. Deceased vs living donor grafts for pediatric simultaneous liver-kidney transplantation: A single-center experience. J Clin Lab Anal. 2020;34:e23219.
10. Nadim MK, Genyk YS, Tokin C, Fieber J, Ananthapanyasut W, Ye W, et al. Impact of the etiology of acute kidney injury on outcomes following liver transplantation: acute tubular necrosis versus hepatorenal syndrome. Liver Transpl. 2012;18:539-48.
11. Lunsford KE, Bodzin AS, Markovic D, Zarrinpar A, Kaldas FM, Gritsch HA, et al. Avoiding Futility in Simultaneous Liver-kidney Transplantation: Analysis of 331 Consecutive Patients Listed for Dual Organ Replacement. Ann Surg. 2017;265:1016-24.
12. Habib S, Habib S, Khan K, Meister E, Rana A, Boyer T. Differential Simultaneous Liver and Kidney Transplant Benefit Based on Severity of Liver Damage at the Time of Transplantation. Gastroenterol Res. 2017;10:106-15.
13. Ekser B, Mangus RS, Fridell W, Kubal CA, Nagai S, Kinsella SB, et al. A Novel Approach in Combined Liver and Kidney Transplantation with Long-term Outcomes. Ann Surg. 2017;265:1000-8.
14. Kim M, Hwang S, Ahn CS, Moon DB, Ha TY, Song GW, et al. Simultaneous liver-kidney transplantation: A single-center experience in Korea. Ann Hepatobiliary Pancreat Surg. 2020;24:454-9.
15. Xiang J, Chen Z, Xu F, Mei S, Li Z, Zhou J, et al. Outcomes of liver-kidney transplantation in patients with primary hyperoxaluria: An analysis of the scientific registry of transplant recipients database. BMC Gastroenterol. 2020;20:208.
16. Di Laudo M, Ravaioli M, La Manna G, Comai G, Cescon M, Del Gaudio M, et al. Combined liver–dual kidney transplant: Role in expanded donors. Liver Transplant. 2017;23:28-34.
17. AbdulRahim N, Anderson L, Kotla S, Liu H, Ariyamuthu VK, Ghanta M, et al. Lack of Benefit and Potential Harm of Induction Therapy in Simultaneous Liver-Kidney Transplants. Liver Transplant. 2019;25:411-24.
18. Ekser B, Kubal CA, Fridell JA, Sharfuddin AA, Taber TE, Lacerda MA, et al. Lack of Benefit and Potential Harm of Induction Therapy in Simultaneous Liver-Kidney Transplants. Liver Transplant. 2019;25:667-8.
19. Taner T, Heimbach JK, Rosen CB, Nyberg SL, Park WD, Stegall MD. Decreased chronic cellular and antibody-mediated injury in the kidney following simultaneous liver-kidney transplantation. Kidney Int. 2016;89:909-17.
20. Cullaro G, Sharma P, Jo J, Rassiwala J, VanWagner LB, Wong R, et al. Temporal Trends and Evolving Outcomes After Simultaneous Liver-Kidney Transplantation: Results from the US SLKT Consortium. Liver Transpl. 2021;27:1613-22.

SECTION 2

Kidney, Pancreas and Small Bowel Transplant

CHAPTER 1

Indications of Kidney Transplantation and Pretransplant Optimization of Recipients Before Transplant

Puneet Bhuwania

INTRODUCTION

Kidney transplantation is the preferred renal replacement therapy for eligible patients with end-stage kidney disease (ESKD), offering superior outcomes in patient survival, quality of life, and cost-effectiveness compared to long-term dialysis.[1] However, the decision to pursue transplantation and the process of preparing a potential recipient involve a complex interplay of medical, psychological, and social factors. This chapter addresses the key clinical considerations in determining transplant candidacy and the essential steps in optimizing potential recipients for successful transplantation.

INDICATIONS FOR KIDNEY TRANSPLANTATION

Primary Indication

End-stage kidney disease, defined as irreversible kidney failure requiring renal replacement therapy, is the primary indication for kidney transplantation. Common etiologies include the following:

- *Diabetic nephropathy:* It is the leading cause of ESKD all around the globe.
- *Hypertensive nephrosclerosis:* It is often associated with long-standing, poorly controlled hypertension.
- Glomerulonephritis
- Polycystic-kidney disease
- Chronic pyelonephritis
- Congenital anomalies of the kidney and urinary tract (CAKUT)[2]

Timing of Transplantation

The optimal timing for kidney transplantation has been a subject of ongoing research and debate.

- *Pre-emptive transplantation:* It is considered when estimated glomerular filtration rate (eGFR) falls below 20 mL/min/1.73 m^2 and there is evidence of progressive and irreversible kidney disease. It is associated with improved graft and patient survival compared to postdialysis transplantation.[3]
- *Early versus late transplantation:*
    - Early transplantation is associated with better outcomes.
    - If dialysis is done before transplantation, it increases the risk of graft failure by 6% and death by 21% post-transplantation each year.[4]

Special Populations

- *Pediatric patients:*
    - Strong candidates due to impact on growth and development
    - Associated with improved cognitive development and quality of life.[5]
- *Elderly patients:*
    - No absolute age cutoff; evaluate based on physiological rather than chronological age.
    - Consider comorbidities and frailty index.[6]
- *Diabetic patients:*
    - May benefit from combined kidney–pancreas transplantation
    - Evaluate for macro- and microvascular complications.[7]

Contraindications

Although ESKD is the primary indication for transplantation, certain conditions may temporarily or permanently contraindicate transplantation.

- *Absolute:*
    - *Active malignancy:* Generally, a cancer-free interval of 2–5 years is recommended, depending on the type and stage of cancer.
    - Severe and irreversible extrarenal disease with limited life expectancy
    - Uncontrolled psychiatric illness interfering with adherence

- *Relative:*
  - Active substance abuse
  - Recurrent nonadherence to medical therapy
  - Lack of adequate social support[8]

PRETRANSPLANT EVALUATION

Once a patient is considered for kidney transplantation, a comprehensive evaluation is necessary to ensure the best possible outcomes. This evaluation typically includes the following:

Comprehensive Medical Assessment

- *Detailed history and physical examination:* A thorough review of the patient's medical history, including the cause of ESKD, comorbidities, prior surgeries, and medication use, is essential. A comprehensive physical examination helps identify any undiagnosed conditions that could affect transplant outcomes.
- *Laboratory testing:* Extensive laboratory testing is performed, including:
  - Blood grouping and human leukocyte antigen (HLA) typing b. Panel-reactive antibody (PRA) testing
  - Comprehensive metabolic panel
  - Complete blood count
  - Coagulation studies
  - Infectious disease screening [e.g., human immunodeficiency virus (HIV), hepatitis B and C, cytomegalovirus (CMV), Epstein–Barr virus (EBV)]
  - Age-appropriate cancer screening[9]

Cardiovascular Evaluation

Cardiovascular disease is the leading cause of morbidity and mortality in transplant recipients. Therefore, a thorough cardiac evaluation is crucial, which may include:

- Electrocardiogram (ECG)
- Echocardiogram
- Stress testing (e.g., myocardial perfusion imaging, stress echocardiography)
- *Coronary angiography in high-risk patients*

Note: The 2012 American Heart Association/American College of Cardiology Foundation scientific statement recommends noninvasive stress testing for all kidney transplant candidates with no active cardiac conditions.[10]

Additional Evaluations

Additional evaluations include the following:

- *Pulmonary:* Chest X-ray and pulmonary function tests
- *Gastrointestinal:* Risk and age-appropriate colorectal cancer screening
- *Urological:* Assessment of lower urinary tract anatomy and function
- *Psychosocial:* Evaluation of mental health, social support, and adherence potential[11]

PRETRANSPLANT OPTIMIZATION

Following the initial evaluation, several steps are taken to optimize the recipient's condition before transplantation.

Cardiovascular Risk Reduction

- *Blood pressure control:*
  - *Target*: <130/80 mm Hg as per Kidney Disease: Improving Global Outcomes (KDIGO) 2021 guidelines[12]
  - Consider renin-angiotensin system (RAS) blockade in proteinuric chronic kidney disease (CKD).
- *Lipid management:*
  - Statins are recommended for most transplant candidates.
  - Target low-density lipoprotein cholesterol (LDL-C) <100 mg/dL.[13]
- *Smoking cessation:*
  - Implement structured cessation programs.
  - Consider pharmacotherapy (e.g., bupropion).[14]
- *Weight management:*
  - Target body mass index (BMI) <30 kg/m^2 as it is associated with increased post-transplant complications.
  - Consider bariatric surgery for morbidly obese candidates (BMI >35 kg/m^2).[15]

Infection Prevention and Management

- *Vaccination:*
  - Administer age-appropriate vaccinations pretransplant.
  - Provide key vaccines like influenza, pneumococcal, hepatitis B, human papillomavirus for eligible candidates.[16]
- *Latent infections:*
  - Screen and treat latent tuberculosis.
  - Consider prophylaxis for pneumocystis pneumonia (PCP) in high-risk candidates.[17]

Diabetes Management

- Individualize glycated hemoglobin (HbA1c) targets based on patient factors.
- Generally, aim for HbA1c <7.5–8.0% in ESKD patients.
- Consider continuous glucose monitoring for brittle diabetics.[18]

Mineral and Bone Disorder Management

- *Control secondary hyperparathyroidism:* Target parathyroid hormone (PTH): The range should be two to nine times the upper limit of normal.
- *Optimize vitamin D status:* Correct 25-hydroxyvitamin D deficiency.
- Manage serum phosphate and calcium levels.[19]

Anemia Management

- *Target hemoglobin:* 9–11 g/dL
- Use erythropoiesis-stimulating agents and iron supplementation as needed.
- Investigate and treat other causes of anemia [e.g., occult gastrointestinal (GI) bleeding].[20]

Nutrition Optimization

- *Protein intake:* 1.2 g/kg/day for dialysis patients
- Manage electrolyte imbalances (potassium and phosphate).
- Ensure adequate calorie intake.
- *Consider dietitian consultation for individualized nutrition plans.*[21]

Psychosocial Support

- Treat depression, anxiety, or other psychiatric conditions.
- Provide substance abuse treatment when indicated.
- Assess and bolster social support systems.
- Implement comprehensive transplant education programs.[22]

Immunological Risk Assessment and Management

- *Human leukocyte antigen antibody assessment:* Identify and characterize anti-HLA antibodies.
- *Desensitization:*
  - Consider for highly sensitized patients.
  - Protocols may include plasmapheresis, intravenous immunoglobulin (IVIG), Rituximab, or Bortezomib.[23]

Dental Evaluation

Comprehensive dental evaluation and treatment of any active oral infection are recommended to reduce the risk of post-transplant infections.[24]

Dialysis Optimization

For patients on dialysis, ensuring adequate dialysis is crucial. This includes:

- Adequate dialysis dose (Kt/V >1.2 for hemodialysis and weekly Kt/V >1.7 for peritoneal dialysis)
- Appropriate dry weight management.
- Vascular access care in hemodialysis patients[25]

SPECIAL CONSIDERATIONS

Pediatric Recipients

Children require special considerations in pretransplant optimization:

- Optimize growth and development.
- Complete age-appropriate vaccinations.
- Provide family education and support.
- Address transition of care for adolescents.[26]

Elderly Recipients

Older transplant candidates may require:

- Conducting frailty assessments (e.g., fried frailty phenotype, short physical performance battery)
- Evaluation of cognitive function
- Considering acceptance of extended criteria donor kidneys[27]

Highly Sensitized Patients

Patients with high levels of anti-HLA antibodies may benefit from:

- Enrolment in kidney paired donation programs
- Implementing desensitization protocols
- Consideration of acceptable mismatch programs[28]

Recurrent Disease Risk

For patients with primary kidney diseases at high risk of recurrence post-transplant:

- Counsel patients with high-risk diseases [e.g., focal segmental glomerulosclerosis (FSGS), atypical hemolytic uremic syndrome (aHUS)] about recurrence risk.
- Develop tailored management plans (e.g., pre-emptive plasma exchange for FSGS).[29]

EMERGING TRENDS AND FUTURE DIRECTIONS

Biomarkers for Transplant Readiness

Research is ongoing to identify biomarkers that could predict transplant outcomes and help in the selection and optimization of recipients. These include markers of immune activation, inflammation, and allograft injury.

Novel Desensitization Protocols

For highly sensitized patients, new approaches to desensitization are being developed, including the use of complement inhibitors and proteasome inhibitors.

Personalized Immunosuppression

Advances in pharmacogenomics and immune monitoring may allow for more tailored immunosuppression regimens, potentially improving outcomes and reducing side effects.

Artificial Intelligence in Recipient Selection

Machine learning algorithms are being developed to assist in the complex decision-making process of recipient selection and donor–recipient matching.

Xenotransplantation Research[30-32]

While still in the experimental stage, xenotransplantation (transplantation of organs from other species, typically pigs) could potentially address organ shortage in the future.

CONCLUSION

Kidney transplantation offers the best outcomes for most patients with ESKD. However, the success of transplantation relies heavily on proper recipient selection and thorough pretransplant optimization. The evaluation and preparation process is complex and multidisciplinary, requiring close collaboration among nephrologists, transplant surgeons, cardiologists, infectious disease specialists, psychiatrists, and other healthcare professionals.

The goal of pretransplant optimization is to ensure that recipients are in the best possible physical and psychological condition at the time of transplantation. This not only improves the chances of a successful transplant but also enhances the recipient's ability to manage the complex care regimen required post-transplantation.

As the field of transplantation continues to evolve, new strategies for expanding access to transplantation and improving outcomes are being developed. These include novel desensitization protocols, expanded criteria donor programs, and advances in immunosuppression. However, the fundamental principles of careful recipient selection and comprehensive pretransplant optimization remain crucial to achieving optimal outcomes in kidney transplantation.

REFERENCES

1. Wolfe RA, Ashby VB, Milford EL, Ojo AO, Ettengar RE, Agodoa LY, et al. Comparison of mortality in all patients on dialysis, patients on dialysis awaiting transplantation, and recipients of a first cadaveric transplant. N Engl. J Med. 1999;341(23):1725-30
2. United States Renal Data System. (2020). USRDS Annual Data Report. [online] USRDS website. Available from https://usrds-adr.niddk.nih.gov/2020. [Last accessed May, 2025].
3. Kasiske BL, Snyder JJ, Matas AJ, Ellison MD, Gill JS, Kausz AT. Preemptive kidney transplantation: the advantage and the advantaged. Journal of the American Society of Nephrology. 2002;13(5):1358-64.
4. Meier-Kriesche HU, Port FK, Ojo AO, Rudich SM, Hanson JA, Cibrik DM, et al. Effect of waiting time on renal transplant outcome. Kidney Int. 2000;58(3):1311-7.
5. Harambat J, van Stralen KJ, Kim JJ, Tizard EJ. Epidemiology of chronic kidney disease in children. Pediatric nephrology. 2012;27:363-73.
6. Knoll GA. Kidney transplantation in the older adult. Am J Kidney Dis. 2013;61(5):790-7.
7. Dean PG, Lund WJ, Larson TS, Prieto M, Nyberg SL, Ishitani MB, et al. Wound-healing complications after kidney transplantation: a prospective, randomized comparison of sirolimus and mycophenolate mofetil. Am J Transplant. 2008;8(11):2277-88.
8. Scandling JD, Busque S, Dejbakhsh-Jones S, Benike C, Sarwal M, Millan MT, et al. Tolerance and withdrawal of immunosuppressive drugs in patients given kidney and hematopoietic cell transplants. American Journal of Transplantation. 2012;12(5):1133-45.
9. Kasiske BL, Zeier MG, Chapman JR, Craig JC, Ekberg H, Garvey CA, et al. KDIGO clinical practice guideline for the care of kidney transplant recipients: a summary. Kidney international. 2010;77(4):299-311.
10. Lentine KL, Costa SP, Weir MR, Robb JF, Fleisher LA, Kasiske BL, et al. Cardiac disease evaluation and management among kidney and liver transplantation candidates: a scientific statement from the American Heart Association and the American College of Cardiology Foundation. J Am Coll Cardiol. 2012;60(5):434-80.

11. Bunnapradist S, Danovitch GM. Evaluation of adult kidney transplant candidates. Am J Kidney Dis. 2007;50(5):890-8.
12. Kidney Disease: Improving Global Outcomes KDIGO Transplant Work Group. KDIGO 2021 Clinical Practice Guideline for the Management of Blood Pressure in Chronic Kidney Disease. Kidney Int. 2021;99(3S):S1-87.
13. Holdaas H, Fellström B, Cole E, Nyberg G, Olsson AG, TR Pedersen, et al. Long-term cardiac outcomes in renal transplant recipients receiving fluvastatin: the ALERT extension study. Am J Transplant. 2005;5(12): 2929-36.
14. Nogueira JM, Haririan A, Jacobs SC, Cooper M, Weir MR. Hepatitis C virus infection in kidney transplantation: risk factors, impact, and management. Am J Transplant. 2010;10(10):2252-7.
15. Gore JL, Danovitch GM, Litwin MS, Pham PT, Singer JS. Disparities in the utilization of live donor renal transplantation. Am J Transplant. 2006;6(8):1932-9.
16. Danziger-Isakov L, Kumar D, Vaccination in solid organ transplantation. Am J Transplant. 2013;13(Suppl 4):S311-7.
17. Subramanian AK, Juliar BE, Becker YT, Sudan DL. Kidney transplantation in HIV-infected recipients: a prospective, multicenter study from the HIV Transplant Study Group. Am J Transplant. 2019;19(8):2262-77.
18. Sharif A, Hecking M, de Vries AP, Porrini E, Hornum M, Rasoul-Rockenschaub S, et al. Proceedings from an international consensus meeting on posttransplantation diabetes mellitus: recommendations and future directions. Diabetes Care. 2014;37(8):2440-6.
19. Kidney Disease: Improving Global Outcomes (KDIGO) CKD-MBD Update Work Group. KDIGO 2017 Clinical Practice Guideline Update for the Diagnosis, Evaluation, Prevention, and Treatment of Chronic Kidney Disease-Mineral and Bone Disorder (CKD-MBD). Kidney Int Suppl. 2017;7(1):1-59.
20. Kidney Disease: Improving Global Outcomes (KDIGO) Anemia Work Group. KDIGO Clinical Practice Guideline for Anemia in Chronic Kidney Disease. Kidney Int Suppl. 2012;2(4):279-335.
21. Ikizler TA, Burrowes JD, Byham-Gray LD, Campbell KL, Carrero JJ, Chan W, et al. Kidney Disease Outcomes Quality Initiative (KDOQI) Clinical Practice Guideline for Nutrition in CKD: 2020 Update. Am J Kidney Dis. 2020;76(3):S1-107.
22. Maldonado JR, Dubois HC, David EE, Sher Y, Lolak S, Dhabhar FS, et al. The Stanford Integrated Psychosocial Assessment for Transplantation (SIPAT): a new tool for the psychosocial evaluation of pre-transplant candidates. Psychosomatics. 2012;53(2):123-31.
23. Jordan SC, Vo AA, Kim IK, Wu P, Toyoda M, Shin B-H, et al. Intravenous immune globulin (IVIG): a multi-targeted biologic for inflammation, autoimmunity and transplantation. N Engl J Med. 2011;365(4):318-26.
24. Guggenheimer J, Moore PA, Rossie K, Myers D, Mongelluzzo MB, Block HM, et al. Insufficient training in oral health care in medical curricula. Oral Surg Oral Med Oral Pathol Oral Radiol Endod. 2007;103(5):587-92.
25. National Kidney Foundation. Clinical practice guidelines for hemodialysis adequacy, update 2006. Am J Kidney Dis. 2006;48(Suppl 1):S2-90.
26. Goldstein SL, Graham N, Burwinkle T, Warady B, Seikaly M, McKenna M, et al. Health-related quality of life in pediatric patients with ESRD. Pediatr Transplant. 2007;11(4):422-7.
27. Pondrom S. News and issues that affect organ and tissue transplantation. Am J Transplant. 2009;9(1):1-2.
28. Vo AA, Lukovsky M, Toyoda M, Wang J, Reinsmoen NL, Lai CH, et al. Rituximab and intravenous immune globulin for desensitization during renal transplantation. N Engl J Med. 2008;359(3):242-51.
29. Djamali A, Kaufman DB, Ellis TM, Zhong W, Matas A, Samaniego M, et al. Am J Transplant. 2014;14(2):255-71.
30. Roedder S, Sigdel T, Salomonis N, Hsieh SC, Dai H, Bestard O, et al. The kSORT assay to detect renal transplant patients at high risk for acute rejection: results of the multicenter AART study. Am J Transplant. 2014;14(5): 1179-89.
31. Loupy A, Lefaucheur C, Vernerey D, Prugger C, van Huyen JPD, Mooney N, et al. Antibody-mediated rejection and the clinical value of kidney allograft histology. N Engl J Med. 2020;383(13):1266-76.
32. Cooper DKC, Ekser B, Ramsoondar J, Phelps C, Ayares D. The role of genetically engineered pigs in xenotransplantation research. Lancet. 2017;389(10070):702-10.

CHAPTER 2

Donor Selection in Kidney Transplant: Cadaver and Living Donor Setting

Puneet Bhuwania

INTRODUCTION

Kidney transplantation is the preferred treatment for patients with end-stage renal disease (ESRD), offering improved quality of life and longevity compared to dialysis.[1] A critical factor in the success of kidney transplantation is the careful selection of suitable donors. This chapter explores the processes and considerations involved in donor selection for both cadaveric and living donor kidney transplants.

The selection of appropriate kidney donors is a complex process that involves medical, ethical, and psychosocial considerations. The primary goal is to ensure the best possible outcomes for both the recipient and, in the case of living donation, the donor. This chapter will delve into the specifics of donor selection in both cadaveric and living donor settings, highlighting the key differences and unique challenges associated with each.

CADAVERIC DONOR SELECTION

Cadaveric donor kidneys, also known as deceased-donor kidneys, come from individuals who have been declared brain dead or have died from circulatory death. The process of selecting and allocating these organs **(Flowchart 1)** is highly regulated and follows strict protocols.[2]

Types of Cadaveric Donors

- *Donation after brain death (DBD):* These donors have suffered irreversible loss of brain function but are maintained on mechanical ventilation to preserve organ function until procurement.[3]
- *Donation after circulatory death (DCD):* These donors have experienced irreversible cessation of circulatory and respiratory functions. DCD kidneys may have a higher risk of delayed graft function but can still provide excellent long-term outcomes.[4]

Initial Donor Screening

The initial screening of potential cadaveric donors involves a thorough review of medical history, physical examination, and laboratory tests. Key factors considered include the following:

- *Age:* While there is no absolute upper age limit, donors over 60 years old are generally considered expanded criteria donors (ECDs).[5]
- *Medical history:* Presence of hypertension, diabetes, or other chronic diseases that may affect kidney function[6]
- *Cause of death:* Certain causes, such as cerebrovascular accidents, may be associated with better kidney quality than others, like prolonged cardiac arrest.[7]
- *Kidney function:* Assessment of serum creatinine, estimated glomerular filtration rate (eGFR), and urine output[8]
- *Infectious disease screening:* Testing for human immunodeficiency virus (HIV), hepatitis B and C, cytomegalovirus (CMV), Epstein–Barr virus (EBV), and other relevant pathogens[9]
- *Malignancy screening:* Careful evaluation to rule out active or recent malignancies that could be transmitted to the recipient[10]

Expanded Criteria Donors

To increase the donor pool, many transplant centers now accept kidneys from ECDs. These include donors:

- Aged 60 years or older
- Aged 50–59 years with at least two of the following: Hypertension, serum creatinine >1.5 mg/dL, or death from cerebrovascular accident[2]

While ECD kidneys may have a higher risk of graft failure compared to standard criteria donor kidneys, they can still provide significant survival benefit for certain recipients, particularly older patients or those with long waiting times.[11]

Flowchart 1: Selection of standard and extended criteria donor in deceased donation.

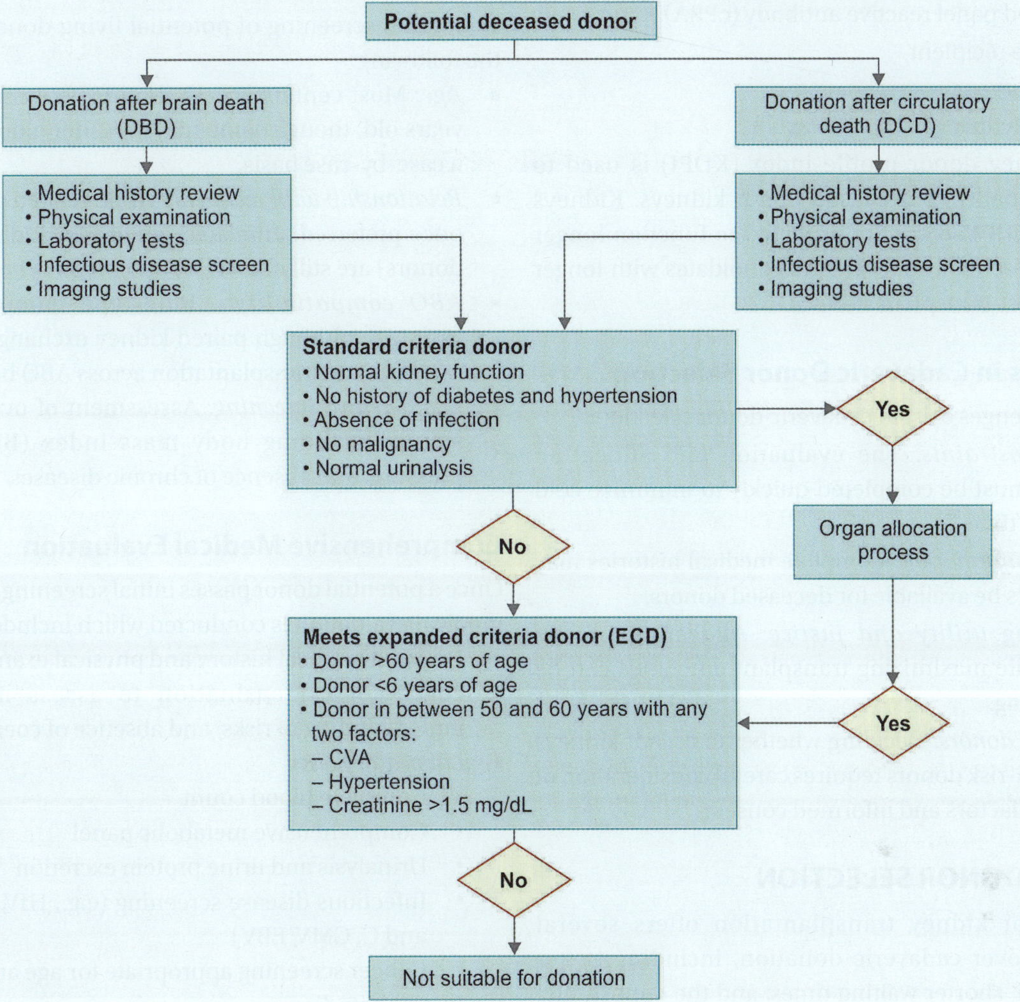

Kidney Biopsy

For donors with risk factors or borderline function, a pretransplant kidney biopsy may be performed to assess organ quality. The biopsy can provide valuable information about glomerulosclerosis, tubular atrophy, interstitial fibrosis, and vascular changes.[12]

Contraindications to Deceased Donor Kidney Donation

- *Absolute contraindications include:*
  - Active malignancy (except for select primary brain tumors)
  - Uncontrolled sepsis
  - HIV infection (in most cases)
  - Prion diseases
- *Relative contraindications include:*
  - Chronic kidney disease
  - Severe atherosclerosis
  - History of treated malignancy
  - Hepatitis B or C infection (may be considered for hepatitis-positive recipients)

Allocation Systems

The allocation of cadaveric kidneys varies with country and region. In the United States, the United Network for Organ Sharing (UNOS) manages the allocation system, while in India, the National Organ and Tissue Transplant Organisation (NOTTO) is the main governing body which has set up a state-wise allocation authority, e.g., zonal transplant coordination center (ZTCC) in Maharashtra. The following factors are considered before organ allocation in a deceased donor-setting:

- Blood-type compatibility
- Human leukocyte antigen (HLA) matching

- Time on the waiting list
- Calculated panel reactive antibody (cPRA)
- Age of the recipient
- Medical urgency
- Pediatric status[13]

The kidney donor profile index (KDPI) is used to assess the quality of deceased donor kidneys. Kidneys with lower KDPI scores are expected to function longer and are preferentially allocated to candidates with longer estimated post-transplant survival.[14]

Challenges in Cadaveric Donor Selection

Several challenges exist in cadaveric donor selection:

- *Time constraints:* The evaluation and allocation process must be completed quickly to minimize cold ischemia time.[15]
- *Limited information:* Complete medical histories may not always be available for deceased donors.
- *Balancing utility and justice:* Allocating organs fairly while maximizing transplant outcomes can be challenging.
- *Marginal donors:* Deciding whether to accept kidneys from high-risk donors requires careful consideration of recipient factors and informed consent.[16]

LIVING DONOR SELECTION

Living donor kidney transplantation offers several advantages over cadaveric donation, including better graft survival, shorter waiting times, and the opportunity for pre-emptive transplantation.[17] However, the selection process for living donors is more complex due to the need to ensure the long-term health and safety of the donor.

Types of Living Kidney Donors

- *Related donors:*
  - First-degree relatives (parents, siblings, children, spouses)
  - Second-degree relatives (grandparents, aunts/uncles, nieces/nephews)
- *Unrelated donors (not approved in India):*
  - Emotionally related (friends)
  - Altruistic (nondirected) donors
- *Paired kidney exchange:* This involves two or more donor–recipient pairs who are incompatible with each other but can "swap" donors to achieve compatible transplants.

Initial Screening

The initial screening of potential living donors includes the following:

- *Age:* Most centers accept donors between 18 and 65 years old, though some may consider older donors on a case-by-case basis.
- *Relationship with recipient:* While related donors were once preferred, unrelated donors (including altruistic donors) are still not widely accepted.
- *ABO compatibility:* Blood-type compatibility is essential, although paired kidney exchange programs can facilitate transplantation across ABO barriers.
- *Basic health screening:* Assessment of overall health status, including body mass index (BMI), blood pressure, and absence of chronic diseases.

Comprehensive Medical Evaluation

Once a potential donor passes initial screening, a thorough medical evaluation is conducted which includes:

- Detailed medical history and physical examination
- Psychological evaluation to assess motivation, understanding of risks, and absence of coercion[18]
- *Laboratory tests:*
  - Complete blood count
  - Comprehensive metabolic panel
  - Urinalysis and urine protein excretion
  - Infectious disease screening (e.g., HIV, hepatitis B and C, CMV, EBV)
  - Cancer screening appropriate for age and gender[19]
- *Imaging studies:*
  - Computed tomography (CT) or magnetic resonance (MR) angiography to assess renal anatomy
  - Renal ultrasound
  - Chest X-ray
- *Cardiovascular evaluation:*
  - Electrocardiogram (ECG)
  - Stress test for older donors or those with risk factors[20]
- *Glomerular filtration rate (GFR) measurement:*
  - 24-hour urine collection for creatinine clearance
  - Nuclear medicine GFR study [e.g., diethylenetriaminepentaacetic acid (DTPA) clearance]

Contraindications to Living Kidney Donation

- *Absolute contraindications include:*
  - Chronic kidney disease (GFR <60 mL/min/1.73 m^2)
  - Uncontrolled hypertension

- Diabetes mellitus
- Significant cardiovascular disease
- Active malignancy
- Chronic infections (HIV, hepatitis B or C)
- Psychiatric conditions that impair decision-making capacity

- *Relative contraindications include:*
  - Obesity (BMI >35 kg/m^2)
  - Kidney stones
  - Family history of kidney disease
  - Mild, controlled hypertension
  - Impaired glucose tolerance

Specific Considerations in Living Donor Evaluation

- *Kidney function:* Donors should have normal kidney function, typically defined as a GFR ≥80 mL/min/1.73 m^2. Some centers may accept donors with GFR ≥60 mL/min/1.73 m^2 if other factors are favorable.[21]
- *Proteinuria:* Significant proteinuria (>500 mg/day) is generally a contraindication to donation.[22]
- *Hypertension:* Well-controlled hypertension in older donors may be acceptable, but uncontrolled or early-onset hypertension is usually a contraindication.[23]
- *Obesity:* While practices vary, many centers exclude donors with BMI >35 kg/m^2 due to increased surgical risks and long-term health concerns.[24]
- *Diabetes:* Diabetes is generally a contraindication to donation, although some centers may consider prediabetic donors with careful counseling.[25]
- *Familial kidney disease:* Careful evaluation is needed for donors with a family history of kidney disease, particularly those related to the recipient.[26]
- *Stone disease:* A history of kidney stones is not an absolute contraindication but requires careful evaluation and counseling.[27]
- *Psychosocial factors:* Assessment of the donor's support system, financial stability, and ability to comply with follow-up care is crucial.

Informed Consent

Obtaining informed consent is a critical part of the living donor evaluation process. Potential donors must be fully informed of:

- The risks of surgery and long-term risks of living with one kidney
- The expected outcomes for the recipient
- The voluntary nature of donation and the right to withdraw at any time
- Alternative treatment options for the recipient[28]

Ethical Considerations

Several ethical issues must be considered in living donor selection:

- *Autonomy:* Ensuring that the donor's decision is voluntary and free from coercion
- *Beneficence:* Weighing the potential benefits to the recipient against the risks to the donor
- *Nonmaleficence:* Minimizing harm to the donor while maximizing benefit to the recipient
- *Justice:* Ensuring fair access to living donation for all potential recipients

Special Situations in Living Donation

- *ABO-incompatible donation:* With advanced desensitization protocols, ABO-incompatible transplantation is now feasible, though it carries higher immunological risks.[29]
- *Paired-kidney exchange:* These programs allow incompatible donor–recipient pairs to be matched with other incompatible pairs, increasing access to living donor transplantation.[30]
- *Altruistic donation:* Nondirected donors require careful psychosocial evaluation to ensure appropriate motivations and expectations.[31]
- *Extended criteria living donors:* Some centers are expanding criteria for living donors (e.g., older age, controlled hypertension) to increase the donor pool, necessitating careful risk–benefit analysis.
- *HLA-sensitized recipients:* Patients with high levels of anti-HLA antibodies (high cPRA) face challenges in finding compatible donors. Strategies to facilitate transplantation in these patients include:
  - Desensitization protocols using plasmapheresis, intravenous immunoglobulin (IVIG), and Rituximab
  - Acceptable mismatch programs to identify donors against whom the recipient has no or low-level antibodies
  - Kidney paired donation to find compatible donors within a larger pool[32]
- *Elderly donors and recipients:* The increasing prevalence of ESRD in older adults has led to more consideration of elderly donors and recipients:
  - *Elderly living donors:* Careful evaluation is crucial, with particular attention to cardiovascular risk and

renal function. Some centers use an age cutoff (e.g., 70 years) for living donation, while others assess on a case-by-case basis.
  - *Elderly recipients:* Outcomes of kidney transplantation in carefully selected elderly recipients can be favorable. The use of ECD or older living donors may be appropriate in this population, balancing the reduced life expectancy of the recipient with the expected graft lifespan.[33]
- *Donor selection in pediatric-kidney transplantation:* Pediatric recipients have unique considerations in donor selection:
  - *Size matching:* The donor kidney should be appropriately sized for the recipient's body. Adult-sized kidneys may be used in children >20 kg, but special surgical techniques may be required.
  - *Living donors:* Parents are often potential donors, but long-term family dynamics and the potential need for retransplantation later in life should be considered.
  - *Immunological factors:* Children may have a more robust immune response, potentially affecting graft survival.[34]

CONCLUSION

Donor selection in kidney transplantation is a complex process that requires careful consideration of medical, surgical, ethical, and psychosocial factors. In the cadaveric donor setting, the focus is on maximizing the utility of a scarce resource while ensuring fair allocation. The evaluation process must be efficient to minimize cold ischemia time and optimize outcomes.

For living donors, the paramount concern is ensuring the long-term health and well-being of the donor while providing the best possible outcome for the recipient. The comprehensive evaluation process and informed consent are crucial to mitigate risks and ensure ethical practice.

As the demand for kidney transplants continues to outpace the supply of available organs, transplant programs face ongoing challenges in expanding the donor pool while maintaining excellent outcomes. Innovations such as expanded criteria donors, donation after circulatory death, and paired exchange programs have helped to increase access to transplantation. However, these advances also bring new complexities to the donor selection process.

Future directions in donor selection may include more sophisticated risk prediction models, incorporation of genomic data, and refinement of allocation algorithms to better match donor kidneys with recipients. Continued research and ethical discourse will be essential to navigate the evolving landscape of kidney transplantation and optimize outcomes for both donors and recipients.

REFERENCES

1. Wolfe RA, Ashby VB, Milford EL, Ojo AO, Ettenger RE, Agodoa LY, et al. Comparison of mortality in all patients on dialysis, patients on dialysis awaiting transplantation, and recipients of a first cadaveric transplant. N Engl J Med. 1999;341(23):1725-30.
2. Metzger RA, Delmonico FL, Feng S, Port FK, Wynn JJ, Merion RM. Expanded criteria donors for kidney transplantation. American Journal of Transplantation. 2003;3:114-25.
3. Wijdicks EF, Varelas PN, Gronseth GS, Greer DM. American Academy of Neurology. Evidence-based guideline update: determining brain death in adults: report of the Quality Standards Subcommittee of the American Academy of Neurology. Neurology. 2010;74(23):1911-8.
4. Incerti D, Summers N, Ton TG, Boscoe A, Chandraker A, Stevens W. The lifetime health burden of delayed graft function in kidney transplant recipients in the United States. MDM policy & practice. 2018;3(1):2381468318781811.
5. Rao PS, Ojo A. The alphabet soup of kidney transplantation: SCD, DCD, ECD—fundamentals for the practicing nephrologist. Clinical Journal of the American Society of Nephrology. 2009;4(11):1827-31.
6. Port FK, Bragg-Gresham JL, Metzger RA, Dykstra DM, Gillespie BW, Young EW, et al. Donor characteristics associated with reduced graft survival: an approach to expanding the pool of kidney donors. Transplantation. 2002;74(9):1281-6.
7. Miranda B, Fernandez-Yañez J, Gonzalez-Posada JM, Naya MT, Meneu-Diaz JC, Sopeña B, et al. Organ donation in Spain. Nephrol Dial Transplant. 2003;18(7):1266-73.
8. Giral M, Foucher Y, Karam G, Vanspauwen V, Daguin P, Abrahamians C, et al. Kidney and patient survival after kidney transplantation: a 10-year multicenter French cohort study. Kidney Int. 2005;67(1):349-57.
9. Fishman JA. Infection in solid-organ transplant recipients. N Engl J Med. 2007;357(25):2601-14.
10. Kauffman HM, McBride MA, Cherikh WS, Spain PC, Marks WH, Roza AM. Transplant tumor registry: donor related malignancies. Transplantation. 2002;74(3):358-62.
11. Merion RM, Ashby VB, Wolfe RA, Distant DA, Hulbert-Shearon TE, Metzger RA, et al. Deceased-donor characteristics and the survival benefit of kidney transplantation. Jama. 2005;294(21):2726-33.
12. Remuzzi G, Cravedi P, Perna A, Dimitrov BD, Turturro M, Locatelli G, et al. Dual Kidney Transplant Group. Long-term outcome of renal transplantation from older donors. N Engl J Med. 2006;354(4):343-52.

13. Organ Procurement and Transplantation Network. (2025). OPTN/UNOS Policy. [online] OPTN website. Available from https://optn.transplant.hrsa.gov/media/1200/optn_policies.pdf. [Last accessed May, 2025].
14. Rao PS, et al. Kidney donor profile index (KDPI): A tool for assessing deceased donor kidney quality. Am J Transplant. 2009;9(7):1567-79.
15. Russo MW, Galanko JA, Zacks SL, Beavers KL, Fried MW, Shrestha R. Impact of donor age and year of transplant on graft survival in liver transplant recipients with chronic hepatitis C. Am J Transplant. 2004;4(7):1133-8.
16. Reese PP, Harhay MN, Abt PL, Levine MH, Halpern SD. New solutions to reduce discard of kidneys donated for transplantation. Journal of the American Society of Nephrology. 2016;27(4):973-80.
17. Ojo AO, Hanson JA, Meier-Kriesche HU, Okechukwu CN, Wolfe RA, Leichtman AB, et al. J Am Soc Nephrol. 2001; 12(3):589-97.
18. Dew MA, DiMartini AF, Dabbs AD, Myaskovsky L, Steel J, Unruh M, et al. Rates and risk factors for nonadherence to the medical regimen after adult solid organ transplantation. Transplantation. 2007;83(7):858-73.
19. Mandelbrot DA, Pavlakis M, Danovitch GM, Johnson SR, Karp SJ, Khwaja K, Hanto DW, Rodrigue JR. The medical evaluation of living kidney donors: a survey of US transplant centers. American Journal of Transplantation. 2007;7(10):2333-43.
20. Sharma S, Elliott PM, Whyte G, Mahon N, Virdee MS, Mist B, et al. Utility of metabolic exercise testing in distinguishing hypertrophic cardiomyopathy from physiologic left ventricular hypertrophy in athletes. J Am Coll Cardiol. 2000;36(3):864-70.
21. Garg AX, Muirhead N, Knoll G, Yang RC, Prasad GV, Thiessen-Philbrook H, et al. Donor Nephrectomy Outcomes Research (DONOR) Network. Proteinuria and reduced kidney function in living kidney donors: a systematic review, meta-analysis, and meta-regression. Kidney international. 2006;70(10):1801-10.
22. Garg AX, Muirhead N, Knoll G, Yang RC, Prasad GV, Thiessen-Philbrook H, et al. Donor Nephrectomy Outcomes Research (DONOR) Network. Proteinuria and reduced kidney function in living kidney donors: A systematic review, meta-analysis, and meta-regression. Kidney Int. 2006;70(10):1801-10.
23. Boudville N, Prasad GV, Knoll G, Muirhead N, Thiessen-Philbrook H, Yang RC, et al. Ann Intern Med. 2006;145(3):185-96.
24. Reese PP, Harhay MN, Abt PL, Levine MH, Halpern SD. Selection and management of the older kidney donor. Am J Transplant. 2009;9(7):1564-6.
25. Ibrahim HN, Foley R, Tan L, Rogers T, Bailey RF, Guo H, et al. Long-term consequences of kidney donation. N Engl J Med. 2009;360(5):459-69.
26. Skrunes R, Tøndel C, Leh S, Larsen KK, Houge G, Davidsen ES, et al. Long-term dose-dependent agalsidase effects on kidney histology in Fabry disease. Clinical Journal of the American Society of Nephrology. 2017;12(9):1470-9.
27. Kasiske BL, Cangro CB, Hariharan S, Hricik DE, Kerman RH, Roth D, et al. The evaluation of renal transplantation candidates: clinical practice guidelines. American journal of transplantation: official journal of the American Society of Transplantation and the American Society of Transplant Surgeons. 2001;1:3-95.
28. Gordon EJ. Informed consent for living donation: a review of key empirical studies, ethical challenges and future research. American Journal of Transplantation. 2012;12(9):2273-80.
29. Montgomery RA, Lonze BE, King KE, Kraus ES, Kucirka LM, Locke JE, et al. Desensitization in HLA-incompatible kidney recipients and survival. N Engl J Med. 2011;365(4):318-26.
30. Segev DL, Gentry SE, Warren DS, Reeb B, Montgomery RA. Kidney paired donation and optimizing the use of live donor organs. JAMA. 2005;293(15):1883-90.
31. Jendrisak MD, Hong B, Shenoy S, Lowell J, Desai N, Chapman W, et al. Altruistic living donors: evaluation for nondirected kidney or liver donation. American Journal of Transplantation. 2006;6(1):115-20.
32. Tullius SG, et al. The influence of age on organ transplantation. Am J Transplant. 2013;13(8):1967-75.
33. Veroux M, Grosso G, Corona D, Mistretta A, Giaquinta A, Giuffrida G, et al. Age is an important predictor of kidney transplantation outcome. Nephrol Dial Transplant. 2012;27(4):1663-71.
34. Van Arendonk KJ, Boyarsky BJ, Orandi BJ, James NT, Smith JM, Colombani PM, et al. National trends over 25 years in pediatric kidney transplant outcomes. Pediatrics. 2014;133(4):594-601.

CHAPTER 3

Postoperative Management of Kidney Transplant Recipients

Sanjay Chaudhary, Pramod Kumar Guru

INTRODUCTION

Kidney transplantation stands as a transformative medical intervention, offering a lifeline to individuals grappling with advanced chronic kidney disease (CKD) including end-stage renal disease (ESRD).[1] This procedure not only enhances the quality of life but also extends longevity compared to other kidney replacement therapies like dialysis.[2] The perioperative phase of transplantation is often challenging due to the high prevalence of medical comorbidities in transplant patients. Common complications include hypotension, delayed graft function (DGF), renal-vascular issues, ureteric surgical problems, and organ rejection, which pose significant difficulties for both the recipient and the transplant team. Studies from transplant and dialysis registries indicate that, within the first 3 months, transplanted patients experience higher mortality rates compared to those on dialysis [heart rate (HR) 2.0, 95% confidence interval (CI) 1.5–2.7, $p < 0.001$]. However, this trend reverses by 6 months, with transplanted patients showing significantly lower mortality rates (HR 0.27, 95% CI 0.16–0.47, $p < 0.001$). By 12 months, transplantation results in an 80% reduction in mortality compared to dialysis.[3] The overall benefit of kidney transplant is indisputable, but so is the importance of attention to nuances of surgical procedure and meticulous postoperative management.

GOALS OF POSTOPERATIVE CARE

Goals of postoperative care are given in **Box 1**. Kidney transplantation success depends on a multidisciplinary team including transplant surgeons, nephrologists, coordinators, pharmacists, dietitians, anesthesiologists, and critical care physicians. This team provides individualized care tailored to each recipient's needs.

This chapter covers key aspects of postoperative management for kidney transplant recipients, including immediate care focused on fluid and hemodynamics, immunosuppressive therapy, graft function monitoring, and complication management. These elements are vital for transplant success and improving recipients' quality of life.

BOX 1: Goals of postoperative care.

- Ensure early graft function and prevent complications such as rejection and infection
- Establish and maintain adequate immunosuppression to prevent rejection while minimizing the risk of adverse effects
- Monitor and manage fluid status, electrolytes, and hemodynamics for optimal kidney allograft function
- Provide comprehensive support, including psychosocial and financial assistance, to address the unique challenges faced by transplant recipients and promote overall well-being

PREOPERATIVE CONSIDERATIONS

Patients awaiting kidney transplantation should be thoroughly investigated and have their cardiovascular status, glycemic control, and hypertension optimized before listing. This preparation is crucial for surgery and ensuring proper allograft function. A comprehensive review of the patient's clinical status through history, physical examination, and necessary tests should be conducted.

Deciding whether to dialyze the patient before surgery is key. It is generally better to correct fluid and electrolyte imbalances preoperatively rather than dealing with a postoperative unstable patient.

Patients on warfarin may need urgent reversal before surgery using vitamin K, fresh frozen plasma, or prothrombin complex concentrate. Directly acting oral anticoagulants (DOACs) should be avoided by transplant candidates.

Pretransplant Dialysis

Many patients require dialysis before transplantation. The choice of dialysis modality is often center-specific, influenced by patient preference and medical factors. Factors like availability, convenience, comorbidities, and socioeconomic conditions guide the choice, rather than transplantation needs. Studies comparing pretransplant dialysis modalities have shown no clear advantage of one over another regarding graft or patient survival.[4,5] A meta-analysis of 26 observational studies involving 269,715 transplant recipients found no significant differences in outcomes between patients who underwent pretransplant peritoneal dialysis and those who underwent pre-transplant hemodialysis. These outcomes included all-cause mortality (HR 0.98, 95% CI 0.85–1.01), death-censored graft failure (HR 0.98, 95% CI 0.85–1.14), graft vessel thrombosis, and post-transplant diabetes mellitus.[6] Pretransplant peritoneal dialysis showed an association with a lower risk for overall graft failure (HR 0.96, 95% CI 0.92-0.99) and DGF (HR 0.73, 95% CI 0.70–0.76). However, it is important to note that the strength of the evidence was rated as very low to low.

Routine hemodialysis within 24 hours prior to kidney transplantation is not recommended, as it may elevate the risk of DGF. This differs from nontransplant surgery, where presurgery dialysis is recommended. Studies also suggest avoiding ultrafiltration within 16–24 hours of transplantation to minimize DGF risk.[7]

Dialysis is sometimes required to correct metabolic issues, like hyperkalemia, that ca not be managed conservatively. To prevent intravascular volume depletion and DGF, ultrafiltration should generally be avoided. Dialysis prescriptions should be tailored to patient needs, considering session length, dialysate composition, avoiding heparin near surgery, and using biocompatible dialyzer membranes to support kidney recovery post-transplant.

INTRAOPERATIVE CONSIDERATIONS

The primary focus of this chapter is not on surgical and anesthetic considerations. However, intraoperative events have profound impact on the patient's postoperative course. Review of the documentation of intraoperative events is essential for optimal postoperative management.

Some of the important intraoperative considerations include:

- *Donor graft and graft perfusion (appearance on cross-clamp release; intraoperative Dopplers):* Transplant surgeons should report any surgical complications or anatomical challenges, such as multiple renal arteries, complex bench surgery, or renal capsule tears, as these details are essential for anticipating perioperative complications. Documenting intraoperative Doppler assessments, when available, is advised to confirm adequate postperfusion flow parameters in the transplanted kidney. If concerns arise about allograft perfusion during the perioperative period or in cases of early unexpected oligoanuria, an early duplex ultrasound should be requested to evaluate flow in the transplant vessels.
- *Hemodynamics:* Significant blood loss, reliance on inotropic support, and intraoperative hemodynamic instability are key indicators of suboptimal organ perfusion and increase the risk of DGF. A central venous catheter is commonly placed during surgery, with central venous pressure (CVP) serving as a valuable metric both intraoperatively and in the immediate postoperative period. However, the limitations of hemodynamic data must be acknowledged. While intraoperative CVP trends can inform fluid management decisions, they should not be the sole determinant of fluid management strategies due to their inconsistent correlation with actual intravascular volume.
- *Kidney function and electrolytes:* Hyperkalemia is common after kidney transplantation surgery, even with preoperative optimization, and is primarily caused by tissue trauma and the absorption of intra-abdominal blood. When potassium levels exceed 6 mmol/L in the immediate postoperative phase, dialysis should be considered, depending on urine output. If graft urine output (adjusted for native residual renal function) exceeds 100 mL/h, medical management with insulin-dextrose infusion and loop diuretics may be appropriate. However, it is important to recognize that intraoperative insulin-dextrose administration often results in rebound hyperkalemia during the postoperative period.
- *Perioperative fluid management:* Effective fluid management during the perioperative period is crucial for maintaining cardiac output, ensuring adequate kidney perfusion, and improving postoperative outcomes. However, there is limited evidence on this topic, and as a result, few guidelines are available to assist clinicians in making decisions at the bedside. A recent randomized trial found that a nonrestrictive intravenous (IV) fluid strategy during high-risk abdominal surgery was at least as effective as a

restrictive strategy in terms of disability-free survival. Furthermore, the restrictive fluid strategy was associated with a higher incidence of acute kidney injury (8.6% compared to 5.0%, $p < 0.001$).[8] In another study involving 66 kidney transplant patients, perioperative goal-directed therapy and stroke volume optimization, in comparison to conventional fluid therapy, effectively influenced the rate of major postoperative complications, reducing the overall morbidity and thus the mortality in patients receiving kidney transplantation.[9] With similarly conflicting data from some other studies, the questions about ideal fluid management strategy are far from settled.

After kidney transplantation, a common approach for postoperative fluid replacement is to replenish the urine output from the previous hour, plus an additional 30 mL to account for insensible losses. During the transplant surgery itself, a loop diuretic and/or mannitol may be used to induce diuresis, with the goal of reducing the need for dialysis. However, it is important to note that this practice has not been shown to improve graft outcomes.[10]

A strong urine output in the early post-transplant phase is an important indicator of graft function. However, in recipients with significant residual renal function, it can be difficult to differentiate between urine produced by the allograft and that from the native kidneys. Oligoanuria, especially when it follows a period of adequate urine output, may indicate DGF or the onset of an early complication. In such cases, performing an urgent bedside ultrasound is a valuable diagnostic tool to assess allograft perfusion and identify potential issues with the ureter or vasculature. Hypoechoic fluid collections observed on the ultrasound could suggest hemorrhage or a urinary anastomotic leak.

There is growing evidence supporting the use of balanced crystalloid solutions over 0.9% saline for IV fluid administration. In the Better Evidence for Selecting Transplant Fluids (BEST-Fluids) study, a pragmatic, registry-embedded, multicenter, double-blind, randomized controlled trial, conducted in 16 hospitals in Australia and New Zealand, 808 deceased donor kidney transplant recipients were involved. The study found that the incidence of DGF was lower in patients who received a balanced crystalloid solution compared to those who received 0.9% saline (30% vs. 40%). The adjusted risk difference was 10.1% (95% CI 3.5–16.6).[11]

Irrespective of the fluid type and volume administered, it goes without saying that regular evaluation of the recipient's fluid status utilizing multiple tools—clinical, hemodynamic, and image-guided—and urine output is vital for maintaining appropriate fluid replacement and preventing volume overload. Nevertheless, reliance solely on traditional parameters and clinical assessment may prove unreliable due to compromised homeostatic mechanisms in end-stage kidney disease (ESKD) and the postischemic transplanted kidney.[12] Once feasible after transplantation, recipients should have their weight checked and compared to their preoperative weight. This comparison provides an objective measure for assessing fluid status.

Important considerations for volume management post-transplant are given in **Box 2**.

BOX 2: Important considerations for volume management post-transplant.

- Optimal perioperative fluid management is crucial for cardiac output, kidney perfusion, and postoperative outcomes
- Limited guidelines exist due to insufficient data
- One should be careful with restrictive fluid strategy in this patient population
- Perioperative goal-directed therapy reduces complications and mortality
- Post-transplant fluid replacement involves replenishing urine output, sometimes using diuretics, but their impact on graft outcomes is uncertain
- Early urine output is vital for graft function assessment, but distinguishing allograft from native urine may be challenging
- Ultrasound is valuable for detecting post-transplant complications such as hemorrhage or leaks
- There is a trend toward favoring balanced crystalloid solutions over 0.9% saline
- Regular fluid status assessment, incorporating various tools, is paramount to optimal volume administration in the perioperative period

POSTOPERATIVE MANAGEMENT

The immediate postoperative period following kidney transplantation is a critical phase that requires vigilant monitoring and management to ensure optimal graft function and minimize complications. This period begins immediately after the surgical procedure and typically extends for the first few days to weeks, depending on the individual patient's recovery trajectory. During this time, the primary goals of care include stabilizing the patient's condition, assessing graft function, managing pain, maintaining fluid and electrolyte balance, and preventing complications such as infection and thrombosis.

- *Vital signs and hemodynamic monitoring:* Close monitoring of vital signs post-kidney transplantation is critical to detect hemodynamic instability or complications such as bleeding or hypotension. Vital signs should be frequently assessed, with any deviations prompting further evaluation. Continuous telemetry may be necessary for high-risk patients.
- *Graft function assessment:* Early assessment is key to detecting complications such as DGF or rejection. Graft function is evaluated through urine output, serum creatinine, and other renal markers. Decreased urine output or increased creatinine may indicate issues requiring further evaluation.
- *Fluid and electrolyte management:* Maintaining balance is vital to prevent complications such as dehydration, electrolyte disturbances, or acute kidney injury. IV fluids and close monitoring of electrolytes such as sodium, potassium, and magnesium are essential. Diuretics may be used cautiously to manage fluid overload.
- *Pain management:* Effective pain management is crucial for comfort and early mobilization. Multimodal analgesia, combining opioids with nonopioid analgesics or regional anesthesia, is commonly used. Pain management should be tailored to the patient's needs while minimizing side effects.
- *Complication prevention:* The postoperative period carries risks such as infections, thrombosis, and rejection. Prophylactic antibiotics and anticoagulant therapy may be used to reduce these risks. Close monitoring for complications and prompt intervention are essential.

Post-transplant Dialysis

The indications for acute dialysis in patients in the immediate transplant period are not different from those for nontransplant patients with acute kidney injury. DGF refers to the need for dialysis during the first postoperative week after kidney transplantation, regardless of the underlying cause. The incidence of DGF is approximately 20%.[13] Studies have shown that DGF is independently associated with a nearly two- to threefold increase in the risk of patient death, graft failure, and death-censored graft failure.[14] The optimal dialysis modality in the postoperative period following kidney transplantation has not been well studied, but most nephrologists prefer hemodialysis. This preference is largely due to concerns about peritoneal membrane disruption and the risk of infection post-transplant. While some patients have successfully used low-volume peritoneal dialysis, it is recommended that the peritoneal dialysis catheter be removed during the transplant surgery. This helps avoid the approximately 5% or greater risk of peritonitis, even in patients who do not require dialysis.[15] The indications for continuous kidney replacement therapies generally remain the same, primarily focused on hemodynamic instability. Regardless of the chosen modality, excessive ultrafiltration should be avoided to prevent ischemic injury to the allograft. Fluid removal should be targeted at no more than 10 mL/kg/hour, and the patient's weight should be maintained within 1–2 kilograms of their dry weight.

GRAFT FUNCTION MANAGEMENT IN KIDNEY TRANSPLANT RECIPIENTS

Graft function management is a cornerstone of post-operative care in kidney transplant recipients, aiming to ensure optimal function of the transplanted kidney while minimizing the risk of complications such as rejection and graft loss. Graft function is primarily assessed through monitoring of renal function parameters, including serum creatinine levels, urine output, and other biochemical markers. Early detection and prompt intervention in case of abnormalities are crucial for preserving graft function and improving long-term outcomes. In this section, we will elaborate on the principles of graft function management, including monitoring strategies, evaluation of graft function, and interventions to address complications.

Acute Allograft Dysfunction

While there is no universally accepted definition for acute allograft dysfunction following kidney transplantation, it is generally characterized by one or more of the following criteria:

- An increase in serum creatinine of ≥25% from baseline within a 1–3 month time period
- Failure of the serum creatinine to decrease following transplantation
- Proteinuria >1 g/day.

Some patients with acute allograft dysfunction may go on to develop DGF. DGF is most commonly defined by one or more of the following criteria:

- The need for at least one dialysis treatment within the 1st week after transplantation
- Low or absent urine output immediately after kidney transplantation

- Failure of the serum creatinine to decrease by >25% within 24 hours of transplant surgery.

Causes of acute allograft dysfunction in the first week post-transplant are given in **Table 1**.

TABLE 1: Causes of acute allograft dysfunction in the first week post-transplant.

Etiology	*Causes/contributing factors*
Postischemic acute tubular necrosis	• Longer cold ischemia time • Prior sensitization in retransplanted patients • Type of dialysis performed immediately prior to transplantation • Quality of the donor (age and history of hypertension) • Preservation of allograft in Euro Collins solution • Severe vascular disease in donor and recipient • Administration of mTOR inhibitors (sirolimus or everolimus) • Laparoscopic donor nephrectomy. • Use of dopamine or pump perfusion in donor management
Hyperacute rejection	Preformed donor-specific anti-HLA antibodies (DSAs), such as ABO isoagglutinins, anti-HLA antibodies, and rarely, antiendothelial antibodies
Fluid loss	Vasodilation caused by anesthesia and cytokine release from induction agents (e.g., antilymphocyte agents) can lead to fluid extravasation and intravascular fluid loss
Surgical complications	*Vascular thrombosis:* Arterial and venous thrombosis, primary and secondary, caused by technical problems (intimal dissection and kinking), hyperacute or unresponsive acute rejection, hypercoagulable state, multiple renal arteries, and unidentified intimal flaps *Fluid collections:* Lymphoceles, urinary leaks (urinomas), and perinephric hematomas *Multiple renal arteries:* Potential infarction due to ligation of small polar vessels
Atheroemboli	Rare, potential source from recipient's native vascular tree or donor's aorta
Calcium oxalate	Deposits causing acute irreversible kidney injury

(HLA: human leukocyte antigen; mTOR: mammalian target of rapamycin)

Prompt evaluation and diagnosis of the cause of allograft dysfunction are crucial, as some causes of acute allograft dysfunction, such as vascular thrombosis, in the immediate postoperative period are associated with a high risk of allograft loss.

Some other conditions that are usually seen past the first week post-transplant and may rarely present earlier include:

- *Acute rejection:* It typically occurs within the first 12 months after kidney transplantation but can also develop later in patients who are nonadherent to their immunosuppression regimen. It should be suspected in any transplant recipient with elevated creatinine levels above their usual baseline, particularly, if accompanied by symptoms such as fever, oliguria, and graft pain or tenderness.

  Histologically, there are 2 forms of acute rejection:

  1. *Cellular (acute T-cell-mediated) rejection:* Marked by the presence of lymphocytes and other inflammatory cells infiltrating the allograft.
  2. *Antibody-mediated rejection (ABMR):* It necessitates morphological evidence of acute tissue injury, the presence of circulating donor-specific antibodies (DSAs), and immunological signs of an antibody-mediated process, such as C4d deposition in the allograft.

     The management of acute rejection should be done in close coordination with transplant nephrologist and nephropathologist.

- Thrombotic microangiopathy
- Recurrent primary disease
- Calcineurin inhibitor toxicity
- Transplant renal artery stenosis
- Postallograft biopsy arteriovenous fistula
- Urinary obstruction
- Infections
- Retained ureteral stent.

POSTOPERATIVE COMPLICATIONS

Early complications are reflective of intraoperative challenges and underlying comorbidities. Because of the denervation of the kidney allograft, symptoms may be minimal to none, and one should maintain a higher degree of vigilance and a lower threshold to initiate investigations in the face of any perceived perturbations.

Hematological and Metabolic Derangements

Electrolyte abnormalities are common early post-transplant. Perioperative hyperkalemia often leads to hypokalemia due to diuretics, polyuria, and large-volume IV fluids. Hypomagnesemia, worsened by calcineurin inhibitor (CNI) therapy, increases diabetes risk. Hypophosphatemia, caused by high fibroblast growth factor 23 (FGF23) and parathyroid hormone (PTH) levels, is almost universal.

To prevent arrhythmias, intravenous electrolytes should keep potassium at 3.5–5 mmol/L and magnesium >0.4 mmol/L. Severe hypophosphatemia (<0.4 mmol/L) may require IV replacement. Oral potassium, magnesium, and sometimes phosphate are often needed post-transplant, despite possible gastrointestinal side effects.

Myelosuppression is common with immunosuppressive therapy, affecting myeloid, lymphoid, and erythroid cells. Investigations focus on identifying the cause, with blood films often helpful.

Postoperative anemia, observed in 40% of kidney transplant recipients, is primarily caused by erythropoietin deficiency, pretransplant anemia, and blood loss. Erythropoiesis-stimulating agents can be helpful in cases of poor graft function. Lymphopenia and neutropenia are commonly the result of bone marrow suppression caused by antiproliferative agents (such as mycophenolate and azathioprine), mTOR inhibitors (like sirolimus and everolimus), and antiviral medications (such as valganciclovir). If neutrophil counts fall below 1,000/μL (1.0×10^9/L), granulocyte colony-stimulating factor (G-CSF) may be used to prevent progression to severe neutropenia (<500/μL or <0.5×10^9/L), which increases the risk of infections and requires reverse barrier nursing. Other potential causes, such as parvovirus B19 and cytomegalovirus (CMV) infection, should also be considered.

Thrombocytopenia is less common but often occurs alongside leukopenia due to bone marrow suppression. In severe cases, the risk of bleeding increases and platelet transfusion may be necessary for invasive procedures if platelet counts drop below <50×10^9/L. Post-transplant thrombocytopenia should prompt investigation for thrombotic microangiopathy (TMA), which can result from the recurrence of primary hemolytic uremic syndrome or new complications. Potential triggers for TMA include medications (such as CNIs, mTOR inhibitors, and valacyclovir) and infections (such as CMV and parvovirus B19), which can cause graft damage.

Postoperative stress, corticosteroids, and cyclosporine or tacrolimus therapy can lead to significant hyperglycemia, even in patients without a prior history of diabetes, with incidence rates ranging from 80–90%. Persistent post-transplant diabetes develops in 10–45% of patients. Hyperglycemia is associated with perioperative rejection and long-term metabolic complications, making capillary glucose monitoring essential. Given the impact of immunosuppressive drugs and metabolic risk factors (such as impaired glucose tolerance, preexisting diabetes, ethnicity, age, and obesity), personalized immunotherapy is necessary to manage these risks effectively.

Hematological and metabolic derangements are given in **Table 2**.

Bleeding and Hemodynamic Issues

Bleeding occurs in up to 15% of kidney transplant cases within the first 48 hours postsurgery. It may present as increased output from the surgical drain, pain or swelling at the transplant site, or a drop in hemoglobin levels on serial blood tests. Risk factors for bleeding include challenging bench surgery (which increases the risk fourfold), uremic platelet dysfunction, and the use of antiplatelet agents or heparin. Notably, each year spent on dialysis adds an additional 2% increased risk of bleeding.[16] Suspicion of hemorrhage should prompt a hematology profile and imaging, in coordination with the transplant surgeon. Perinephric hematomas can often be identified via ultrasound, but deep or retroperitoneal hemorrhage may require computed tomography (CT) for accurate detection. A perinephric hematoma can compress the allograft, impairing perfusion and leading to increased diastolic pressures, even with normal arcuate artery blood flow. Managing bleeding involves optimizing intravascular volume through red blood cell transfusions. However, the risk of allosensitization and the formation of DSAs with blood product administration should be considered. Surgical intervention decisions should always be made in close collaboration with the transplant surgeon.

Perioperative hypotension may suggest decreased intravascular volume, anesthetic-induced vasoplegia, or myocardial dysfunction. If hypotension persists despite adequate fluid replacement, temporary vasopressor or inotropic support may be necessary. Hypovolemia, even in the absence of hypotension, can increase the risk of DGF and poor outcomes. Due to the high prevalence of coronary artery disease in patients with ESKD, it is

TABLE 2: Hematological and metabolic derangements.

Condition	Causes	Management	Notes
Hyperkalemia	Perioperative period	–	Often followed by hypokalemia
Hypokalemia	Diuretics, polyuria, and large-volume IV fluids	Maintain potassium at 3.5–5 mmol/L and oral replacement	Common after hyperkalemia
Hypomagnesemia	CNI therapy	Maintain serum magnesium >0.4 mmol/L and oral replacement	Increases post-transplant diabetes risk
Hypophosphatemia	High FGF23 and PTH levels	IV replacement if severe (<0.4 mmol/L) and oral replacement	Nearly universal, rarely severe
Myelosuppression	Immunosuppressive therapy	Investigate underlying cause and blood films	Affects myeloid, lymphoid, and erythroid cells
Postoperative anemia	Erythropoietin deficiency, pretransplant anemia, and blood loss	Erythropoiesis-stimulating agents	Seen in 40% of kidney recipients
Lymphopenia and neutropenia	Antiproliferative agents (mycophenolate and azathioprine), mTOR inhibitors (sirolimus and everolimus), and valganciclovir	G-CSF if neutrophils <1,000/μL (1.0×10^9/L), reverse barrier nursing if <500/μL (0.5×10^9/L), check for infections (parvovirus B12 and CMV)	Increases severe infection risk
Thrombocytopenia	Bone marrow suppression	Platelet transfusion if <50×10^9/L for invasive procedures and check for TMA	Less common, increases bleeding risk
Thrombotic microangiopathy	CNI therapy, mTOR inhibitors, valacyclovir, and infections (CMV and parvovirus B19)	Check for primary hemolytic uremic syndrome recurrence and new triggers	Potential for graft damage and kidney injury
Hyperglycemia	Postoperative stress, corticosteroids, cyclosporine, and tacrolimus	Monitor capillary glucose levels and individualize immunotherapy	80–90% incidence post-transplant, persistent in 10–45%, linked to rejection, and metabolic issues

(CMV: *cytomegalovirus*; CNI: calcineurin inhibitor; FGF23: fibroblast growth factor 23; G-CSF: granulocyte colony-stimulating factor; IV: intravenous; mTOR: mammalian target of rapamycin; PTH: parathyroid hormone; TMA: thrombotic microangiopathy)

crucial to rule out ischemic myocardial damage through electrocardiography (ECG) and cardiac enzyme assays.

Renal Vascular Complications

If sudden oliguria or anuria develops in a recipient with previously good postoperative urine output, transplant vessel pathology should be suspected. Early vascular issues can stem from vessel kinking, anatomical abnormalities, or thrombosis. Diagnosis often relies on duplex ultrasound and close collaboration with transplant surgeons.

Renal transplant artery or vein thrombosis, though rare (2–3% incidence), typically occurs within the first week after transplantation. Artery thrombosis usually presents with sudden oligoanuria, while vein thrombosis may cause swelling, pain, and hematuria. Risk factors include low perfusion pressures, hypotension, donor-related issues, and recipient thrombophilia. Urgent renal duplex ultrasonography is critical for diagnosis, and sudden anuria requires immediate surgical review to prevent graft loss.[17]

Renal transplant artery stenosis, usually a later complication, can also occur perioperatively, presenting with hypertension, allograft dysfunction, and fluid overload. Risk factors include donor atherosclerosis and challenging bench surgery. Diagnosis is made through duplex scanning, which reveals increased velocity at the anastomotic sites and flow differences between the aorta and the transplant artery.

Intermittent vessel kinking caused by allograft nephroptosis can be difficult to diagnose due to its positional nature. Nonprone duplex scans and CT angiography are useful in identifying positional vessel compression or kinking.[18]

Ureteric Complications

Ureteric pathology is more common than vascular issues in kidney transplantation but rarely impacts graft survival. The most frequent early urological complication is a urine leak (with an incidence of 8%), followed by later ureteric stenoses. Vesicoureteric reflux and urolithiasis are less common. Ureteric leaks typically occur within the first few weeks post-transplant and present with localized pain, increased surgical drain output, or a peritransplant collection on imaging. Risk factors include recipient age, pretransplant urological issues, immunosuppressive therapy, and donor-related factors. If a urine leak is suspected, fluid from the drain or collection should be tested for creatinine to distinguish between serous or lymphatic fluid and urine. Significant leaks may cause apparent graft function deterioration due to the reabsorption of urinary creatinine and urea.

Managing urine leaks usually involves consulting with a transplant urologist. Minor leaks can often be managed conservatively with bladder decompression via an indwelling catheter and ureteric stenting to promote healing. Larger leaks may require contrast-enhanced CT, percutaneous nephrostomy, or surgical repair.[19]

IMMUNOSUPPRESSIVE THERAPY IN KIDNEY TRANSPLANT RECIPIENTS

Immunosuppressive therapy is crucial in kidney transplantation, preventing graft rejection and supporting long-term survival. Since the 1960s, advancements have improved outcomes and reduced acute rejection, though balancing rejection prevention and minimizing side effects remains challenging. This section covers the principles of immunosuppressive therapy, including agent types, induction and maintenance strategies, drug level monitoring, and side effect management.

Types of Immunosuppressive Agents

These agents target various immune system components to suppress the alloimmune response against the transplant:

- *CNIs:* Tacrolimus and cyclosporine block T-cell activation by inhibiting the calcineurin pathway.
- *Antiproliferative agents:* Mycophenolate mofetil (MMF) and azathioprine inhibit lymphocyte proliferation by disrupting deoxyribonucleic acid (DNA) synthesis.
- *Corticosteroids:* Prednisone or methylprednisolone provide anti-inflammatory effects and reduce acute rejection risk.
- *Biologic agents:* Basiliximab, antithymocyte globulin (ATG), and others target specific cytokines or receptors, offering intense early immunosuppression.

Induction Therapy

Administered before or after transplantation, induction therapy uses potent agents such as basiliximab and ATG to prevent acute rejection and reduce the need for high-dose maintenance drugs. It is often combined with corticosteroids and CNIs.

Maintenance Immunosuppression

Maintenance immunosuppression aims to prevent rejection with minimal long-term side effects. Common regimens include CNIs (e.g., tacrolimus), antiproliferative agents (e.g., MMF), and corticosteroids, with options for steroid-sparing or alternative agents based on individual factors.

Monitoring Drug Levels

Therapeutic drug monitoring is vital to balance effective immunosuppression and toxicity. CNIs have a narrow therapeutic index, so regular blood level checks and dosage adjustments are necessary. Monitoring for drug interactions is also crucial.

Management of Side Effects

Immunosuppressants can cause nephrotoxicity, hypertension, dyslipidemia, diabetes, and infections. Close monitoring and proactive management, including dose adjustments, alternative agents, and adjunctive therapies, are essential. Patient education and lifestyle changes, such as diet and exercise, help mitigate side effects and improve overall health.

CONCLUSION

The postoperative management of kidney transplant patients is a multifaceted and dynamic process that requires a comprehensive, patient-centered approach. While few patients require management in an intensive care unit, it is important for the critical care team to be familiar with the patient population and the nuances of management of kidney transplant recipients. Vigilant monitoring, timely intervention, and interdisciplinary collaboration are paramount to ensure optimal outcomes. The success of a kidney transplant not only hinges on the surgical procedure itself but also on the meticulous perioperative care, which includes hemodynamic optimization, close monitoring, immunosuppressive therapy, infection prevention, management of comorbidities, and patient education. By adhering to evidence-based protocols and staying attuned to the individual needs of each patient, healthcare providers can significantly enhance graft survival and improve the quality of life for transplant recipients. As advancements in medical technology and pharmacology continue to evolve, the future of postoperative management promises even greater strides toward achieving long-term success in kidney transplantation.

REFERENCES

1. Suthanthiran M, Strom TB. Renal transplantation. N Engl J Med. 1994;331(6):365-76.
2. Port FK, Wolfe RA, Mauger EA, Berling DP, Jiang K. Comparison of survival probabilities for dialysis patients vs cadaveric renal transplant recipients. JAMA. 1993;270(11):1339-43.
3. McDonald, SP Russ GR. Survival of recipients of cadaveric kidney transplants compared with those receiving dialysis treatment in Australia and New Zealand, 1991-2001. Nephrol Dial Transplant. 2002;17(12):2212-9.
4. Snyder JJ, Kasiske BL, Gilbertson DT, Collins AJ. A comparison of transplant outcomes in peritoneal and hemodialysis patients. Kidney Int. 2002;62(4):1423-30.
5. Goldfarb-Rumyantzev AS, Hurdle JF, Scandling JD, Baird BC, Cheung AK. The role of pretransplantation renal replacement therapy modality in kidney allograft and recipient survival. Am J Kidney Dis. 2005;46(3):537-49.
6. Ngamvichchukorn T, Ruengorn C, Noppakun K, Thavorn K, Hutton B, Sood MM, et al. Association between pretransplant dialysis modality and kidney transplant outcomes: A systematic review and meta-analysis. JAMA Netw Open. 2022;5(10):e2237580.
7. Kikić Z, Lorenz M, Sunder-Plassmann G, Schillinger M, Regele H, Györi G, et al. Effect of hemodialysis before transplant surgery on renal allograft function—a pair of randomized controlled trials. Transplantation. 2009;88(12):1377-85.
8. Myles PS, Bellomo R, Corcoran T, Forbes A, Peyton P, Story D, et al. Restrictive versus liberal fluid therapy for major abdominal surgery. N Engl J Med. 2018;378(24):2263-74.
9. Cavaleri M, Veroux M, Palermo F, Vasile F, Mineri M, Palumbo J, et al. Perioperative goal-directed therapy during kidney transplantation: An impact evaluation on the major postoperative complications. J Clin Med. 2019;8(1):80.
10. Weimar W, Geerlings W, Bijnen AB, Obertop H, van Urk H, Lameijer LD, et al. A controlled study on the effect of mannitol on immediate renal function after cadaver donor kidney transplantation. Transplantation. 1983;35(1):99-101.
11. Collins MG, Fahim MA, Pascoe EM, Hawley CM, Johnson DW, Varghese J, et al. Balanced crystalloid solution versus saline in deceased donor kidney transplantation (BEST-Fluids): A pragmatic, double-blind, randomised, controlled trial. Lancet. 2023;402(10396):105-17.
12. Calixto Fernandes MH, Schricker T, Magder S, Hatzakorzian R. Perioperative fluid management in kidney transplantation: A black box. Crit Care. 2018;22(1):14.
13. Irish WD, Ilsley JN, Schnitzler MA, Feng S, Brennan DC. A risk prediction model for delayed graft function in the current era of deceased donor renal transplantation. Am J Transplant. 2010;10(10):2279-86.
14. Tapiawala SN, Tinckam KJ, Cardella CJ, Schiff J, Cattran DC, Cole EH, et al. Delayed graft function and the risk for death with a functioning graft. J Am Soc Nephrol. 2010;21(1):153-61.
15. Warren J, Jones E, Sener A, Drage M, Taqi A, Griffin S, et al. Should peritoneal dialysis catheters be removed at the time of kidney transplantation? Can Urol Assoc J. 2012;6(5):376-8.
16. Hernández D, Rufino M, Armas S, González A, Gutiérrez P, Barbero P, et al. Retrospective analysis of surgical complications following cadaveric kidney transplantation in the modern transplant era. Nephrol Dial Transplant. 2006;21(10):2908-15.
17. Bakir N, Sluiter WJ, Ploeg RJ, van Son WJ, Tegzess AM. Primary renal graft thrombosis. Nephrol Dial Transplant. 1996;11(1):140-7.
18. Dosch AR, Pahl M, Reddy U, Foster CE 3rd, Ichii H. Post-transplantation nephroptosis causing recurrent episodes of acute renal failure and hypertension secondary to intermittent vascular torsion of intraperitoneal renal allograft. J Surg Case Rep. 2017;2017(5):rjx033.
19. Branchereau J, Karam G. Management of urologic complications of renal transplantation. European Urology Supplements. 2016;15(9):408-14.

CHAPTER 4

ABO Incompatible Kidney Transplant: Challenges in Management

Bharat V Shah, Madhavi A Dadwe

INTRODUCTION

In patients with end-stage renal failure, kidney transplantation offers a considerable survival advantage compared to hemodialysis. The organ can come from a deceased (usually brainstem dead) donor or a living related donor (LRD). The deceased donor program is still not well developed in our country, with organ donation rates of <1 per million population. Therefore, we still depend on LRD in our country.

Historically, LRD kidney transplantation across ABO blood group barriers resulted in a high incidence of early graft loss due to antibody-mediated rejection (ABMR), making ABO incompatibility (ABOi) an absolute contraindication. However, in 1981, Slapak et al. documented the successful reversal of acute ABMR in an unintended ABOi kidney transplant using plasmapheresis (PP).[1]

Subsequently, Alexandre et al. from Belgium reported positive outcomes in ABOi kidney transplantation following a desensitization protocol that included repeated PP and splenectomy—aimed at depleting antibody-secreting B cells—along with intensified post-transplant immunosuppression.[2,3] Over time, advancements in desensitization strategies have refined this approach, replacing splenectomy with rituximab for B-cell depletion and incorporating immunoadsorption (IA) for selective antibody removal. These improvements have significantly expanded the global adoption of ABOi kidney transplantation. As a result, the acceptance of ABOi donors has increased the living donor pool by approximately 20–25%.

CHALLENGES IN ABO INCOMPATIBILITY KIDNEY TRANSPLANT

Challenges in ABOi kidney transplant are as follows

- *Accurate determination of anti-blood group antibody titers (ABGAT):* Anti-A and/or -B antibodies are present in the recipients with A, B, or O blood group. These antibodies can bind to blood group antigens expressed on the endothelial cells of kidney grafts. If anti-blood group antibodies are not accurately determined and if their levels are high at the time of transplant, they will bind to blood group antigens and activate complement, leading to hyper-acute or acute ABMR.[4,5]
- Blood group O individuals have higher antibody titers against blood group A and B. Hence, recipients of blood group O have higher chances of ABMR.[6]
- *Desensitization:* It is a procedure to reduce ABGAT to acceptable levels before kidney transplant.[7] It can be difficult to desensitize people who produce very high levels of anti-ABO antibodies. If the blood group antibodies are not adequately depleted, it can lead to hyperacute or acute ABMR.
- Preoperative desensitization is expensive because it involves the use of B-cell depleting agent (rituximab) and use of apheresis.[8] The higher the level of antibodies, more the requirement for apheresis and greater the expense.
- Plasma exchange (PEX) is the most common apheresis method used for removal of blood group antibodies. Since this procedure also results in loss of coagulation factors, ABOi transplants may be associated with intra and postoperative bleeding events.
- ABOi kidney transplants are associated with increased risk of ABMR because of preexisting blood group antibodies. If these antibodies are not adequately removed or if they rebound in the early period after transplant, they can lead to acute ABMR.
- Since the process of removal of anti-blood group antibodies requires aggressive immunosuppression, there is an increase in the risk of infection and possibly malignancy.

ABO INCOMPATIBILITY TRANSPLANT PROTOCOL FOR MANAGEMENT

Measurement of Anti-Blood Group Antibody Titers

The immunoglobulin G (IgG) and immunoglobulin M (IgM) anti-blood group antibody titers are determined at baseline and after antibody removal. Accurate measurement is important for successful ABOi kidney transplantation. If the titer is underestimated compared to the actual titer of patient, it can lead to rejection. There are three common methods of measuring ABGAT: (1) Conventional tube method, (2) column agglutination technique (CAT), and (3) flow cytometry.[9] Tube method is less precise and subjective;[10] CAT provides more standardized and objective results; flow cytometry is highly sensitive and specific, but requires expensive equipment and highly trained personnel, and hence, not routinely used.[11] We use CAT for the measurement of ABGAT, and for decision-making, only IgG antibody titers are used. Desensitization is done if baseline IgG ABGAT are >1:32. Many centers aim for a lower titer while some centers in Japan accept titers of 1:64.

Desensitization

Desensitization is a procedure done to reduce the ABGAT to desired level before kidney transplant. The protocol commonly includes B-cell depletion with rituximab and antibody depletion by apheresis. The apheresis technique is divided into two basic types (1) nonselective or (2) selective.[12]

Plasma exchange is a nonselective apheresis technique that involves separating plasma from whole blood through centrifugation or filtration, followed by its removal and replacement with albumin or fresh frozen plasma.[13,14] However, PEX has a notable drawback, as it leads to the loss of coagulation factors, albumin, and essential immunoglobulins with antibacterial and antiviral properties. On the other hand, its advantage lies in its ability to eliminate harmful antibodies, including anti-human leukocyte antigen (anti-HLA) antibodies and complement components involved in allograft injury mediated by anti-blood group antibodies. Additionally, PEX is a cost-effective, widely accessible, and rapidly deployable apheresis technique.[15-17]

An alternative to PEX is double-filtration plasmapheresis (DFPP), where plasma is initially separated using a plasma separator and then passed through a plasma fractionator that selectively removes gamma globulins. This method ensures the removal of immunoglobulins while preserving other essential blood components. A study by Han et al. demonstrated the success of ABO-incompatible kidney transplants following a preconditioning regimen incorporating DFPP and rituximab.[18]

The most selective apheresis technique is ABO-specific IA. In this method, separated plasma is processed through an antigen-specific absorber containing immobilized blood group A or B antigens on a Sepharose matrix before being reinfused into the patient. This approach effectively removes ABO antibodies while preserving vital plasma components. Additionally, IA can lower complement component levels, helping to prevent ABMR associated with ABO-incompatible transplantation, thereby enhancing treatment efficiency.[19,20]

At our center, the apheresis technique used is PEX, when ABGATs are <1:512. It is generally carried out on alternate days, starting 1 week before an elective transplant. If the ABGATs do not fall down to the desired level, PP is continued until titers drop to an acceptable level. The replacement solution used is albumin and/or donor blood group or AB group plasma. IAs + PEX is done when the titers are >1:512. Desensitization is considered successful if ABGAT drops to <1:32.

Some centers administer intravenous immunoglobulins (IVIg) following PEX before ABO-incompatible kidney transplantation to mitigate the risk of an early post-transplant rebound in anti-A/B antibodies.[21,22] IVIg infusion is also thought to help reduce infection risk by replenishing depleted immunoglobulins. However, it is important to note that IVIg preparations contain IgG antibodies targeting A/B antigens, which may inadvertently raise anti-A/B antibody titers after administration.

In our desensitization protocol **(Fig. 1)**, rituximab (200 mg) dose is administered on day 14. Prednisolone

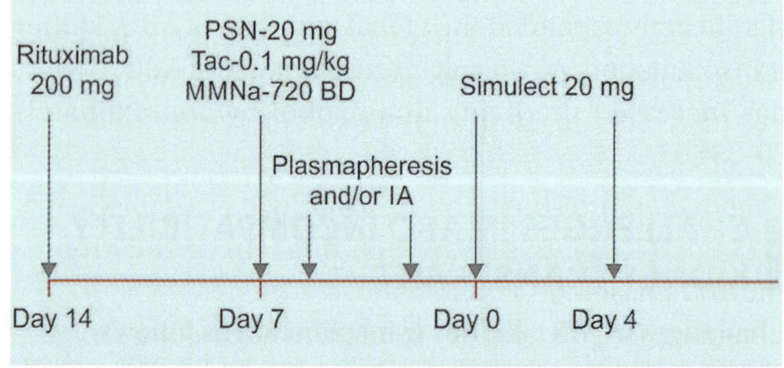

Fig. 1: Desensitization protocol. (IA: immunoadsorption; MMNa: mycophenolate mofetil sodium salt; PSN: prednisolone; Tac: tacrolimus)

20 mg, tacrolimus (0.1 mg/kg), and mycophenolate sodium salt (720 mg twice a day) are initiated on the day 7. PEX alone is done when ABGATs are <1:512. It is carried out on alternate days, starting 1 week before the planned transplant till titers drop to an acceptable level. The replacement solution used is albumin and/or donor blood group or AB group plasma.

Immunoadsorptions along with PEX are done when the titers are >1:512. Desensitization is considered successful if ABGAT drops to <1:32.[20,23]

Induction and Post-transplant Immunosuppression

Patients who successfully undergo desensitization proceed to kidney transplantation. Induction therapy, a form of immunosuppression given at the time of transplantation, helps minimize the risk of allograft rejection. Antithymocyte globulin (thymoglobulin), a T cell-depleting agent, is the preferred choice for induction; however, it is avoided when rituximab, a B cell-depleting agent, is used to prevent excessive immunosuppression. In such cases, basiliximab, an interleukin-2 receptor antagonist (IL-2 RA), is the preferred alternative, administered as a 20 mg dose with a repeat on day 4.

For maintenance immunosuppression, the standard regimen includes tacrolimus at 0.1 mg/kg in two divided doses, adjusted to maintain a trough level of 5–10 ng/mL, along with mycophenolate sodium at 720 mg twice daily, modified based on white blood cell count. Prednisolone is tapered gradually, typically reaching a dose of 5 mg per day by 1-month post-transplant.

Monitoring of Anti-Blood Group Antibody Titers

During the desensitization period, ABGAT are monitored on specific days following PP or IA. Post-transplant, monitoring is conducted daily or on alternate days for the 1st week, followed by twice-weekly checks in the 2nd week, and weekly assessments for the subsequent 4 weeks. Additional testing is performed if clinically indicated. Beyond 6 weeks, ABGAT is only checked when necessary, as accommodation typically occurs between 3 and 6 weeks post-transplant.

Accommodation refers to the phenomenon where ABO-incompatible kidney grafts continue to function effectively despite elevated anti-A/B antibody titers. While it is generally believed to occur within 1 to 4 weeks after ABO-incompatible transplantation, our experience suggests that it can develop even earlier, sometimes within the 1st week. This early post-transplant period is particularly critical, as the risk of acute ABMR remains high if antibody titers are elevated. Thus, we do not try to deplete antibodies if they rise, even in the first week, if the graft function is stable.[21,24,25]

OUTCOME OF ABO INCOMPATIBLE KIDNEY TRANSPLANTS

The outcome today is almost similar to that of ABO-compatible (ABOc) kidney transplants. In our experience,1-,5- and 9-year patient survival was 98%, 85.4%, and 73%, respectively (98%, 91%, and 80% in ABO compatible transplants) **(Fig. 2)** and death-censored graft survival was 93%, 84% and 84% (97%, 84%, and 74% in ABO compatible transplants), respectively **(Fig. 3)**.

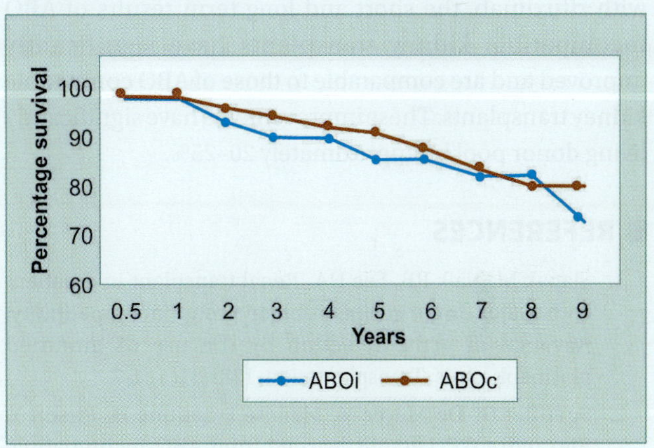

Fig. 2: Patient survival in ABO incompatible and ABO compatible transplants. (ABOc: ABO compatible; ABOi: ABO incompatible)

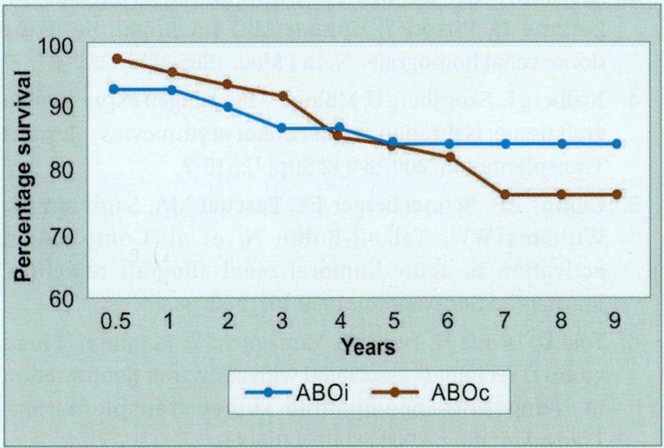

Fig. 3: Graft survival in ABO incompatible and ABO compatible transplants. (ABOc: ABO compatible; ABOi: ABO incompatible)

Acute rejection rates have been reported to be higher with ABOi transplants compared to ABOc kidney transplants, but these are treatable and overall graft survival rates are similar.

The incidence of infectious complications after ABO-incompatible kidney transplantation remains a subject of debate.

Despite the use of desensitization protocols in ABO-incompatible transplants, there is no statistically significant difference in malignancy risk between ABO-incompatible and ABOc transplant recipients.

There are conflicting results of infectious complications after ABOi kidney transplantation.

CONCLUSION

With effective desensitization which includes removal of blood group antibodies and depletion of B cells with rituximab, the short and long term results of ABO incompatible kidney transplants have significantly improved and are comparable to those of ABO compatible kidney transplants. These improvements have significantly living donor pool by approximately 20–25%.

REFERENCES

1. Slapak M, Naik RB, Lee HA. Renal transplant in a patient with major donor-recipient blood group incompatibility: Reversal of acute rejection by the use of modified plasmapheresis. Transplantation. 1981;31(1):4-7.
2. Squifflet JP, De Meyer M, Malaise J, Latinne D, Pirson Y, Alexandre GP. Lessons learned from ABO-incompatible living donor kidney transplantation: 20 years later. Exp Clin Transplant. 2004;2(1):208-13.
3. Alexandre GP, De Bruyere M, Squifflet JP, Moriau M, Latinne D, Pirson Y. Human ABO-incompatible living donor renal homografts. Neth J Med. 1985;28(6):231-4.
4. Rydberg L, Skogsberg U, Mölne J. ABO antigen expression in graft tissue: Is titration against donor erythrocytes relevant? Transplantation. 2007;84(12 Suppl):S10-2.
5. Collins AB, Schneeberger EE, Pascual MA, Saidman SL, Williams WW, Tolkoff-Rubin N, et al. Complement activation in acute humoral renal allograft rejection. Journal Am Soc Nephrol. 1999;10(10):2208-14.
6. Toki D, Ishida H, Horita S, Yamaguchi Y, Tanabe K. Blood group O recipients associated with early graft deterioration in living ABO-incompatible kidney transplantation. Transplantation. 2009;88(10):1186-93.
7. Salvadori M. Strategies for access to kidney transplantation for highly sensitized and incompatible patients. Transplantology. 2023;4(2):85-9.
8. Ramos EJ, Pollinger HS, Stegall MD, Gloor JM, Dogan A, Grande JP. The effect of desensitization protocols on human splenic B-cell populations in vivo. Am J Transplant. 2007;7(2):402-7.
9. Chung Y, Ko DH. Laboratory support of ABO antibody monitoring for ABO-incompatible solid organ transplantation. Korean J Transplant. 2022;36(2):99.
10. Bachegowda LS, Cheng YH, Long T, Shaz BH. Impact of uniform methods on interlaboratory antibody titration variability: Antibody titration and uniform methods. Arch Pathol Lab Med. 2017;141(1):131-8.
11. Won D, Kim BC. Optimized flow cytometry to measure anti-ABO immunoglobulin G. Lab Med. 2012;43(6):281-90.
12. Vrielink H, le Poole K. Plasmapheresis in ABO incompatible kidney transplant. Transfus Apher Sci. 2023;62(2):103673.
13. Hanaoka A, Naganuma T, Takemoto Y, Uchida J, Nakatani T, Kabata D, et al. Efficacy of selective plasma exchange as pre-Transplant apheresis in ABO-incompatible kidney transplantation. Ren Replace Ther. 2019;5(1).
14. O'Donghaile D, Kelley W, Klein HG, Flegel WA. Recommendations for transfusion in ABO-incompatible hematopoietic stem cell transplantation. Transfusion (Paris). 2012;52(2):456-8.
15. Melexopoulou C, Filiopoulos V, Marinaki S. Therapeutic apheresis in renal transplantation: An update. Transfus Apher Sci. 2024;63(1):103844.
16. Orandi BJ, Montgomery RA, Segev DL. Kidney Transplants from HLA-Incompatible Live Donors and Survival. N Eng J Med. 2016;375(3):286-9.
17. Connelly-Smith L, Alquist CR, Aqui NA, Hofmann JC, Klingel R, Onwuemene OA, et al. Guidelines on the use of therapeutic apheresis in clinical practice—Evidence-based approach from the Writing Committee of the American Society for Apheresis: The Ninth Special Issue. J Clin Apher. 2023;38(2):77-278.
18. Han S, Hwang E, Park S, Park U, Kim H, Cho W. Clinical outcomes of ABO-incompatible kidney transplant with rituximab and double-filtration plasmapheresis. Exp Clin Transplant. 2014;12(5):401-4.
19. Genberg H, Kumlien G, Wennberg L, Tyden G. The efficacy of antigen-specific immunoadsorption and rebound of anti-A/B antibodies in ABO-incompatible kidney transplantation. Nephrol Dial Transplant. 2011;26(7):2394-400.
20. Tydén G, Kumlien G, Genberg H, Sandberg J, Lundgren T, Fehrman I. ABO incompatible kidney transplantations without splenectomy, using antigen-specific immunoadsorption and rituximab. Am J Transplant. 2005;5(1):145-8.

21. Salvadori M, Tsalouchos A. Current protocols and outcomes of ABO-incompatible kidney transplantation. World J Transplant. 2020;10(7):191-205.
22. Shehata N, Palda VA, Meyer RM, Blydt-Hansen TD, Campbell P, Cardella C, et al. The use of immunoglobulin therapy for patients undergoing solid organ transplantation: An evidence-based practice guideline. Transfus Med Rev. 2010;24 Suppl 1:S7-27.
23. Salvadori M, Tsalouchos A. Therapeutic apheresis in kidney transplantation: An updated review. World J Transplant. 2019;9(6):103.
24. Dorling A. Transplant accommodation: Are the lessons learned from xenotransplantation pertinent for clinical allotransplantation? Am J Transplant. 2012;12(3):545-53.
25. Salama AD, Delikouras A, Pusey CD, Cook HT, Bhangal G, Lechler RI, et al. Transplant accommodation in highly sensitized patients: a potential role for Bcl-xL and alloantibody. Am J Transplant. 2001;1(3):260-9.
26. Lentine KL, Axelrod D, Klein C, Simpkins C, Xiao H, Schnitzler MA, et al. Early clinical complications after ABO incompatible live donor kidney transplantation: a national study of Medicare-insured recipients. Transplantation. 2014;98(1):54-65.

Pancreatic Transplantation: Patient Selection, Preoperative Assessment, Surgical Challenges, Postoperative Management from an Intensive Care Perspective

Neha Bhatt, Somnath Chattopadhyay

INTRODUCTION

There have been many novel advancements in the medical management of diabetes mellitus (DM). Development of newer insulin analogs, continuous glucose monitoring technology and advanced insulin delivery systems such as glucose-responsive "smart" insulin pens have made self-management of disease easier and more effective. Despite this, many patients still suffer from poor glycemic control, dangers of hypoglycemia unawareness, and the risk of progression of secondary complications of DM.

To effectively cure diabetes, it is necessary to restore both insulin production as well as glucose-dependent insulin secretion.[1] Hence, when offered to a select group of diabetic individuals, pancreas transplantation offers the advantages of better glycemic control, improved quality of life, delay in progression, and in certain circumstances, even improvement in secondary complications of DM.

Pancreas transplant (PT) is most commonly offered to a uremic and diabetic individual as a simultaneous pancreas–kidney transplant (SPK) transplant. Less commonly, it is performed as a pancreas after kidney transplant (PAK) in an individual who is now nonuremic after undergoing a kidney transplant in the past. Rarely, it can be performed as a pancreas transplant alone (PTA) in patients suffering from acute life-threatening complications of DM.

Nearly 90% of PTs in the United States and around the world are performed as SPK, with the rest being performed as PTA or sequential PAK transplant.[2]

INDICATIONS

As indicated in the latest Organ Procurement and Transplant Network (OPTN) policy,[3] a patient is eligible for PT enlistment upon fulfilling *at least one* of the following conditions:

- Diagnosis of DM, which is dependent on insulin therapy, along with complications difficult to manage on conventional therapy
- Requires transplantation of pancreas as part of a multiple organ transplant for technical reasons
- Rare cases of severe pancreatic exocrine insufficiency, not managed by dietary supplements

PATIENT SELECTION AND OPTIMAL PROCEDURE

Selecting the optimal procedure for the patient depends on the *indication* for transplant, *recipient's condition,* and *organ availability.*

American Diabetes Association (ADA) guidelines[4] recommend PT with a kidney transplant in the following circumstances.

- *Insulin-requiring diabetic patient with chronic kidney disease (CKD) stage 4 or 5 [glomerular filtration rate (GFR) <20 mL/min or dialysis dependence] without excessive risk for dual transplant, in whom the surgery is not otherwise contraindicated.*

  Most of these patients will undergo simultaneous dual transplant (SPK). Some may receive it as a PAK transplant (a fragile recipient who underwent a living donor kidney transplant as a bridge to PAK or as definitive therapy when a suitable kidney alone was available).

  The benefits of a PT are not only the restoration of beta cell mass and endogenous insulin production but also a self-regulated insulin secretion driven by blood glucose levels, albeit at the cost of surgical morbidity and the need for lifelong immunosuppression. This "risk–reward ratio" is most favorable for a diabetic individual requiring a kidney transplant for end-stage renal disease.

  A prototype recipient for PT is hence a patient with uremia (GFR <20 mL/min) and type 1 diabetes mellitus (T1DM), without detectable C-peptide, who is suffering from poor metabolic control and/or progressive secondary complications of diabetes on insulin therapy.

The successful addition of a pancreas to a kidney transplant improves patient's survival, will restore normoglycemia, and may improve kidney survival. SPK has shown better patient survival than either kidney transplant alone or dialysis.[5,6]

The pancreas graft survival rate is based on insulin independence. Pancreas allograft survival has shown to be better when done simultaneously with a kidney transplant. Unadjusted 5-year pancreas graft survival are 71% (SPK), 65% (PAK), and 58% (PTA),[7] respectively. More recently, 10-year actual insulin independence rates have been reported to exceed 80% in SPK and 60% in PTA.[8,9]

C-peptide is a 31-amino-acid peptide that is cleaved from the proinsulin molecule, resulting in the secretion of equimolar quantities of insulin and C-peptide from the beta cells of the islets during insulin secretion. Normal fasting C-peptide level is 0.9–1.8 ng/mL and a level <0.6 ng/mL is consistent with beta cell failure, as seen in T1DM.

While the PT is most commonly offered to the T1DM patient, where the basic defect is autodestruction of islet cells resulting in insulinopenia (and hence absence of C-peptide), highly selected individuals with type 2 diabetes mellitus (T2DM) may also benefit from augmentation of insulin production from PT.

Also, it is now accepted that there is considerable overlap in the phenotypes of T1DM and T2DM, and hence, a pretransplant measurable value of C-peptide may not be accurate marker for presence of T2DM, more so in the presence of kidney disease as the kidney itself is the major site of C-peptide catabolism. United Network for Organ Sharing (UNOS)/OPTN guidelines[10] have recently removed both C-peptide and body mass index (BMI) from their selection criteria for PT, thus extending the benefit of PT to more patients with T2DM

In the UK[11] National Health Service Blood and Transplant (NHSBT) policy, a patient with T2DM can be listed for PT when:

- The disease is insulin-dependent (and not getting managed with medicines and lifestyle changes).
- BMI is <30 kg/m^2 at the time of listing (overtly obese may have a component of insulin resistance, and hence, respond poorly to PT).

A prototype T2DM patient who is offered a PT is an individual aged 55–60 years, with insulin-dependent diabetes for a minimum of 3–5 years, total daily insulin dose <1 units/kg/day or 100 units/day, not overtly obese, without any major cardiovascular disease, and otherwise fulfilling criteria for SPK/PAK transplant.

- *In the absence of indications for kidney transplantation, PTA should only be considered a therapy in patients who exhibit one of these three criteria:*
  1. A history of frequent, acute, and severe metabolic complications (hypoglycemia unawareness, hyperglycemia, and ketoacidosis) requiring medical attention
  2. Clinical and emotional problems with exogenous insulin therapy that are so severe as to be incapacitating
  3. Consistent failure of insulin-based management to prevent complications

  In recipients of solitary pancreas grafts (PAK and PTA), accurate estimate of renal function is mandatory, as there is a risk of development or exacerbation of renal dysfunction with calcineurin-based immunosuppression. This risk is reduced when the baseline GFR is ≥60–70 mL/min[12] or >35–40 mL/min if already on a calcineurin inhibitor after kidney transplant.

A prototype patient for PTA is a young (<50 years), nonobese individual without any major cardiovascular disease, who has suffered from multiple episodes of hypoglycemia unawareness. The patient should have stable renal function and the benefit of transplant should outweigh the risk of deterioration in renal function from lifelong immunosuppression therapy.

To summarize, all pancreas transplant (PT) recipients have complicated, typically long-standing, insulin dependent diabetes (T1DM >>T2DM), and most are uremic or posturemic. The remaining patients are individuals suffering from brittle diabetes, typically plagued by unawareness of hypoglycemic events, and/or having progressive extrarenal complications.[13]

CONTRAINDICATIONS

While ABO compatibility and a negative crossmatching is ensured to proceed with transplant, presence of any of the below conditions in a recipient is considered a contraindication:

- Age >65–70 years
- BMI >35 kg/m^2
- Insufficient cardiovascular functional reserve
- Severe peripheral (aortoiliac) vascular disease

- Ongoing, untreated substance abuse (drug, alcohol, and tobacco)
- Ongoing, untreated psychiatric illness or non-compliance
- Active, untreated infection
- Malignancy (other than localized basal cell or squamous cell skin cancer)
- Poor overall functional performance status (severe malnutrition, frailty, or dementia)

PREOPERATIVE EVALUATION

A comprehensive medical evaluation **(Table 1)** of the preoperative patient is performed by a multidisciplinary team of endocrinologists, nephrologists, transplant surgeons, and anesthetists.

The team confirms the diagnosis of insulin-requiring DM, determines the patient's ability to withstand the operative procedure and long-term immunosuppression, establishes the absence of any contraindication, and documents end-organ complications for future tracking after transplantation.[14]

The degree of nephropathy (decides the type of transplant), cardiovascular risk, pulmonary function, and overall functional and performance status are assessed.

Cardiac status is assessed meticulously, as significant and often silent coronary artery disease is not uncommon in this population. At a minimum, two-dimensional (2D) Echo and pharmacological stress test are performed. Selective high-risk candidates will require coronary angiography. Coronary angiographic evidence of significant noncorrectable coronary artery disease, ejection fraction below 30–40%, a recent history of myocardial infarction or congestive heart failure, and right ventricular end-diastolic pressure >45–50 mm Hg are contraindications.[15]

An endocrinology opinion is taken for perioperative management. Psychiatric evaluation is performed to ensure that the patient is capable of post-transplant care and compliance with lifelong immunosuppression therapy. Neurology, infectious disease, urology, and ophthalmology clearance is done when indicated.

TABLE 1: Recipient evaluation.

Standard blood tests	• Complete blood count with differential and platelet count • Coagulation studies with thrombophilia screen • Biochemistry including liver and renal function tests, serum amylase, and lipase levels • Endocrine and metabolic workup including glycosylated hemoglobin and C-peptide levels, thyroid function tests, lipid, and iron profiles
Tumor markers	• PSA levels in males above age 45 years • CA 125 in females • CEA, CA 19–9 in both
Serology and immunological evaluation	• ABO blood type and HLA tissue type • Viral titers (Epstein–Barr virus, herpes simplex virus, varicella-zoster virus, human immunodeficiency virus, hepatitis B virus, hepatitis C virus, and *Cytomegalovirus*) • Venereal disease research laboratory/fluorescent treponemal antibody test for syphilis
Urinary evaluation	Urine analysis with culture, 24-hour urine for creatinine and protein clearance (or spot urine protein/creatinine ratio with calculated GFR)
Cardiac evaluation	• 2D Echo • Pharmacological stress test • Coronary angiography in selective cases
Pulmonary evaluation	• Chest radiograph and pulmonary function test
Imaging studies	• Abdominal ultrasound, abdominal and pelvic computerized tomographic scan • Doppler for aortoiliac and carotid vessels
Gynecological evaluation	• Mammography for women above the age of 40 years • Pelvic examination with pap smear

(CA: cancer antigen; CEA: carcinoembryonic antigen; GFR: glomerular filtration rate; HLA: human leukocyte antigen; PSA: prostate-specific antigen)

SURGICAL CHALLENGES

The whole pancreas with an attached duodenal segment is an established graft now. Surgery is most commonly performed using a lower midline intraperitoneal approach, while surgeons prefer placing the pancreas on the right side since the vena cava is on the right and exposure of right iliac vessels is easier and more superficial. The pancreas is transplanted on the distal inferior vena cava (IVC)/right common iliac vein and right common iliac artery/distal aorta followed by the kidney transplanted more distally on the right external iliac vein and artery or on the opposite side.[16]

In an SPK, the kidney can be placed on the ipsilateral or contralateral side. Using the right side for both minimizes vascular dissection, decreases operative time, and also preserves the left side for the future.

Gentle pancreatic tissue handling during procurement and grafting is a must to prevent trauma, inadvertent hematomas, and the risk of postoperative pancreatitis. Compared with the kidney, the pancreas is very sensitive to ischemia–reperfusion injury and is usually placed first to minimize the cold ischemia time (CIT) to <12 hours. This will minimize complications of graft pancreatitis and early thrombosis.[17]

In a PAK transplant too, the pancreas is preferably placed intraperitoneally on the right side, while the kidney remains more distal and extraperitoneal on the right iliac vessels.[18]

The propensity for graft thrombosis is a unique challenge in PT. It is seen more frequently in pancreas than any other solid organ transplant owing to an inherently low-flow microcirculatory system derived from splenic and mesenteric circulation. In addition, there are the risks of vascular diseases, atherosclerotic vessels, and hypercoagulable state, typically seen in long-standing diabetes. Uremia, associated with its antiplatelet and anticoagulant effects, in fact, protects against early graft thrombosis—an advantage that is lost in the setting of PAK or even a preemptive SPK. Hence, most centers include a thrombophilia screening in pretransplant evaluation and perioperative use of anticoagulation in the form of unfractionated heparin or low molecular weight heparin for a variable period up to 2–4 weeks followed by the use of aspirin.

The main variations in surgical technique are in regard to the site for venous drainage (either systemic or portal) and the site for exocrine secretions through the pancreatic duct (either urinary or enteric).

Portal Versus Systemic Venous Drainage

In portal venous drainage, the portal vein of the pancreas allograft is drained into the recipient's splanchnic venous system (usually the superior mesenteric vein), resulting in "portal hyperinsulinemia". Systemic venous drainage, on the other hand, utilizes the recipient's iliac vein or distal IVC, resulting in insulin release into the systemic circulation, bypassing the first-pass metabolism in the liver. Theoretically, portal circulation sounds more physiological, although no consistent long-term metabolic and immunologic benefits of this technique have been seen.[19]

Bladder Versus Enteric Drainage of Exocrine Secretions

Historically, the pancreatic exocrine secretions via the pancreatic duct were drained by anastomosing the allograft duodenum to the urinary bladder. Urinary amylase was easily measured as a marker of pancreas graft rejection. However, bladder drainage was associated with a high incidence of urinary [urinary tract infection (UTI), bleeding] and metabolic (dehydration, bicarbonate loss, and metabolic acidosis) complications. Enteric drainage into the proximal recipient jejunum or using a Roux-en-y limb prevents these complications, and is hence, preferable **(Fig. 1)**.

The combination of systemic venous outflow and enteric exocrine drainage is currently most prevalent and seen in majority of cases.

POSTOPERATIVE COMPLICATIONS

The fragility of a diabetic and uremic patient, concomitant comorbidities, postoperative complications of graft pancreatitis and vascular thrombosis in a low-flow system, and the need for stronger immunosuppression are unique to PT and contribute to increased operative morbidity.

Complications are also more common and severe in SPK compared to kidney transplants alone during the first-year post-transplant. Longer postoperative stay, more frequent early rehospitalizations, and higher perioperative morbidity, and early mortality are seen post SPK.[20,21] Increased complexity of surgery and use of stronger immunosuppression are important causes.

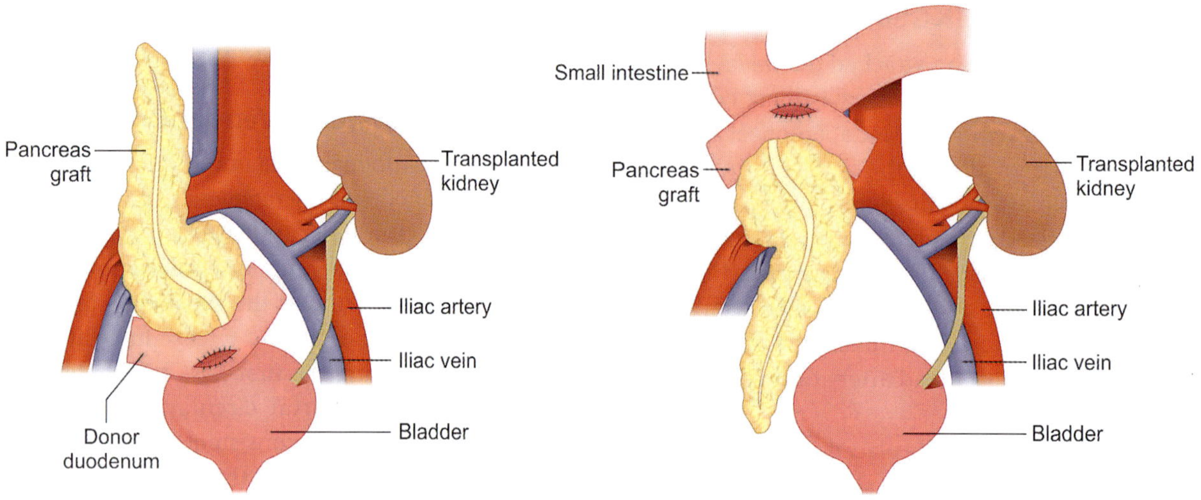

Fig. 1: Bladder and enteric drained pancreas graft.

Pancreas Failure

United Network for Organ Sharing (UNOS) defines pancreas failure as the presence of any one of below criteria:[22-23]

- A recipient's transplanted pancreas is removed.
- A recipient reregisters for a pancreas.
- A recipient registers for an islet transplant after receiving a PT.
- A recipient's insulin use is ≥0.5 units/kg/day for 90 consecutive days.
- A recipient dies.

Early (within the first 3 months) technical failure rate is seen in about 5% for SPK, 5.5% for PAK, and 7% for PTA recipients, as reported in the US. It results in graft loss in 5–8% patients.

Graft vascular thrombosis is the most common cause of early technical failure, accounting for 80% of graft losses seen, and usually, needs a graft pancreatectomy.[24,25] Rest 20% of early graft losses are secondary to infections, pancreatitis, anastomotic leaks, bleeding, and primary nonfunction.

From 3 to 12 months, the most common causes of graft loss are rejection and infections.[24]

Pancreas Graft Thrombosis

Risk of vascular thrombosis in PT is the highest among all solid organ transplants due to an inherently low flow circulation. It is seen in 5–10% of cases. Venous thrombosis is twice as common as arterial. Risk factors include donor age >50, donor hemodynamic instability, obese donor, traumatic graft procurement, technical factors, increased CIT, ischemia-reperfusion injury, postoperative graft pancreatitis, and PTA or PAK transplant.

Clinical presentation includes abdominal pain, tenderness, sudden increase in serum glucose level or increase in insulin requirement, and dark massive hematuria (bladder-drained grafts). Biochemical markers include increased serum amylase/lipase levels and decreased urinary amylase (bladder drained pancreas). Diagnosis is usually confirmed on color Doppler ultrasound. It is an easily available, noninvasive, and less costly investigation. If clinical and Doppler evaluation are suggestive of thrombosis, it should be confirmed with CT angiography. Treatment is often graft pancreatectomy. In nonocclusive or partial thrombosis, anticoagulation or thrombolysis may be tried.

Graft Pancreatitis

Graft pancreatitis is seen in 10–20 % of patients post-PT. Risk factors are ischemia-reperfusion injury, prolonged CIT (>12 hours), hypotension, traumatic graft procurement, reflux associated with bladder drainage, and certain medicines.

Clinical presentation of graft pancreatitis includes abdominal pain, graft tenderness, nausea, vomiting, ileus, or change in bowel habit or hemodynamics. Biochemical markers include elevation of serum amylase and lipase, although the levels correlate poorly with the severity of allograft pancreatitis. A computed tomography (CT) scan with intravenous (IV) contrast of the abdomen should be performed to assess the pancreas and look for signs of inflammation such as graft edema/peripancreatic fluid or necrosis. Management is stopping oral intake and use of supplemental parenteral nutrition. Recurrent pancreatitis secondary to bladder drainage of the pancreas may necessitate conversion to enteric drainage.

Anastomotic Leaks

Leaks can happen at the anastomotic site for drainage of pancreatic exocrine secretions. Presentation includes abdominal pain/tenderness, change in character of abdominal drain, or signs of infection such as tachycardia, fever, hypotension, peritonitis, etc. Biochemical markers include leukocytosis, neutrophilia, thrombocytosis, thrombocytopenia, raised C-reactive protein (CRP), etc. Bladder-drained pancreas leak at the site of duodeno-cystostomy and can be managed conservatively by draining the bladder using the urinary catheter. Enteric drained pancreas leak at the duodeno-enteric anastomosis. These are managed with in situ surgical drains or addition of percutaneous catheter drainage in collections. Broad spectrum antibiotics and antifungals are continued. Peritonitis may necessitate relaparotomy and control of leak or graft takedown.

Bleeding

Bleeding, usually seen in the early postoperative period, is most commonly due to the use of anticoagulation. It may be from the surgical site, pancreatic duct anastomosis, or iliac artery pseudoaneurysms. It is manifested by hematuria in bladder-drained grafts, gastrointestinal bleed in enteric-drained grafts, sanguineous postoperative drains, change in hemodynamics, and fall in hemoglobin levels. CT angiography assists in diagnosis. Management includes supportive blood transfusion, adjusting anticoagulation, endovascular therapies, endoscopy, and bleed control or rarely even relaparotomy.

Metabolic

Metabolic complications are seen commonly with bladder-drained grafts, resulting in acute bicarbonate loss, normal anion gap metabolic acidosis, hyponatremia, and acute dehydration. Refractory metabolic disturbance may require conversion to enteric drainage of the exocrine pancreas.

Infections

Patient has propensity to develop various bacterial, fungal, and viral infections due to the immunosuppressed state. The dominant bacterial flora involved in postoperative infections includes gram-negative bacteria *(Escherichia coli, Klebsiella pneumoniae, and Pseudomonas)* and Group-D streptococci (*Enterococcus faecium* and *Enterococcus faecalis*). Fungal strains include *Candida* species. Abdominal infections can be superficial or deep space, usually as a result of leak/collection. While superficial infections are easily treated, deep-space infections are associated with a high rate of graft loss and increased mortality. Management includes intravenous broad-spectrum antibiotics and percutaneous drainage. Rarely, relaparotomy and even graft pancreatectomy may be required. Bladder-drained grafts have higher risk of UTIs. Late infections can be acquired, opportunistic, *Cytomegalovirus* (CMV)-related, or even BK virus nephropathy in the transplanted kidney.

Rejection

Acute rejection is seen in about 10–12% of cases of SPK/PAK and about 20% of cases of PTA. It can occur any time after the transplant but is most common in the first 3–6 months. Patients can be asymptomatic or present with abdominal pain, fever, tenderness, ileus, or altered bowel function. *The most common presentation is a new elevation in serum amylase and lipase, often in an asymptomatic patient.* The sensitivity of both to detect acute rejection is 70 % and 50%, respectively.[26]

In the case of SPK, rising serum creatinine can be a marker for pancreas rejection since there is a concordance in kidney and pancreas rejection in about 60% of cases. In 20% of cases, there may be isolated rejection of either organ. Elevated fasting glucose, glycosylated hemoglobin, and a decrease in fasting C-peptide level are usually late findings of acute rejection and happen when significant graft destruction has already happened. Also, it lacks specificity as elevated glucose levels can be secondary to medications. A combined interpretation of all these basic blood tests is useful in diagnosing rejection, especially in the asymptomatic patient. Imaging in the form of CT scan can show nonspecific findings of swelling of the pancreas and surrounding fat stranding, but is important to rule out other intra-abdominal pathologies such as leaks, collections, etc. In the case of nonspecific imaging findings, a pancreatic biopsy can be diagnostic, especially for

T-cell-mediated rejection. Antibody-mediated rejection is diagnosed with histopathology in addition to the presence of donor-specific antibodies (DSA) and C4d positivity.

Treatment of borderline biopsy-proven acute rejection is augmenting immunosuppression by increasing dosages of glucocorticoids and tacrolimus in addition to mycophenolate mofetil. Grade I/II/III rejection requires the addition of rabbit antithymocyte globulin (r-ATG).

Outcomes depend upon the severity and time of detection, as well as the promptness and intensity of therapy. Early diagnosis and treatment of pancreas allograft rejection result in the preservation of graft endocrine function.[22,27,28]

Malignancy

This is a late complication as a result of chronic immunosuppressive use. The most common cancers that occur in transplant patients secondary to chronic immunosuppression are skin cancers followed by post-transplant lymphoproliferative disorder (PTLD). Non-Hodgkin lymphoma is the most common PTLD. Treatment of PTLD is effective, especially with the use of rituximab.

CRITICAL CARE MANAGEMENT IN THE INTRAOPERATIVE AND POSTOPERATIVE PERIOD

Pancreas transplant is a technically demanding procedure with critical vascular anastomosis and reconstruction for pancreatic exocrine drainage. Despite undergoing many technical evolutions, it still has one of the highest complication rates for any solid organ transplant.

As discussed, complications unique to PT include a high incidence of early graft failure secondary to vascular thrombosis and postoperative pancreatitis secondary to ischemia–reperfusion injury.

Postoperatively, the patient needs initial management in the intensive care unit (ICU). In the ICU, most patients are extubated within the first 24 hours postsurgery. Pancreas allograft function is monitored closely by measuring both serum and drain fluid amylase, serum lipase, frequent blood glucose charting, and the need for exogenous insulin requirement. Serum creatinine helps monitor the function of graft kidney. Ultrasound color Doppler is performed regularly in the initial days to check for graft vascularity and look for edema/fluid collection around graft. If the graft is difficult to visualize, as in cases of obese individuals or gas over shadowing the graft, a CT abdomen with contrast may be done to rule out thrombosis or allograft pancreatitis.

Instituting optimal fluid therapy, good glycemic control, antibiotic prophylaxis, anticoagulation, and using a carefully balanced induction immunosuppression regimen constitute the corner-stones of critical care management in the postoperative patient.

Fluid Therapy

Intravascular fluid status plays a critical role. While hypovolemia would lead to hypoperfusion and propensity for graft thrombosis, hyperperfusion comes with the perils of tissue edema and problems of anastomotic healing. Optimal fluid and electrolyte balance is must. All patients have central venous monitoring and an arterial line, which is maintained from the intraoperative period. Blood pressure (BP) should be maintained above a systolic pressure of 110 mm Hg, accompanied by a target central venous pressure (CVP) of 8–10 mm Hg. Crystalloid and colloid infusions (including human albumin) should be used to optimize the CVP.

Glycemic Control

Society for Critical Care Medicine recommends maintenance of glucose level below 180 mg/dL for patients in the ICU. Shokouh-Amiri et al.[29] describe the use of insulin infusion (1 I.U/mL) started at a basal rate of 0.2–0.3mL/kg/h to achieve a targeted sugar level of <150 mg/dL in the intraoperative period. Sugar is checked every 2 hours and the drip rate is adjusted accordingly **(Table 2)**. Insulin independence is expected from the time of allograft reperfusion.[29] However, the stress of surgery and use of immunosuppressive medications (steroids/tacrolimus) may result in hyperglycemia and use of supplemental insulin in initial few days. Postoperative monitoring includes checking the blood glucose every 2 hours for the first few days; and use of exogenous insulin, if needed, should be given every 2 hours to maintain euglycemia. Once the steroids are tapered off, the need for supplemental insulin decreases. *A sudden increase in insulin requirement is considered a red flag.* Graft should be evaluated to rule out thrombosis or allograft pancreatitis requiring immediate intervention to prevent graft loss.

Bowel Rest and Antibiotic Prophylaxis

The patient is kept on bowel rest and nasogastric tube drainage till the return of bowel function.

TABLE 2: Blood glucose level and corresponding titration of the insulin drip.

Blood glucose (mg/dL)	*Infusion rate*
<50	Stop insulin
50–75	Decrease drip by 50%
75–100	Decrease drip by 25%
100–150	No change
150–175	Increase rate 2 mL/h
175–200	Increase rate 4 mL/h
200–225	Increase rate 6 mL/h
225–250	Increase rate 8 mL/h + check ketones

In bladder-drained allografts, the Foley catheter is kept in situ for 10–14 days. In enteric drained grafts, the abdominal drain is kept till one is reasonably sure of healing at the duodenojejunostomy anastomotic site.

Most units give some form of prophylactic broad-spectrum antibacterial, antifungal, and antiviral (CMV) prophylaxis in the initial postoperative period when immunosuppression is highest and the patient is recovering from surgical stress. CMV positive donor and CMV negative recipient are independent risk factors for CMV infection and need prophylaxis with ganciclovir/valganciclovir.

Anticoagulation

Graft thrombosis is a dreaded complication, often resulting in early graft loss. The inherent hypercoagulable state of diabetics, coupled with low flow system of pancreas allograft, contribute to increased risk. Hence, most units use some form of anticoagulation in the postoperative period. The choice, dose, and duration of anticoagulant is variable, often finely balancing the risk of thrombosis and postoperative bleeding. Common regimens include the use of low-molecular-weight heparin (dalteparin and enoxaparin) or infusion of unfractionated heparin titrated to target activated partial thromboplastin time (APTT) of 60–70 seconds. At discharge, patient may be switched to aspirin 75 mg a day for up to 3–6 months depending on risk assessment.

Immunosuppression

Induction therapy is intravenous methylprednisolone (10 mg/kg) bolus along with T cell-depleting agent [either rabbit antithymocyte globulin (rATG)-thymoglobulin or alemtuzumab]. In high-risk cases, a nondepleting interleukin-2 (IL2) receptor antagonist can be used. *Maintenance therapy* includes the use of a calcineurin inhibitor (tacrolimus > cyclosporine), an antimetabolite (mycophenolate mofetil > azathioprine), and tapering doses of glucocorticoids. Regular monitoring of tacrolimus or cyclosporine level is done to maintain it in the therapeutic range. Owing to the higher immunogenicity of the pancreas, PAK transplant patients need higher levels of immunosuppression than they were previously on.

Rejection episodes are identified by an increase in serum creatinine (in SPK recipients), a decrease in urinary amylase (in recipients with bladder drainage), an increase in serum amylase, and in the later stages, an increase in serum glucose levels. In cases where a kidney transplant biopsy would not be helpful (PAK or PTA), a percutaneous/endoscopic biopsy of the pancreas can be obtained under ultrasound or CT guidance or via cystoscopy in bladder-drained allografts.

A fine balance must be maintained with regards to immunosuppression to protect the graft against rejection as well as to prevent life-threatening infections due to excessive immunosuppression in the postoperative patient.

OUTCOMES

Unadjusted 5-year pancreas graft survival are 71% (SPK), 65% (PAK), and 58% (PTA),[7] respectively. More recently, 10-year actual insulin independence rates have been reported to exceed 80% in SPK and 60% in PTA.[8,9]

Five-year patient survival rates for PAK, PTA, and SPK are 88.6%, 94.6%, and 92.7%, respectively.[30] PTA recipients have the best patient survival of the three groups, presumably due to the lack of significant renal insufficiency in this group. 5-year survival rates for pancreas recipients with T1DM and T2DM are comparable at 92.7% and 91.6%, respectively.[30]

Outcomes for kidney allografts after SPK are outstanding, with 1-, 5-, and 10-year all-cause kidney failure at 4.2%, 13.2%, and 33.4%, respectively.[30] Long-term kidney allograft success rate after PAK with a deceased donor kidney are also good, with 1-, 5-, and 10-year all-cause kidney graft failure of 2.4%, 13.1%, and 38.1%.[30]

Patient mortality remained low for all categories of PT recipients at 1 year, at 3.5%, 1.8%, and 2.6% for PAK, PTA, and SPK, respectively, for transplants performed in 2018-19.[30] 10-year mortality rates among 2010-11 transplant recipients were 20.3%, 17.5%, and 20.9% for PAK, PTA, and SPK, respectively, likely reflecting cardiovascular comorbidities in the population.[5]

Restoration of normoglycemia after PT has also shown to have beneficial effects on long-term complications of DM. Retinal lesions in diabetic retinopathy have shown stabilization and delay in progression in presence of a normally functioning graft.[31] In SPK, normoglycemia protects the new graft from nephropathy. Peripheral and autonomic neuropathies improve or stabilize in most PT recipients. This is demonstrated by improvements in nerve conduction velocity, gastric function, cardiac function, and a beneficial effect on microcirculatory blood flow.[29]

CONCLUSION

Pancreas transplant is a worthy option for the treatment of beta-cell penic diabetes, especially as a dual organ transplant (SPK) in uremic patients in whom it should be performed preemptively rather than late for best results.[13] In patients with stable renal function post kidney transplant, PT (PAK) can be considered with the expected benefits of insulin-free life as well as delayed progression of secondary diabetic complications. PTA is an option in a cohort of diabetic patients suffering from recurrent life-threatening complications of brittle diabetes and hypoglycemia unawareness, albeit at the cost of some deterioration of renal function in the long run due to the use of chronic immunosuppression.

REFERENCES

1. Singh A, Afshan N, Singh A, Singh SK, Yadav S, Kumar M, et al. Recent trends and advances in type 1 diabetes therapeutics: A comprehensive review. Eur J Cell Biol. 2023;102(2):151329.
2. Kandaswamy R, Stock PG, Miller J, White J, Booker SE, Israni AK, et al. OPTN/SRTR 2020 Annual Data Report: Pancreas. Am J Transplant. 2022;22 Suppl 2:137-203.
3. Organ Procurement and Transplantation Network. (2025). Policies. [online] Available from https://optn.transplant.hrsa.gov/media/eavh5bf3/optn_policies.pdf.
4. Robertson RP, Davis C, Larsen J, Stratta R, Sutherland DE; American Diabetes Association. Pancreas and islet transplantation in type 1 diabetes. Diabetes Care. 2006; 29(4):935.
5. Tydén G, Tollemar J, Bolinder J. Combined pancreas and kidney transplantation improves survival in patients with end-stage diabetic nephropathy. Clin Transplant. 2000; 14(5):505-8.
6. Ojo AO, Meier-Kriesche HU, Hanson JA, Leichtman A, Magee JC, Cibrik D, et al. The impact of simultaneous pancreas-kidney transplantation on long-term patient survival. Transplantation. 2001;71(1):82-90.
7. Gruessner AC, Gruessner RW. Pancreas transplant outcomes for United States and non-United States cases as reported to the United Network for Organ Sharing and the International Pancreas Transplant Registry as of December 2011. Clin Transpl. 2012:23-40.
8. Marchetti P, Occhipinti M, Rondinini L, Mariotti R, Amorese G, Barsotti M, et al. Metabolic and cardiovascular effects of beta cell replacement in type 1 diabetes. Intern Emerg Med. 2013;8 Suppl 1:S55-6.
9. Boggi U, Vistoli F, Amorese G, Giannarelli R, Coppelli A, Mariotti R, et al. Long-term (5 years) efficacy and safety of pancreas transplantation alone in type 1 diabetic patients. Transplantation. 2012;93(8):842-6.
10. Organ Procurement and Transplantation Network. (2018). Policies. Changes to waiting time criteria for kidney pancreas candidates. [online] Available from https://optn.transplant.hrsa.gov/policies-bylaws/public-comment/changes-to-waiting-time-criteria-for-kidney-pancreas-candidates.
11. NHSBT. (2024). Pancreas Transplantation. Patient Selection Policy 185/6. [online] Available from https://nhsbtdbe.blob.core.windows.net/umbraco-assets-corp/17326/pancreas-selection-policy-pol185.pdf
12. Kim SJ, Smail N, Paraskevas S, Schiff J, Cantarovich M. Kidney function before pancreas transplant alone predicts subsequent risk of end-stage renal disease. Transplantation. 2014;97(6):675-80.
13. Boggi U, Vistoli F, Egidi FM, Marchetti P, De Lio N, Perrone V, et al. Transplantation of the pancreas. Curr Diab Rep. 2012;12(5):568-79.
14. Stratta RJ, Taylor RJ, Wahl TO, Duckworth WC, Gallagher TF, Knight TF, et al. Recipient selection and evaluation for vascularized pancreas transplantation. Transplantation. 1993;55(5):1090-6.
15. Stratta RJ, Farney AC, Orlando G, Rogers J. Pancreas Transplantation for Type 2 Diabetes Mellitus: Who and Why? Curr Transpl Rep. 2015;2:149-58.
16. Fridell JA, Shah A, Milgrom ML, Goggins WC, Leapman SB, Pescovitz MD. Ipsilateral placement of simultaneous pancreas and kidney allografts. Transplantation. 2004; 78(7):1074-6.
17. Rudolph EN, Dunn TB, Sutherland DER, Kandaswamy R, Finger EB. Optimizing outcomes in pancreas transplantation: Impact of organ preservation time. Clin Transplant. 2017;31(9).
18. Yin H, Arpali E, Leverson GE, Sollinger HW, Kaufman DB, Odorico JS. Ipsilateral versus contralateral placement of the pancreas allograft in pancreas after kidney transplant recipients. Clin Transplant. 2018;32(8):e13337.
19. Petruzzo P, Laville M, Badet L, Lefrançois N, Bin-Dorel S, Chapuis F, et al. Effect of venous drainage site on insulin

action after simultaneous pancreas-kidney transplantation. Transplantation. 2004;77(12):1875-9.

20. Gruessner RW, Sutherland DE, Gruessner AC. Mortality assessment for pancreas transplants. Am J Transplant. 2004;4(12):2018-26.
21. Gruessner AC, Gruessner RW. Pancreas transplantation of US and Non-US Cases from 2005 to 2014 as Reported to the United Network for Organ Sharing (UNOS) and the International Pancreas Transplant Registry (IPTR). Rev Diabet Stud. 2016;13(1):35-58.
22. OPTN/UNOS Pancreas Transplantation Committee. (2015). Definition of Pancreas Graft Failure. [online] Available from https://optn.trans plant.hrsa.gov/media/1572/policynotice_20150 701_pancreas.pdf.
23. Stratta RJ, Farney AC, Fridell JA. Analyzing outcomes following pancreas transplantation: Definition of a failure or failure of a definition. Am J Transplant. 2022;22:1523-6.
24. Grochowiecki T, Gałązka Z, Madej K, Frunze S, Nazarewski S, Jakimowicz T, et al. Multivariate analysis of complications after simultaneous pancreas and kidney transplantation. Transplant Proc. 2014;46(8):2806-9.
25. Manrique A, Jiménez C, López RM, Cambra F, Morales JM, Andrés A, et al. Relaparotomy after pancreas transplantation: Causes and outcomes. Transplant Proc. 2009; 41(6):2472-4.
26. Sugitani A, Egidi MF, Gritsch HA, Corry RJ. Serum lipase as a marker for pancreatic allograft rejection. Clin Transplant. 1998;12(3):224-7.
27. Gruessner AC, Sutherland DE. Pancreas transplant outcomes for United States (US) and non-US cases as reported to the United Network for Organ Sharing (UNOS) and the International Pancreas Transplant Registry (IPTR) as of June 2004. Clin Transplant. 2005;19(4):433-55.
28. Morel P, Brayman KL, Goetz FC, Kendall DM, Moudry-Munns K, Chau C, et al. Long-term metabolic function of pancreas transplants and influence of rejection episodes. Transplantation. 1991;51(5):990-1000.
29. Shokouh-Amiri MH, Stratta RJ, Latif KA, Gaber O. Glucose control during and after pancreatic transplantation. Diabetes Spectr. 2002;15(1):49-53.
30. HRSA. (2020). OPTN/SRTR 2020 Annual Data Report: Pancreas. [online] Available from https://srtr.transplant.hrsa.gov/annual_reports/2020/Pancreas.aspx.
31. Lombardo C, Perrone VG, Amorese G, Vistoli F, Baronti W, Marchetti P, et al. Update on pancreatic transplantation in the management of diabetes. In: Feingold KR, Ahmed SF, Anawalt B, et al., editors. Endotext [Internet]. South Dartmouth (MA): MDText.com, Inc.; 2021. Available from: https://www.ncbi.nlm.nih.gov/books/NBK278979/.

CHAPTER 6

Intestinal Transplantation

Hirak Pahari, Shikhar Tripathi, Samiran Nundy

INTRODUCTION

Intestinal transplantation (ITx), over the past few decades, has risen as a pivotal treatment modality over the past few decades, offering a life-saving option to patients suffering from irreversible intestinal failure (IF). This procedure is particularly critical for cases where severe sequelae and complications develop in patients who have underwent long-term parenteral nutrition (PN), such as intestinal failure-associated liver disease (IFALD), recurrent central venous catheter infections, or loss of central venous access.[1] Additionally, factors such as recurrent sepsis, thrombosis of the central veins, and severe liver disease heighten the risk.[2] What is to be marked here is that it is crucial to identify and manage these risk factors at an earlier stage to prevent the progression to end-stage IF and the subsequent need for transplantation.[3]

The evolution of ITx into a standard treatment for specific cases, traversing through the junction of being an experimental procedure, is a testament to the advancements in medical and surgical management.

The incidence of IF requiring ITx is relatively low compared to other forms of organ failure, such as kidney or liver failure. This is partly due to the rarity of conditions that lead to end-stage IF. These conditions include short bowel syndrome, chronic intestinal pseudo-obstruction, and congenital abnormalities such as gastroschisis and volvulus, which are more common in pediatric populations. In adults, IF is often the result of Crohn's disease, ischemic bowel disease, or complications from surgeries for desmoid tumors or radiation enteritis.[4,5] In contrast, pediatric cases are more commonly due to congenital conditions such as gastroschisis, volvulus, and necrotizing enterocolitis.[6] Short bowel syndrome, often resulting from extensive surgical resection, is the leading cause of IF in both adults and children, accounting for approximately 68% of ITx cases.[7]

The demand for ITx has been increasing, driven by several factors. Advances in the management of IF with PN have improved survival rates, allowing more patients to live longer with PN. However, as these patients survive longer on PN, they are at increased risk of developing life-threatening complications that make ITx necessary. Additionally, improvements in surgical techniques and postoperative care, including better immunosuppression regimens, have contributed to increased patient and graft survival, making ITx a more viable option.[8]

Despite these advancements, the global number of ITx procedures remains relatively limited. Due to the complex nature of the post-transplant complications and their management and the need for lifelong commitment from the recipient and their social support, most centers opt for transplant as the final option in a cascade of treatment options ranging from intravenous hydration, total parenteral nutrition (TPN), partial PN, teduglutide, and bowel lengthening procedures. There is also a limitation due to the scarcity of suitable donor organs and the complexity of the surgical procedure itself in certain cases with a prior surgical history. Donor availability is a major bottleneck, with many patients on waiting lists for extended periods before a suitable match is found. Moreover, the high level of expertise required to perform ITx and manage postoperative care restricts the procedure to specialized centers, predominantly in developed countries. As a result, there are regional variations in the availability and outcomes of ITx, reflecting disparities in healthcare infrastructure, the prevalence of IF, and access to specialized care.[9]

These regional disparities are particularly evident when comparing ITx data from developed and developing countries. In regions with well-established organ transplant programs, such as North America and Europe, ITx is more frequently performed, and outcomes tend to be better due to the availability of multidisciplinary teams and advanced postoperative care. In contrast, in many developing countries, the procedure is less accessible, with the most integral factor being lack of organ donation, for instance, in India, the National Organ and Tissue Transplant Organization (NOTTO), India, reported just 22 cases of ITx between 2013 and 2022.[7,10]

Efforts to increase awareness and improve access to ITx in underrepresented regions are ongoing. These include initiatives to enhance organ donation rates, train healthcare professionals in transplant surgery, and establish more specialized transplant centers globally. However, overcoming these challenges requires a coordinated effort involving policy changes, investment in healthcare infrastructure, and international collaboration.

PATIENT SELECTION

Indications for ITx primarily involve patients with irreversible IF who have developed life-threatening complications from long-term PN. The most common indications include IFALD, frequent and severe catheter-related sepsis, loss of central venous access, and severe dehydration despite aggressive management.[4] Additionally, poor quality of life (QoL) resulting from chronic dependence on PN and frequent hospitalizations are increasingly considered when evaluating candidates for ITx. Recent studies have shown that ITx can significantly improve QoL in patients with these severe complications, making it an important factor in patient selection.[5] **Table 1** categorizes pediatric and adult indications for ITx.

The contraindications for ITx include the presence of significant comorbidities that would preclude the patient from tolerating major surgery and long-term immunosuppression. Active, uncontrolled infections or malignancies that cannot be fully resected during the transplant process are also contraindications.[11] Other considerations include psychosocial factors, such as the lack of a strong postoperative support network, which are critical for the success of post-transplant care. Anatomical challenges, such as extensive thrombosis of the inferior vena cava (IVC) or portal vein, can complicate the transplant procedure and are considered relative contraindications.[12] Opiate dependence is also common in these patients, and early rehabilitation should be considered to optimize outcomes.[13]

In India, the guidelines for organ transplantation, including ITx, are governed by the Transplantation of Human Organs and Tissues Act (THOTA) of 1994, which provide the legal framework for organ donation in India, including the recognition of brain death.[14] According to these guidelines, patient selection for ITx must adhere to strict criteria, ensuring that candidates have exhausted all other treatment options and that the benefits of transplantation outweigh the risks.[15] Additionally, the donor selection process must comply with stringent regulations to ensure that the organs are sourced ethically and safely. **Table 2** summarizes the NOTTO criteria for donor selection for ITx.

Donor evaluation for ITx involves a comprehensive assessment to ensure the donor organ's suitability and compatibility with the recipient. Factors such as donor age (if a living donor), blood type, and tissue matching are critical considerations. Donors must be free from transmissible infections and have no history

TABLE 1: Indications for ITx or MVTx.

Adult	*Pediatric*
Crohn's disease	Intestinal atresia
Superior mesenteric artery thrombosis	Gastroschisis
Diffuse portomesenteric thrombosis	Crohn's disease
Trauma	Microvillus involution disease
Desmoid or neuroendocrine tumors	Necrotizing enterocolitis
Volvulus	Midgut volvulus
Chronic intestinal pseudo-obstruction	Chronic intestinal pseudo-obstruction
Massive resection secondary to tumors	Massive resection secondary to tumors
Radiation enteritis	Hirschsprung disease

(ITx: intestinal transplantation; MVTx: multivisceral transplant)

TABLE 2: NOTTO criteria for deceased and living donor ITx.

Deceased donor	*Living donor*
Blood group compatible	Blood group compatible
Age <45 years	Age <50 years
Minimal inotropic requirement	Complement-dependent cytotoxicity and flow crossmatch negative
Negative blood cultures	
Complement-dependent cytotoxicity and flow crossmatch negative	
The donor weight should be 20% less than recipient weight	

(ITx: intestinal transplantation; NOTTO: National Organ and Tissue Transplant Organization)

of malignancies that could compromise the recipient's health post-transplant.[8] Additionally, the anatomical suitability of the donor intestine is evaluated to ensure a successful transplantation procedure. Recent advances in donor management, including the use of extended criteria donors, have expanded the pool of available organs, although they come with increased risks.[7]

Graft selection in ITx is a critical decision that hinges on the underlying cause of IF and the overall condition of the patient's native organs. The type of graft selected directly impacts the surgical approach, potential complications, and the long-term outcomes for the patient. The three primary graft types used in ITx are—(1) isolated intestinal transplant, (2) combined liver–intestine transplant (CLITx), and (3) multivisceral transplant (MVTx). Each has specific indications based on the extent of organ failure and the presence of other systemic conditions. **Flowchart 1** summarizes the decision-making process for graft selection in ITx.

Isolated intestinal transplantation (IITx) is indicated for patients with irreversible IF who do not exhibit significant liver disease. This option is typically preferred when the patient's liver function is preserved, making it unnecessary to transplant additional organs. Isolated intestinal transplants involve only the small intestine and are most commonly performed in cases where the underlying cause of IF is limited to the gastrointestinal (GI) tract, such as short bowel syndrome or chronic intestinal pseudo-obstruction. The procedure involves anastomosing the donor intestine to the recipient's mesenteric vessels, with the reestablishment of continuity between the graft and the recipient's GI tract. This type of graft is associated with a relatively high 1-year survival rate, particularly in specialized centers with extensive experience in ITx.[16]

Combined liver–intestine transplant is recommended for patients who suffer from both IF and significant liver disease (IFALD). This approach addresses the dual organ failure by transplanting both the liver and small intestine *en bloc*, which has been shown to improve overall outcomes and survival rates compared to isolated intestinal transplants in this patient population. The combined graft is particularly beneficial in reducing the immunogenicity of the transplant, as the liver is believed to exert a protective effect on the intestine, potentially lowering the risk of rejection.[17] This procedure is more complex than IITx, involving multiple anastomoses and the careful management of both hepatic and intestinal vascular structures.

Multivisceral transplant is indicated for patients with extensive abdominal organ failure, including the stomach, pancreas, liver, and small intestine. This procedure is generally reserved for patients with multiple organ failures, such as those with Gardner's syndrome, extensive desmoid tumors, or mesenteric vascular thrombosis leading to widespread abdominal ischemia. MVTx involves the *en bloc* transplantation of all the affected organs and requires a highly coordinated surgical approach to reestablish the necessary vascular and biliary connections.[4] MVTx offers

Flowchart 1: Summary of decision making in graft selection for ITx.

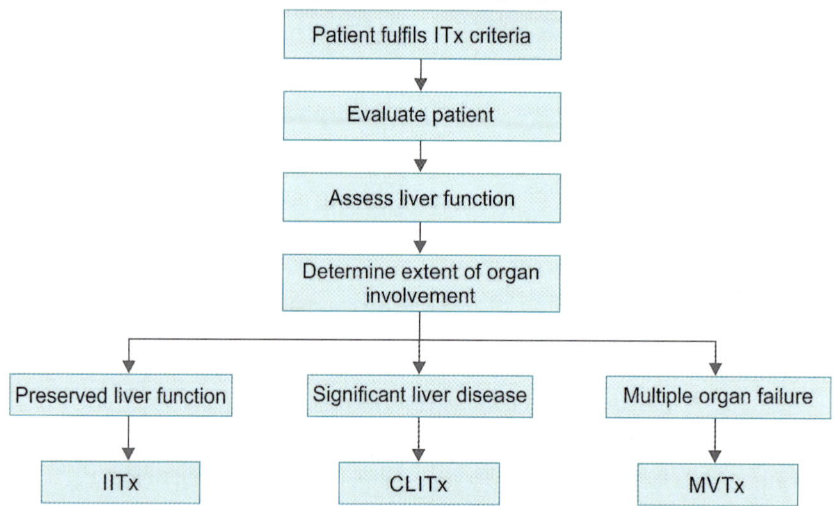

(CLITx: combined liver-intestine transplant; IITx: isolated intestinal transplantation; ITx: intestinal transplantation; MVTx: multivisceral transplant)

a lifesaving option for patients with complex conditions that cannot be managed with less extensive grafts. The survival rates for MVTx have improved significantly in recent years due to advances in surgical techniques, better immunosuppressive protocols, and enhanced postoperative care, with approximately 70% of recipients surviving at 1 year in high-volume centers.[18]

SURGICAL PROCEDURES

Isolated Intestinal Transplantation

The surgical approach for IITx begins with a midline laparotomy, which provides optimal exposure to the abdominal cavity. The donor's small intestine is perfused with a cold preservation solution, most commonly the University of Wisconsin (UW) solution, to reduce ischemic injury and prolong graft viability during the surgical process.[11] The small intestine is then carefully removed and flushed with the preservation solution to prepare it for transplantation.

The vascular anastomoses are crucial and typically involve connecting the donor's superior mesenteric artery (SMA) to the recipient's SMA or aorta, depending on the recipient's vascular anatomy **(Fig. 1A)**. The venous outflow is typically managed by anastomosing the donor's portal vein to the recipient's portal vein or IVC, ensuring adequate venous drainage and reducing the risk of venous thrombosis **(Fig. 1B)**.[8] The continuity of the GI tract is restored by performing an anastomosis between the donor intestine and the recipient's native GI tract both proximally and distally, often involving the jejunum and ileum of the donor graft respectively. A short segment of the Donor colon may sometimes be used to preserve the ileocolic valve function.

To facilitate postoperative monitoring and manage potential complications, a temporary stoma, preferably a chimney or loop ostomy, is frequently created. An end ostomy is used when the distal native bowel is not available for reconstruction. This allows for easy access to the graft for surveillance and biopsy, which are essential for early detection of rejection and other complications.[7]

The outcomes of IITx have improved significantly with advances in surgical techniques and immunosuppression protocols. However, the success of the procedure is highly dependent on meticulous surgical execution and postoperative management. 1-year survival rates for IITx are generally favorable, particularly in experienced transplant centers, with outcomes closely tied to the volume and expertise of the surgical team.[4] Early referral to a specialized transplant center is recommended to optimize outcomes, particularly for patients with rapidly progressing disease or severe TPN-related complications.

Combined Liver–Intestine Transplantation

In cases where the patient has concomitant liver disease, particularly IFALD, a CLITx is indicated. This complex procedure addresses both liver and IF, offering a comprehensive solution for patients at high risk of mortality due to dual organ failure.

The procedure begins with a midline incision to access the abdominal cavity. The donor organs, including the liver and small intestine, are perfused with a cold preservation solution and then excised *en bloc*. After preparing the recipient's abdomen by removing the native liver and

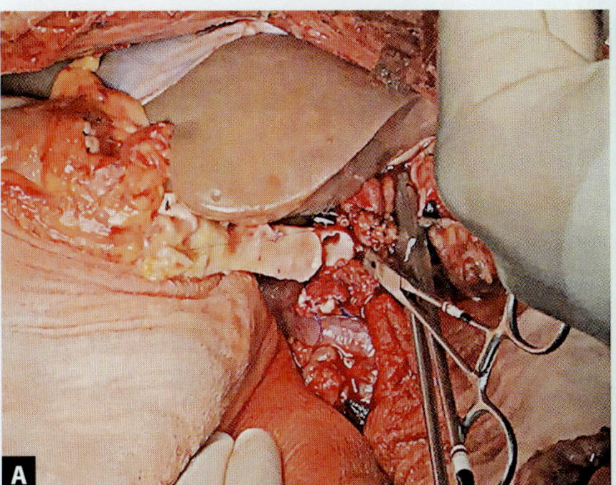

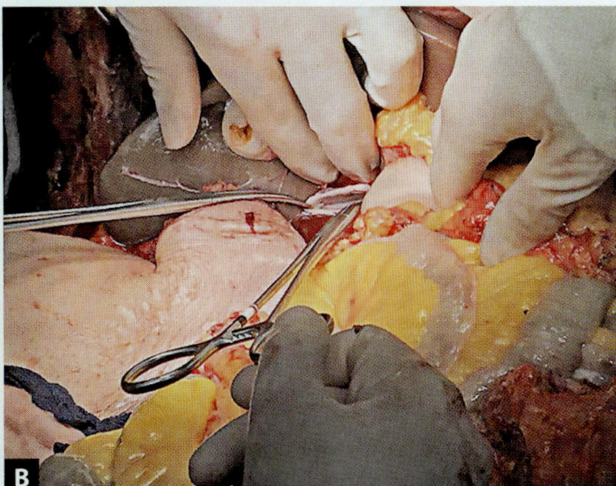

Figs. 1A and B: (A) Anastomosis of donor SMA extension to graft extension from supraceliac aorta for an isolated intestinal graft. (B) Venous anastomosis from donor SMV to recipient SMV. (SMA: superior mesenteric artery; SMV: superior mesenteric vein)

intestines, the transplant surgeon begins with the vascular anastomoses. The hepatic vein (or IVC) and aorta of the donor including both celiac artery and SMA are connected to the recipient's IVC and aorta respectively, ensuring the proper blood supply to the liver and intestinal graft.[19]

The biliary reconstruction is a critical step in CLITx, with a duct-to-duct anastomosis often performed if the recipient's bile duct is intact. In cases where the bile duct is compromised, a Roux-en-Y hepaticojejunostomy is performed to ensure adequate bile drainage.[18] Following vascular and biliary anastomoses, the small intestine is connected to the GI tract to restore continuity.

The CLITx is associated with improved outcomes for patients with IFALD compared to isolated intestinal transplants, due in part to the protective immunological effect the liver graft has on the intestine, which may reduce the risk of acute rejection.[17] However, the procedure is technically demanding, requiring a highly experienced surgical team and a multidisciplinary approach to manage the complex postoperative care.

Multivisceral Transplantation

The operation for MVTx begins with a wide midline incision to allow complete access to the abdominal cavity. The donor's abdominal organs, typically including the stomach, duodenum, pancreas, liver, and small intestine, are harvested *en bloc* and perfused with a preservation solution to maintain viability during the complex surgical process **(Figs. 2A and B)**.[20]

The recipient's native organs are then removed, and the donor graft is positioned within the abdominal cavity. Vascular anastomoses are performed with the donor's aorta connected to the recipient's aorta, and the donor's IVC connected to the recipient's IVC. This ensures adequate arterial inflow and venous outflow for all the transplanted organs.[4] The GI continuity is restored by anastomosing the donor stomach and intestines to the recipient's GI tract, often involving a series of complex anastomoses to reestablish the digestive pathway. A pyloroplasty must be performed if the donor stomach is used.

In cases where the pancreas and spleen are involved with disease or where complete replacement of abdominal organs is necessary, a full MVTx with splenectomy and pancreatectomy is performed. This approach is essential in patients with extensive malignancies or severe pancreatitis affecting these organs.[21] However, in certain cases, especially when pancreatic function is preserved and there are no tumors involving the pancreas or spleen, a MVTx can be performed that spares these native organs. The preservation of the spleen and pancreas can reduce surgical complexity and postoperative complications, particularly those related to pancreatic leaks and infections.[22,23]

Multivisceral transplant is a lifesaving procedure for patients with extensive organ involvement, but it carries significant risks due to the complexity of the surgery and the potential for postoperative complications. Nevertheless, survival rates have improved significantly with advances in surgical techniques and immunosuppression, with high-volume centers reporting 1-year survival rates of

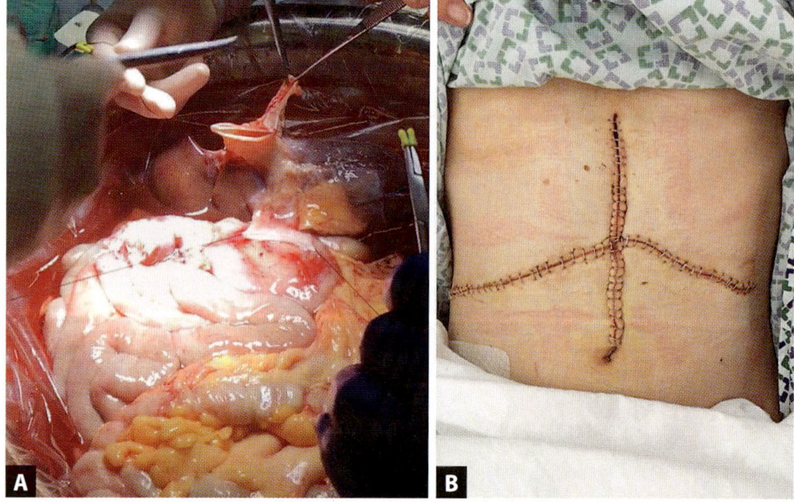

Figs. 2A and B: (A) A multivisceral graft including liver, pancreas, stomach, and small bowel, with donor IVC being prepared on the back table. (B) Incision for a MVTx. (IVC: inferior vena cava; MVTx: multivisceral transplant)

around 70%.[24] The success of MVTx is closely linked to the surgical expertise of the transplant team and the comprehensive management of postoperative care, including vigilant monitoring for rejection and infections.

Figure 3 describes the various surgical procedures and **Table 3** summarizes the indications for the surgical procedures along with their considerations.

Other composite grafts including the intestine, which are rarely used for transplantation, include modified multivisceral grafts (without the liver), pancreas and intestinal grafts, intestine and kidney transplantation, stomach-sparing multivisceral graft, etc. The exact requirement depends on the recipient's needs and the feasibility and complexity of the surgical procedure involved.

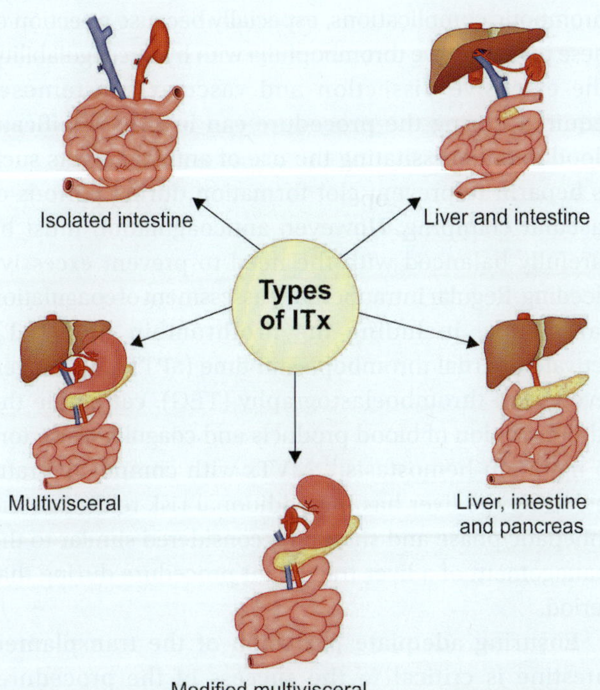

Fig. 3: Surgical procedures for ITx. (ITx: intestinal transplantation)

Living Donor Intestinal Transplant

The living donor intestinal transplant (LDIT) is less common but represents an important option, especially in regions with limited access to deceased donor organs. The donor, typically a close relative, undergoes extensive preoperative evaluation to ensure suitability. The surgical procedure involves resecting a portion of the donor's small intestine, usually the ileum based on the ileocolic vessels, which is then transplanted into the recipient. The operation for the recipient follows the same principles as deceased donor transplants, with careful vascular and GI anastomoses.[25] Living donor transplants carry the benefit of reduced cold ischemia time but require a rigorous selection process to minimize donor risk.[6] In India, the first LDIT was reported in 2012, which was performed using 200 cm of small intestine graft that was based on the continuation of the superior mesenteric vessels beyond the ileocolic branch.[26]

Surgical Challenges

Surgical challenges in ITx are numerous and include managing previous abdominal operations, which often result in extensive adhesions, increasing the difficulty of the procedure. Vascular complications, such as thrombosis or narrowing of the anastomoses, are significant risks that require careful intraoperative assessment and immediate intervention if detected.[12] Postoperative complications, such as leaks at the anastomotic sites, are also a concern and necessitate close postoperative monitoring and early intervention if complications arise.[13] Additionally, the risk of rejection remains high, particularly in the early postoperative period, making vigilant monitoring and prompt treatment of any signs of rejection crucial.[4] Yet, another challenge that persists, especially in adult patients, due to "loss of domain", is abdominal wall closure, where the abdominal contents exceed the capacity of the abdominal cavity, making closure without tension difficult.

TABLE 3: Summary of surgical procedures.

Surgical procedure	*Indication*	*Procedure*	*Consideration*
Isolated intestinal transplant	IF without liver disease	Small intestine transplant with vascular and gastrointestinal anastomoses	Temporary stoma for postoperative surveillance
Combined liver–intestine transplant	IF with significant liver disease	*En bloc* liver and intestine transplant with vascular and biliary anastomoses	Complex procedure, improved survival with dual graft
Multivisceral transplant	Failure of multiple abdominal organs	*En bloc* transplantation of stomach, pancreas, liver, and small intestine	High complexity, requires extensive surgical expertise

(IF: intestinal failure)

This situation often arises following multiple surgeries or in cases with large grafts, leading to an increased risk of wound dehiscence and hernias. In pediatric recipients, the small abdominal cavity presents a different challenge, with limited space to accommodate the transplanted graft without compromising organ perfusion or function. Techniques such as component separation, use of biological meshes, or staged closure may be required to achieve optimal outcomes. In select cases, especially where significant abdominal wall defects exist or when primary closure is not feasible due to loss of domain or infection, an associated abdominal wall transplant may be performed alongside ITx.[27] This procedure involves transplanting a segment of the donor's abdominal wall to provide adequate coverage and support for the transplanted organs, preventing complications such as herniation and infection. This approach is particularly beneficial in patients with extensive previous surgeries or those with large grafts requiring additional space and protection, ultimately improving the overall success and functionality of the transplantation.

Intraoperative Management

Intraoperative management during ITx is a critical component that significantly influences the surgical outcome and long-term success of the procedure. Given the complexity and risks associated with ITx, intraoperative care requires a highly coordinated, multidisciplinary approach that includes surgeons, anesthesiologists, perfusionists, and nursing staff. The main goals during the operation are to maintain stable hemodynamics, ensure adequate perfusion to the transplanted organs, manage fluid and electrolyte balance, and prevent complications such as coagulopathy, hypothermia, and excessive blood loss.

Maintaining stable hemodynamics is paramount during ITx due to the extensive nature of the surgery, which often involves major vascular manipulation and significant fluid shifts. Continuous monitoring of blood pressure, heart rate, central venous pressure (CVP), and cardiac output is essential. Advanced monitoring techniques, such as the use of pulmonary artery catheters or transesophageal echocardiography (TEE), can provide real-time data on cardiac function and fluid status, allowing for precise adjustments in fluid administration and the use of vasoactive medications as needed.[28] Blood products, including packed red blood cells, fresh frozen plasma, and platelets, should be readily available to manage intraoperative hemorrhage and maintain adequate oxygen delivery to tissues.

The management of fluids and electrolytes is another crucial aspect of intraoperative care. Given the potential for significant blood loss and fluid shifts, careful administration of crystalloids, colloids, and blood products is necessary to maintain intravascular volume and prevent hypovolemia. Intraoperative monitoring of electrolytes is essential to prevent arrhythmias and other complications.[20] Additionally, the use of goal-directed fluid therapy, which tailors fluid administration based on dynamic parameters such as stroke volume variation, can optimize tissue perfusion and reduce the risk of complications related to fluid overload or deficit.

Coagulation status must be meticulously monitored during ITx due to the high risk of both bleeding and thrombotic complications, especially because a section of these patients have thrombophilia with hypercoagulability. The extensive dissection and vascular anastomoses required during the procedure can lead to significant blood loss, necessitating the use of anticoagulants such as heparin to prevent clot formation during periods of vascular clamping. However, anticoagulation must be carefully balanced with the need to prevent excessive bleeding. Regular intraoperative assessment of coagulation parameters, including the prothrombin time (PT), activated partial thromboplastin time (aPTT), fibrinogen levels, and thromboelastography (TEG), can guide the administration of blood products and coagulation factors to maintain hemostasis.[11] MVTx with composite grafts including the liver has the additional risk related to the anhepatic phase and should be considered similar to the management of a liver transplant procedure during that period.

Ensuring adequate perfusion of the transplanted intestine is critical to the success of the procedure. Intraoperative Doppler ultrasound is commonly used to assess the patency of vascular anastomoses and confirm blood flow through the graft. This real-time imaging allows the surgical team to detect any vascular complications, such as thrombosis or kinking of vessels, which can be promptly addressed to prevent graft ischemia.[16] In some centers, near-infrared spectroscopy (NIRS) or intraoperative indocyanine green (ICG) angiography may also be employed to evaluate graft perfusion and guide surgical decisions.[24]

Hypothermia is a common concern during lengthy surgeries such as ITx and can lead to coagulopathy,

TABLE 4: Standard immunosuppressive agents used in ITx.

Agent	*Mechanism of action*	*Indication*	*Side effects*
Tacrolimus (CNI)	Inhibits T-cell activation	First-line for preventing acute rejection	Nephrotoxicity, hyperglycemia, neurotoxicity
Mycophenolate mofetil (MMF)	Inhibits lymphocyte proliferation	Combined with CNI to prevent rejection	Gastrointestinal upset, myelosuppression
Corticosteroids	Broad immunosuppression and anti-inflammatory	Early post-transplant, gradually tapered	Hyperglycemia, hypertension, osteoporosis
Antithymocyte globulin (induction)	Polyclonal antibody	Induction in high-risk patients	Profound lymphopenia, increased infection risk
Basiliximab (induction)	Blocks IL-2 receptor on activated T-cells	Induction therapy to reduce early rejection	Infusion reactions, hypersensitivity
Alemtuzumab (induction)	Depletes T- and B-lymphocytes	Induction in high-risk patients	Profound lymphopenia, increased infection risk

(CNI: calcineurin inhibitor; IL-2: interleukin-2; ITx: intestinal transplantation)

increased blood loss, and delayed wound healing. Active warming techniques, including the use of forced-air warming blankets, warmed intravenous fluids, and warming devices for the abdominal cavity, are employed to maintain normothermia throughout the procedure. Thorough irrigation of the abdominal cavity with warm saline before closure further aids in preventing hypothermia-induced complications.[29]

The role of the anesthesiologist in ITx is crucial, with a focus on managing the delicate balance between sedation, pain control, and hemodynamic stability. Given the extensive nature of the surgery, patients typically require deep sedation and muscle relaxation to facilitate surgical exposure and manipulation. The anesthetic plan should also consider the potential for significant blood loss and the need for rapid transfusion, necessitating large-bore intravenous access and possibly central venous catheterization.[18] Additionally, anesthetic agents that minimize cardiovascular depression are preferred to maintain stable hemodynamics throughout the procedure.

POSTOPERATIVE MANAGEMENT

Immunosuppression

Immunosuppression plays a pivotal role in the success of ITx, as it prevents graft rejection—a major cause of graft loss and patient morbidity. The immune system's inherent tendency to recognize the transplanted intestine as foreign necessitates a robust and carefully managed immunosuppressive regimen to achieve long-term graft survival while minimizing the risk of opportunistic infections and other complications associated with immunosuppression. **Table 4** summarizes the standard immunosuppressive agents used in ITx, and **Flowchart 2** summarizes the systematic strategy utilized in administering immunosuppressive agents in ITx.

The cornerstone of immunosuppressive therapy in ITx includes a combination of calcineurin inhibitors (CNIs), corticosteroids, and antiproliferative agents. Tacrolimus, a CNI, is often the preferred agent due to its superior efficacy in reducing acute rejection episodes compared to cyclosporine. Tacrolimus works by inhibiting T-lymphocyte activation, a critical step in the immune response to the graft.[4,5] The therapeutic trough levels of tacrolimus are meticulously adjusted based on the time elapsed since transplantation and the individual patient's risk of rejection. Typically, trough levels are maintained between 10 and 15 ng/mL during the first 3 months post-transplant, gradually tapering to 5–10 ng/mL thereafter.[11] The most frequent administrative route is sublingual, although IV tacrolimus is preferred in other countries especially in pediatric recipients.

Corticosteroids are integral to the immunosuppressive regimen, particularly in the early post-transplant period. They function by broadly suppressing the immune response, reducing inflammation, and mitigating the risk of acute rejection. Corticosteroids are usually initiated at high doses immediately after transplantation and then tapered to minimize the long-term adverse effects, such as hyperglycemia, hypertension, and osteoporosis.[30] Long-term corticosteroid use is often avoided due to these potential side effects, with many centers aiming to wean patients off steroids within the 1st year if the patient remains stable.

Flowchart 2: Immunosuppressive strategy in ITx.

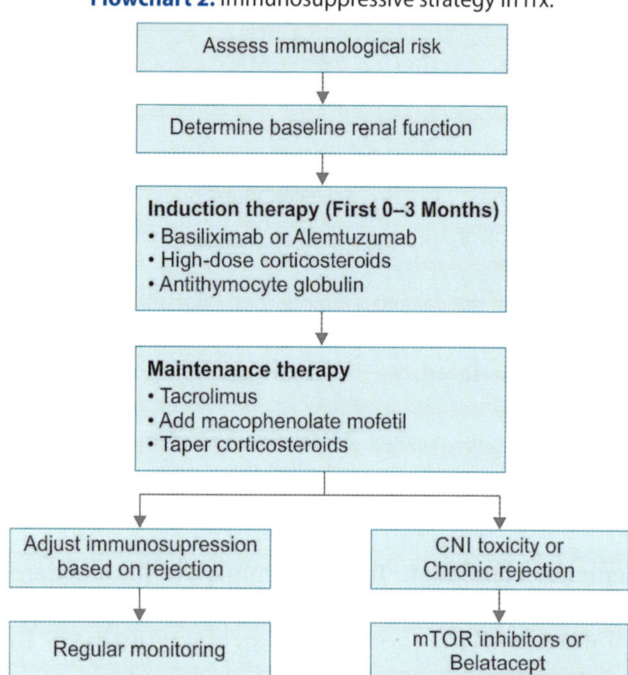

(CNI; calcineurin inhibitor; ITx: intestinal transplantation)

Antiproliferative agents such as mycophenolate mofetil (MMF) or azathioprine are often included in the regimen to provide additional suppression of T- and B-cell proliferation. MMF, in particular, is favored for its selective inhibition of lymphocyte proliferation, which contributes to the overall reduction in rejection rates without causing significant nephrotoxicity—a crucial consideration given the renal side effects associated with CNIs.[20] However, many centers tend to avoid it due to its GI side effect profile.

In addition to maintenance immunosuppression, many centers employ induction therapy to provide intense immunosuppression during the immediate post-transplant period, when the risk of acute rejection is highest. Antithymocyte globulin (ATG, a polyclonal antibody), basiliximab (an anti-CD25 monoclonal antibody), and alemtuzumab (a monoclonal antibody targeting CD52 on lymphocytes) are commonly used induction agents. The choice of induction therapy depends on the center's protocol and the patient's immunological risk profile.

The management of immunosuppression in ITx is complex and must be tailored to each patient's risk factors, including their immunological profile, history of rejection, and comorbid conditions. Long-term immunosuppression increases the risk of infections, post-transplant lymphoproliferative disorder (PTLD), and other malignancies, new-onset diabetes after transplant (NODAT) among others, necessitating vigilant monitoring and adjustments to the immunosuppressive regimen.[31] Opportunistic infections, such as cytomegalovirus (CMV), are of particular concern and often require prophylactic antiviral therapy or preemptive treatment based on regular monitoring of viral loads.[32]

Fluid and Electrolyte Management

Postoperative fluid and electrolyte management is vital due to the large fluid shifts and potential for dehydration, especially in patients with high-output stomas. Patients often require aggressive fluid replacement and electrolyte supplementation to maintain homoeostasis.[4] They are at a high risk for significant fluid shifts, particularly due to the presence of high-output stomas or newly transplanted bowel segments that may initially demonstrate poor absorptive capacity. These factors can lead to substantial fluid losses, which, if not adequately replaced, can result in hypovolemia, hypotension, and renal insufficiency.[5,11] Hyponatremia can occur due to excessive sodium loss from high-output stomas or diarrhea, while hyperkalemia may result from renal insufficiency or the use of certain medications such as potassium-sparing diuretics or CNIs (e.g., tacrolimus).[4,16] Hypomagnesemia is another common issue, often exacerbated by the use of diuretics and tacrolimus, which increases renal magnesium excretion. Persistent electrolyte imbalances can lead to severe complications such as cardiac arrhythmias, muscle weakness, and metabolic acidosis, which necessitate prompt and precise correction. **Table 5** summarizes the electrolyte imbalances in ITx along with their management.

The management of these fluid losses is complicated by the need to avoid both under- and over-resuscitation, as excessive fluid administration can exacerbate edema, compromise wound healing, and impair graft perfusion. In surgical practice, the following strategies are utilized for fluid and electrolyte management:

- *Intravenous fluid replacement:* In the immediate postoperative period, intravenous fluids are the mainstay of therapy. The choice of fluid—whether crystalloids, colloids, or a combination—depends on the patient's clinical status and electrolyte needs. Balanced crystalloids such as lactated Ringer's or PlasmaLyte are often preferred to minimize the risk of hyperchloremic acidosis, a condition that can exacerbate postoperative complications.[24] The rate of fluid administration is guided by continuous hemodynamic monitoring, urine output, and frequent assessments of blood pressure, CVP, and lactate levels.

- *Electrolyte monitoring and supplementation:* Daily monitoring of serum electrolytes is essential in the early postoperative period, with more frequent assessments required if the patient exhibits signs of instability or electrolyte imbalances. Sodium and potassium levels are particularly critical, and supplementation should be tailored to the individual needs of the patient. Oral or enteral supplementation is preferred as bowel function returns, but intravenous replacement is often necessary in the early stages, especially in cases of significant depletion.[20] Magnesium and calcium levels should also be closely monitored, with magnesium sulfate or calcium gluconate administered as needed to correct deficiencies.
- *Transition to oral/enteral fluids:* As bowel function gradually improves, there is a shift from intravenous to oral or enteral fluid and electrolyte supplementation. This transition must be carefully managed to ensure that the patient's intake meets their ongoing needs while avoiding fluid overload. Patients with functioning grafts but persistent high-output stomas may require ongoing oral rehydration solutions containing sodium, potassium, and bicarbonate to maintain electrolyte balance and prevent dehydration.[18]

Rejection

Rejection remains one of the most formidable challenges in the management of ITx. The immune system's natural response to foreign tissue makes rejection a significant risk, requiring vigilant monitoring and prompt intervention. **Flowchart 3** summarizes the management of rejection in ITx.

Rejection in ITx can manifest in various forms, including acute cellular rejection (ACR), antibody-mediated rejection (AMR), and chronic rejection (CR). Each type poses distinct challenges, with ACR being the most common form in the early post-transplant period. AMR, although less frequent, involves the presence of donor-specific antibodies (DSAs) and can lead to more severe graft damage if not promptly treated. CR, characterized

TABLE 5: Electrolyte imbalances in ITx and their management.

Imbalance	*Cause*	*Management*
Hyponatremia	High-output stomas, diarrhea	IV saline, oral rehydration solutions
Hyperkalemia	Renal insufficiency, medications (CNIs)	IV insulin and glucose, potassium binders
Hypomagnesaemia	Diuretics, tacrolimus use	IV magnesium sulfate, oral magnesium supplements
Metabolic acidosis	Bowel losses, kidney dysfunction	IV bicarbonate, oral bicarbonate supplements

Flowchart 3: Management of rejection in intestinal transplantation.

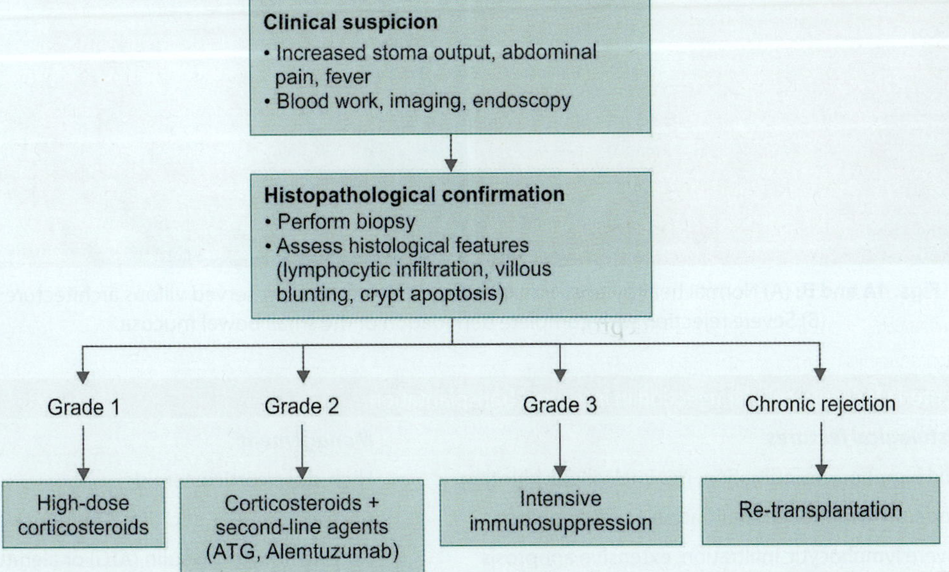

by progressive fibrosis and loss of graft function, remains the most challenging to manage and is often irreversible, frequently necessitating graft enterectomy with or without re-transplantation.[5,16]

Rejection is often suspected based on clinical signs, such as increased stoma output, abdominal pain, fever, and, in some cases, GI bleeding. These symptoms, while indicative, are nonspecific and can overlap with other post-transplant complications, such as infections. Ileoscopy or endoscopy and biopsy are indicated to confirm the diagnosis. The findings of villous blunting, ulceration, and mucosal sloughing are indicative of rejection unless proven otherwise **(Figs. 4A and B)**. Therefore, the gold standard for confirming rejection is endoscopic biopsy of the transplanted intestine.

The Banff criteria (summarized in **Table 6**), initially developed for kidney transplantation, have been adapted and expanded for the assessment of rejection in intestinal transplants, providing a standardized framework for diagnosing and grading the severity of ACR. It provides a histopathological grading system for ACR, which is vital for determining the severity of rejection and guiding treatment decisions. Key histological features include:

- *Lymphocytic infiltration:* The presence of lymphocytes within the epithelium and lamina propria is a hallmark of ACR. The degree of infiltration correlates with the severity of rejection, ranging from mild (Grade 1) to severe (Grade 3).[11,20]
- *Villous blunting:* This refers to the flattening and shortening of the intestinal villi, which are critical for nutrient absorption. Villous blunting reflects ongoing tissue damage and is a key feature in the Banff grading system.
- *Crypt apoptosis:* Apoptosis, or programmed cell death, of the crypt epithelial cells is another significant indicator of rejection. Extensive crypt apoptosis is often associated with more severe grades of rejection and may precede more widespread tissue damage.[29]

The Banff criteria also include considerations for the presence of edema, ulceration, and hemorrhage, which are associated with more advanced or severe rejection. Each of these histological findings contributes to the overall Banff score, guiding the intensity of the immunosuppressive therapy required to manage the rejection.[4]

The management of ACR involves a stepwise approach, starting with high-dose corticosteroids as the first line of therapy. Corticosteroids, due to their potent anti-inflammatory effects, are effective in reversing mild-to-moderate ACR. In cases where ACR is resistant to steroids or in more severe cases, additional immunosuppressive

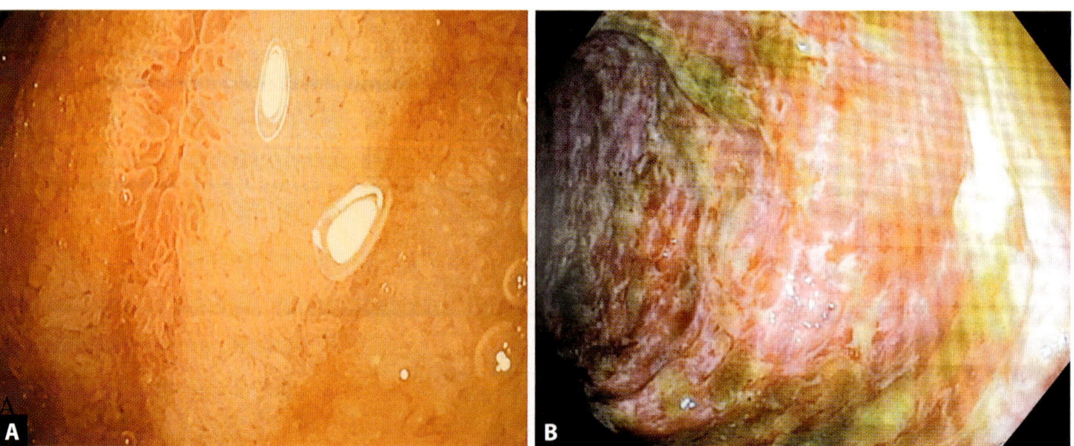

Figs. 4A and B: (A) Normal healthy post-transplant small bowel with preserved villous architecture; (B) Severe rejection with complete denudation of the small bowel mucosa.

TABLE 6: Banff criteria for acute cellular rejection in intestinal transplantation.

Grade	***Histological features***	***Management***
Grade 1	Mild lymphocytic infiltration, minimal villous blunting	High-dose corticosteroids
Grade 2	Moderate lymphocytic infiltration, crypt apoptosis	Corticosteroids + additional immunosuppressants
Grade 3	Severe lymphocytic infiltration, extensive apoptosis	Antithymocyte globulin (ATG) or alemtuzumab

agents such as ATG or alemtuzumab may be administered.[7,28] These agents work by depleting T-cells, thereby reducing the immune response against the graft. On the other hand, CR remains a significant challenge and is characterized by progressive graft fibrosis and eventual loss of function. Unlike ACR, CR is more insidious and resistant to conventional immunosuppressive therapies. The management of CR is often more complex, and once diagnosed, it typically leads to a decline in graft function. Strategies for managing CR include optimizing immunosuppression, treating any underlying AMR, and, in some cases, considering retransplantation as a last resort.[18] In our experience, ACR often involves the distal graft first, but this is not absolute. In irreversible cases, total graft enterectomy may be done to facilitate the withdrawal of immunosuppressants.

Infections

Infections are a leading cause of morbidity and mortality following ITx, and managing these risks is a critical component of postoperative care. The complexity of ITx, combined with the heavy immunosuppression required to prevent rejection and the high bacterial load associated with the transplanted intestine, makes recipients particularly vulnerable to a broad spectrum of infections, including bacterial, viral, and fungal infections. Prophylactic strategies, early diagnosis, and targeted treatment are essential to improve patient outcomes.

Bacterial Infections

Bacterial infections are most common during the early postoperative period, primarily due to the invasive nature of the surgery, the use of central venous catheters, and the immunosuppressive regimen. Broad-spectrum antibiotic prophylaxis is typically administered immediately after surgery to cover gram-positive, gram-negative, and anaerobic bacteria, aiming to prevent early onset infections.[5] The choice of antibiotics is guided by local microbiological data and patient-specific risk factors, including prior colonization with multidrug-resistant organisms.

Central venous catheter care is paramount in preventing catheter-related bloodstream infections (CRBSIs), which are a significant source of morbidity. Rigorous aseptic techniques during catheter insertion and maintenance, along with early removal of catheters when no longer clinically indicated, are critical strategies.[4] Line-related sepsis is an emergency and patient may present in shock—urgent resuscitation and establishment of new venous access, and removal of existing line is the treatment protocol.

When bacterial infections do occur, targeted antibiotic therapy based on culture and sensitivity results is essential. Common pathogens include *Enterococcus* spp., *Pseudomonas aeruginosa*, and *Klebsiella pneumoniae*, among others. Multidrug-resistant organisms, such as vancomycin-resistant *Enterococci* (VRE) and extended-spectrum beta-lactamase (ESBL)-producing Enterobacteriaceae, pose significant challenges and may require the use of newer antibiotics such as linezolid or ceftazidime-avibactam.[11]

Viral Infections

Viral infections are a major concern in the post-transplant period, particularly due to the use of intense immunosuppression that increases susceptibility to opportunistic viral pathogens. CMV and Epstein–Barr virus (EBV) are the most commonly encountered viral pathogens in ITx recipients.

Prophylactic antiviral therapy is a cornerstone of viral infection management. Valganciclovir is routinely administered for the first 6–12 months post-transplant to prevent CMV reactivation. Regular monitoring of CMV viral load through polymerase chain reaction (PCR) assays is critical for the early detection of viral reactivation, allowing for prompt intervention before clinical symptoms develop.[16] CMV disease, if it occurs, may require intravenous ganciclovir, and in cases of resistance, alternative therapies such as foscarnet or cidofovir may be necessary.[33]

The EBV-associated PTLD is another significant risk. Prophylactic or preemptive strategies, including close monitoring of EBV viral loads, reduction in immunosuppression, and, in some cases, administration of rituximab (an anti-CD20 monoclonal antibody), are employed to manage this risk.[34]

Fungal Infections

Fungal infections, particularly invasive candidiasis and aspergillosis, are life-threatening complications in ITx recipients, given the high immunosuppressive burden and the potential for fungal colonization of the transplanted bowel. Prophylactic antifungal therapy is standard practice during the early postoperative period, typically including agents such as fluconazole or echinocandins such as caspofungin or micafungin.[35]

Invasive candidiasis is the most common fungal infection, often associated with central venous catheters, broad-spectrum antibiotics, and TPN. Echinocandins are often preferred for treatment due to their efficacy against *Candida* species, including those resistant to fluconazole. In cases of invasive aspergillosis, voriconazole or liposomal amphotericin B are the agents of choice, particularly in patients with significant neutropenia or other risk factors for mold infections.[36]

Other Complications

Intestinal transplantation can be associated with a variety of complications that impact patient outcomes. Vascular graft thrombosis is a serious concern, where clots form in the transplanted vessels, potentially leading to graft ischemia and loss, necessitating urgent anticoagulation or surgical intervention.[11] GI bleeding, often due to anastomotic ulceration or mucosal ischemia, requires endoscopic or surgical management to control bleeding and prevent further morbidity.[16] Chylous ascites, resulting from lymphatic leakage, is managed with dietary modifications and drainage procedures to reduce fluid accumulation. Enteric leaks, presenting as leakage of intestinal contents, can cause peritonitis and require prompt surgical repair.[4] Wound dehiscence involves the reopening of the surgical incision, posing a risk for infection and requiring secondary closure techniques. Stomal complications, such as retraction or parastomal hernia, can affect function and QoL, often necessitating surgical revision **(Figs. 5A and B)**.[5] Additionally, graft-versus-host disease (GVHD), though rare, may occur when donor immune cells attack the recipient's tissues and is managed with intensified immunosuppression.[7] Disease recurrence is a potential issue in recipients with dysmotility, neuroendocrine tumors, or Crohn's disease, but has not shown to be of any impact in patient survival.[37,38] Each of these complications underscores the need for careful surgical technique, vigilant postoperative care, and timely intervention to improve patient and graft survival.

Stoma Closure

The decision to close a stoma following ITx is complex and should be individualized based on the patient's clinical status, graft function, and risk of complications. Stoma closure may be considered to enhance QoL, reduce complications associated with long-term stoma use, such as skin irritation, and improve fluid and electrolyte balance. However, it is essential to ensure that the graft has demonstrated reliable function without signs of rejection or infection. If closure is deemed appropriate, timing is critical; it is typically recommended to wait at least 6–12 months post-transplant to allow sufficient time for the graft to stabilize and any complications to resolve. Delaying closure can minimize the risk of surgical complications and ensure a better long-term outcome, but decisions should always be made in the context of multidisciplinary

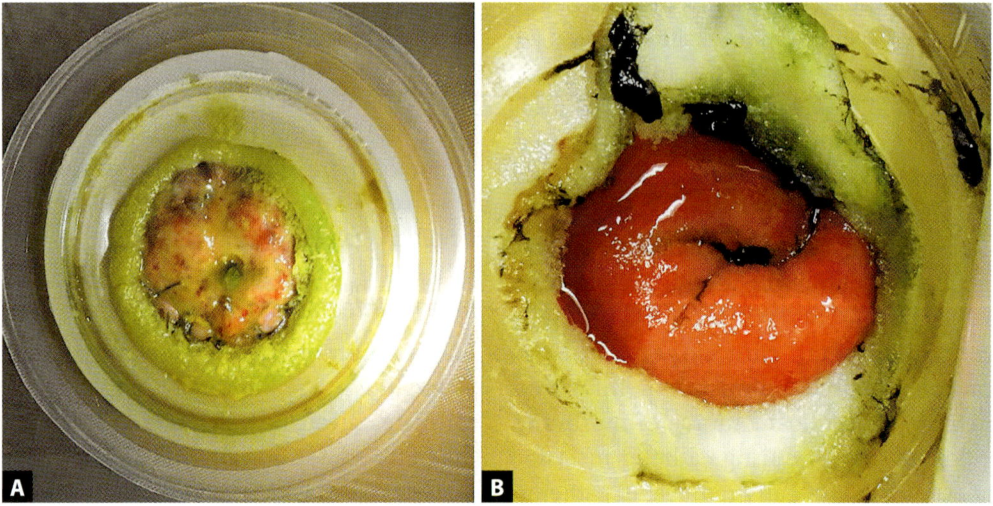

Figs. 5A and B: (A) Stomal rejection. (B) Stomal congestion and oozing.

care, balancing the benefits of stoma closure against potential risks.[39]

Patient and Graft Survival

The survival of both patients and grafts following ITx has seen remarkable improvements over the past few decades, yet significant challenges remain. Advances in surgical techniques, immunosuppression, and postoperative care have contributed to these improved outcomes, but the procedure continues to be associated with high morbidity and mortality rates, particularly in the long term. Understanding the factors that influence survival, the complications that arise, and the strategies to mitigate these risks is crucial for optimizing outcomes in this complex patient population. **Table 7** summarizes key factors influencing morbidity and mortality in ITx.

One-year graft survival rates for ITx are reported to be approximately 70–80%, with patient survival rates slightly higher. These outcomes are a testament to the advancements in surgical techniques and the optimization of immunosuppressive regimens. However, long-term survival rates present a more challenging picture. 5-year survival rates range between 50 and 60%, depending on various factors including the underlying disease, patient demographics, and the experience of the transplant center.[5,16] The variability in survival rates underscores the complexity of managing these patients and the significant impact of early and late complications on long-term outcomes.

Long-term survival in ITx patients is closely associated with the level of care provided by experienced, multidisciplinary teams. Centers that specialize in intestinal and multivisceral transplantation typically have better outcomes due to their ability to manage the complex needs of these patients. This includes not only surgical expertise but also specialized knowledge in immunosuppression management, infection control, nutritional support, and long-term follow-up care.[24,32,40] The involvement of a multidisciplinary team that includes transplant surgeons, gastroenterologists, infectious disease specialists, dietitians, and psychologists is critical for addressing the full spectrum of challenges faced by ITx recipients.

Transplant Enterectomy (Indications)

Transplant enterectomy, the surgical removal of the transplanted intestine, may be indicated in cases of severe graft rejection or recurrent life-threatening infections that are unresponsive to medical management.[41] This procedure is often considered as a last resort when the graft is no longer viable, and the patient's life is at risk. Partial enterectomy may be an option for a graft partially affected with infection or irreversible rejection. Post enterectomy, patients typically return to TPN, can stop immunosuppressants, and can be evaluated for potential retransplantation.[42] **Table 8** summarizes the indications for transplant enterectomy.

Surveillance

Ongoing surveillance post-transplant is essential for early detection of rejection, infection, and other complications. Regular endoscopic evaluations with biopsies of the graft are the cornerstone of surveillance, allowing for early identification of rejection.[8] Additionally, monitoring of immunosuppressant drug levels, routine blood tests, and imaging studies are used to assess graft function and detect complications early.[5] Surveillance is lifelong, and protocols typically include frequent monitoring in the 1st-year post-transplant, with the frequency decreasing as the patient stabilizes.[43]

TABLE 7: Key factors influencing morbidity and mortality in intestinal transplantation.

Factor	*Impact*	*Management*
Acute cellular rejection	Leading cause of early graft loss	Prompt diagnosis and aggressive immunosuppression
Chronic rejection	Progressive graft dysfunction	Close monitoring, potential retransplantation
Infections	Major cause of mortality post-transplant	Prophylaxis, early detection, tailored antimicrobial therapy
Immunosuppression-related complications	Long-term morbidity including nephrotoxicity, PTLD	Tailored immunosuppressive regimens, regular monitoring
Graft-related complications	Includes GVHD, graft failure	Early intervention, consideration of retransplantation

(GVHD: graft-versus-host disease; PTLD: post-transplant lymphoproliferative disorder)

TABLE 8: Key indications for transplant enterectomy in ITx.

Indication	*Clinical presentation*	*Management*
Severe graft rejection	Persistent, refractory to immunosuppression, graft dysfunction	High-dose steroids, ATG, alemtuzumab, consider enterectomy
Recurrent life-threatening infections	Sepsis, persistent infection despite antibiotics, diffuse CMV enteritis	Remove graft, initiate TPN, evaluate for retransplantation
Graft-versus-host disease (GVHD)	Symptoms of GVHD unresponsive to treatment	Remove graft, supportive care, consider enterectomy
Intestinal graft failure	Nonfunctional graft, perforation, and bleeding	Emergency surgery, remove graft, initiate TPN

(ATG: antithymocyte globulin; CMV: cytomegalovirus; ITx: intestinal transplantation; TPN: total parenteral nutrition)

CONCLUSION

Intestinal transplantation represents a transformative yet complex solution for patients with irreversible IF who have exhausted all other treatment options. Over the past few decades, advancements in surgical techniques, immunosuppressive protocols, and postoperative care have significantly improved patient and graft survival rates, making ITx a viable option for a growing number of patients. However, the procedure remains associated with substantial risks, including graft rejection, infection, and complications related to immunosuppression. These challenges underscore the importance of multidisciplinary care and vigilant monitoring to optimize outcomes. As access to ITx expands globally, particularly in developing regions, ongoing efforts to enhance organ donation rates, establish specialized transplant centers, and train healthcare professionals are essential. Despite the challenges, ITx offers a life-saving option for many patients, and with continued advancements, the outlook for these patients will continue to improve. The future of ITx lies in refining patient selection criteria, improving donor availability, and developing more effective immunosuppressive strategies to minimize complications and enhance long-term survival. In summary, while ITx has transitioned from an experimental procedure to a standard of care for select patients, ongoing research and innovation are crucial to furthering its success and accessibility worldwide.

REFERENCES

1. Kumpf VJ. Parenteral nutrition-associated liver disease in adult and pediatric patients. Nutr Clin Pract. 2006; 21(3):279-90.
2. Reyes JD. Intestinal transplantation: an unexpected journey. J Pediatr Surg. 2014;49(1):13-8.
3. Staun M, Pironi L, Bozzeti F, Baxter J, Forbes A, Joly F, et al. ESPEN guidelines on parenteral nutrition: Home parenteral nutrition (HPN) in adult patients. Clin Nutr. 2009;28(4):467-479.
4. Kaufman SS, Atkinson JB, Bianchi A, Goulet OJ, Grant D, Langnas AN, et al. Indications for pediatric intestinal transplantation: a position paper of the American Society of Transplantation. Pediatr Transplant. 2001;5(2):80-7.
5. Fishbein TM. Intestinal transplantation. N Engl J Med. 2009;361(10):998-1008.
6. Iyer KR. Surgical management of short bowel syndrome. JPEN J Parenter Enteral Nutr. 2014;38(1 Suppl):53S-59S.
7. Selvaggi G, Tzakis AG. Indications and contraindications to intestinal and multivisceral transplantation. In: Sudan D (ed). Intestinal and Multivisceral Transplantation. Cham: Springer; 2018. p. 13-25.
8. Grant D, Abu-Elmagd K, Mazariegos G, Vianna R, Langnas A, Mangus R, et al. Intestinal transplant registry report: Global activity and trends. Am J Transplant. 2015;15(1):210-9.
9. Pironi L, Joly F, Forbes A, Colomb V, Lyszkowska M, Baxter J, et al. Long-term follow-up of patients on home parenteral nutrition in Europe: Implications for intestinal transplantation. Gut. 2011;60(1):17-25.
10. National Organ and Tissue Transplant Organization (NOTTO). Data for Organ Donation and Transplantation (2013-2022). [online] Available from https://notto.gov.in. [Last accessed May, 2025]
11. Abu-Elmagd KM, Costa G, Bond GJ, Soltys K, Sindhi R, Wu T, et al. Five hundred intestinal and multivisceral transplantations at a single center: Major advances with new challenges. Ann Surg. 2009;250(4):567-81.
12. Ojo AO, Held PJ, Port FK, Wolfe RA, Leichtman AB, Young EW, et al. Chronic renal failure after transplantation of a nonrenal organ. N Engl J Med. 2003;349:931-40.
13. Taha AM, Sharif K, Johnson T, Clarke S, Murphy MS, Gupte GL. Long-term outcomes of isolated liver transplantation for short bowel syndrome and intestinal failure-associated liver disease. J Pediatr Gastroenterol Nutr. 2012;54:547-51.
14. Ministry of Health and Family Welfare, Government of India. The Transplantation of Human Organs and Tissues

Act, 1994 (Amended 2011). [online] Available from https://main.mohfw.gov.in/sites/default/files/THOTA_0.pdf.
15. National Organ and Tissue Transplant Organization (NOTTO). Guidelines for organ transplantation in India. [online] Available from https://notto.gov.in.
16. Vianna RM, Mangus RS, Tector AJ. Current status of small bowel and multivisceral transplantation. Adv Surg. 2008;42:129-50.
17. Cruz RJ Jr, Costa G, Bond GJ, Soltys K, Rubin E, Humar A, et al. Modified multivisceral transplantation with spleen-preserving pancreaticoduodenectomy for patients with familial adenomatous polyposis "Gardner's syndrome". Transplantation. 2011;91:1417-23.
18. Starzl TE, Todo S, Fung J, Demetris AJ, Venkataramman R, Jain A. FK 506 for liver, kidney, and pancreas transplantation. Lancet. 1989;2:1000-4.
19. Kato T, Tzakis A, Levi D, Defaria W, Selvaggi G, Weppler D, et al. 100 multivisceral transplants at a single center. Ann Surg. 2006;242:480-90.
20. Mangus RS, Tector AJ, Kubal CA, Fridell JA, Vianna RM. Multivisceral transplantation: Expanding indications and improving outcomes. J Gastrointest Surg. 2013;17(1):179-86.
21. Pironi L, Arends J, Bozzeti F, et al. ESPEN guidelines on chronic intestinal failure in adults. Clin Nutr. 2016; 35:247-307.
22. Matsumoto CS, Kaufman SS, Fishbein TM. Inclusion of the colon in intestinal transplantation. Curr Opin Organ Transplant. 2011;16:312-315.
23. Pomp A, Stein JP, Esquivel CO, Cuerda C, Gillanders L, Jeppesen PB, et al. Multivisceral transplantation for en-bloc resection of abdominal tumors. Arch Surg. 2000; 135: 1208-13.
24. Ramisch D, Rumbo C, Echevarria C, Moulin L, Niveyro S, Orce G, et al. Long-Term Outcomes of Intestinal and Multivisceral Transplantation at a Single Center in Argentina. Transplant Proc. 2016;48(2):457-62.
25. Gruessner RW, Sharp HL. Living-related intestinal transplantation: First report of a standardized surgical technique. Transplantation. 1997;64:1605-7.
26. Kumaran V, Mehta NN, Varma V, Pandey S, Rao PS, Nath B, et al. Living donor intestinal transplant using a standardized technique: first report from India. Indian J Gastroenterol. 2012;31:179-85.
27. Levi DM, Tzakis AG, Kato T, Madariaga JR, Mittal NK, Ricordi C, et al. Transplantation of the abdominal wall. Lancet. 2003;361:2173-6.
28. Langnas AN, Goulet OJ, Quigley EM. Intestinal Transplantation in Children: Update 2011. Pediatr Transplant. 2012;16:107-21.
29. Reyes J, Mazariegos GV, Abu-Elmagd K, Macedo C, Bond GJ, Murase N, et al. Intestinal transplantation under tacrolimus monotherapy after perioperative lymphoid depletion with rabbit antithymocyte globulin. Am J Transplant. 2005;5:1430-6.
30. DiBenedetto LM, DiBenedetto G, Bertozzi N, Gatti G, Aquinati A, Baldini A. Management of abdominal wall defects following intestinal transplantation: the use of component separation technique and mesh reinforcement. Transplant Proc. 2005;37:1384-6.
31. Fishbein TM, Matsumoto CS. Intestinal transplantation: Evaluation of graft immunogenicity and chronic rejection. Curr Opin Organ Transplant. 2010;15(3):342-6.
32. Stanley K, Friehling E, Ranganathan S, Mazariegos G, McAllister-Lucas LM, Sindhi R. Post-transplant lymphoproliferative disorder in pediatric intestinal transplant recipients: A literature review. Pediatr Transplant. 2018; 22(5):e13211.
33. Kotton CN. CMV: Prevention, diagnosis and therapy. Am J Transplant. 2013;13:24-40.
34. Green M, Michaels MG. Epstein-Barr virus infection and posttransplant lymphoproliferative disorder: Epstein-Barr virus viral load testing and other diagnostic methods. Clin Microbiol Rev. 2013;26(1):89-109.
35. Gavaldà J, Meije Y, Fortún J, Roilides E, Saliba F, Lortholary O, et al. ESCMID Study Group for Infections in Compromised Hosts. Invasive fungal infections in solid organ transplant recipients. Clin Microbiol Infect. 2014;20(Suppl 7):27-48.
36. Florescu DF, Sandkovsky U. Fungal infections in intestinal and multivisceral transplant recipients. Curr Opin Organ Transplant. 2015;20(3):295-302.
37. Monu G, Amanda P, Elizabeth L, Jennifer R, Hirak P, Yasser F, et al. 230.7: Disease Recurrence After Intestinal and Multivisceral Transplantation. Transplantation. 2019; 103(7S2):S7.
38. Fahad H, Abu-Elmagd K, Lashner B, Fiocchi C. Recurrence of Crohn's Disease After Small Bowel Transplantation: Fact or Fiction. Inflamm Bowel Dis. 2020;26(1):21-3. Erratum in: Inflamm Bowel Dis. 2020;26(4):e29.
39. Moon JI, Zhang H, Waldron L, Iyer KR. "Stoma or no stoma": First report of intestinal transplantation without stoma. Am J Transplant. 2020;20:3550-7.
40. Timpone JG Jr, Girlanda R, Rudolph L, Fishbein TM. Infections in intestinal and multivisceral transplant recipients. Infect Dis Clin North Am. 2013;27(2):359-77.
41. Gerlach UA, Vrakas G, Sawizki B, Macedo R, Reddy S, Friend PJ, et al. Abdominal wall transplantation: Skin as a sentinel marker for rejection. Am J Transplant. 2016;16(6):1892-900.
42. Nagai S, Mangus RS, Anderson E, Ekser B, Kubal CA, Fridell JA, et al. Intestinal graft failure: Should we perform the allograft enterectomy before or with re-transplantation? Transplantation. 2017;101(2):411-20.
43. Pironi L, Baxter JP, Lauro A, Guidetti M, Agostini F, Zanfi C, et al. Assessment of quality of life on home parenteral nutrition and after intestinal transplantation using treatment-specific questionnaires. Am J Transplant. 2012; 12:S60-6.

Index

Page numbers followed by *b* refer to box, *f* refer to figure, *fc* refer to flowchart, and *t* refer to table.

D

H

I

J

K

L

M

N

R

S

T

U

V

W

X

Y

Z